PSYCHIATRIC REHABILITATION OF CHRONIC MENTAL PATIENTS

PSYCHIATRIC REHABILITATION OF CHRONIC MENTAL PATIENTS

Edited by

Robert Paul Liberman, M.D.

1400 K Street, NW
Washington, D.C. 20005

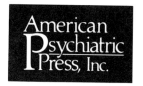

Library of Congress Cataloging-in-Publication Data

Psychiatric rehabilitation of chronic mental patients.

Includes bibliographies and index.
1. Mentally ill—Rehabilitation. 2. Chronically ill—Rehabilitation. I. Liberman, Robert Paul, 1937–   .
[DNLM: 1. Chronic Disease—rehabilitation. 2. Mental Disorders—rehabilitation. WM 29.1 P974]
RC480.53.P78   1987   616.89   87-1492
ISBN 0-88048-201-X

Until attention and energy are focused on the seriously mentally ill, they will continue to be with us—gazing vacantly at the bare walls of deteriorating state hospitals, living in roach-infested boarding houses, haunting back alleys of the inner city like some modern twilight zone. They stand mute, their backs to the walls of vacant buildings, the gargoyles of our civilization.

E. Fuller Torrey and Sidney M. Wolfe
Care of the Seriously Mentally Ill

CONTENTS

LIST OF CONTRIBUTORS

All affiliations are with the Department of Psychiatry of the University of California at Los Angeles School of Medicine, the Brentwood Division of the West Los Angeles Veterans Administration Medical Center, and Camarillo State Hospital.

Harvey E. Jacobs, Ph.D. Assistant Research Psychologist

Timothy G. Kuehnel, Ph.D. Assistant Research Psychologist

Robert Paul Liberman, M.D. Professor of Psychiatry

David Lukoff, Ph.D. Assistant Research Psychologist

Catherine C. Phipps, M.S. Staff Research Associate

Joseph Ventura, M.A. Staff Research Associate

Byron Wittlin, M.D. Associate Clinical Professor of Psychiatry

FOREWORD

lthough persons suffering from severe mental illnesses with residual long-term disabilities have been with us since time immemorial, it took a radical socio-politico-economic movement—deinstitutionalization—to focus professional and public attention on their plight. In the 32 years since the depopulation of our states' mental hospitals began, we have witnessed both the horrors of an unplanned, thoughtless public policy and the fruits of an intensive scientific effort beginning to address an overwhelming problem. Specifically, on the negative side, we are shocked as our cities' streets teem with thousands of homeless severely mentally ill persons, our jails bulge with psychotic individuals charged with largely "nuisance" crimes, and our nursing homes swell to more than 50 percent occupancy by severely and chronically mentally ill persons. But on a positive note, we are heartened by an increased degree of public attention, professional concern, service innovation, training effort, and research agenda devoted to this population.

Psychiatric rehabilitation has a long and distinguished history. But like many other endeavors related to the chronically mentally ill, its service programs developed more rapidly and fully than its body of literature, research base, and training programs—until relatively recently. Now, however, there are three nationally recognized comprehensive centers devoted to this field—of which the one co-sponsored by the University of California at Los Angeles, the Brentwood Veterans Administration Hospital, and the Camarillo State Hospital is a shining example. Robert Liberman and his colleagues have strived to develop a series of innovative service and training programs, with rigorous evaluative and research components, that has as its basis an understanding of the value of work, family, and social relations in patients' lives; that consists of logical and interrelated modules; that focuses on the practical, graspable, and doable; and that is readily transferable.

The fruits of their labors are displayed in this book, a work that is

- full of definitions, specifics, and examples;
- replete with case vignettes that sound like the people we know and work with;
- constructive in providing learning exercises for us and our patients without sounding like a cookbook;
- complete in its functional assessment approach;
- compelling in its argument for a comprehensive, multidisciplinary, and multidimensional approach; and
- eminently clear and readable.

Dr. Liberman and his colleagues have written a wonderful, useful book; a one-of-a-kind endeavor that will be of immense value to all concerned with the rehabilitation, treatment, and care of the chronically mentally ill for many years to come.

John A. Talbott, M.D.
Professor and Chairman
Department of Psychiatry
University of Maryland School of Medicine, Baltimore

Past President
American Psychiatric Association

PREFACE

Why should another book on the chronic mental patient be published? The professional literature is crowded with books, articles, and even entire journals devoted to the problems and care of the chronically mentally ill. Moreover, the authors of this volume do not believe in the redeeming value of books for mental health practitioners. Books look impressive on library shelves, and they embellish the curriculum vitas of their authors, but they are rarely read. Each article in a scientific journal, for example, is read by less than 200 people on the average. Even if journals and books are read, the readers are usually not students preparing to enter a profession or the practitioners in the "trenches" with the patients. Most studies of professional practice indicate that adoption of innovations and changes in practice occurs through personal influence and face-to-face contact with teachers, mentors, and colleagues.

Thus, there should be good reason to foist yet another book describing the plight of the chronic mental patient upon the professional public. One reason for this book lies in its content and format. Rather than elaborate on the psychopathology, the social disability, or the societal burden posed by chronic and severe mental illness, this book presents practical answers to those seeking help to treat and rehabilitate the chronically mentally ill. Each chapter provides highly detailed prescriptions for assessment and treatment techniques and does so with case examples and learning exercises for the reader. No conventional textbook, this volume is a clarion call for action and intervention.

It began as an experiment in active-directive teaching. At the Clinical

Research Center for Schizophrenia and Psychiatric Rehabilitation at the University of California at Los Angeles and the Brentwood Division of the West Los Angeles Veterans Administration Medical Center, a plan was hatched to design and offer an intensive workshop experience for postgraduate students in psychiatry, psychology, social work, and nursing as well as mental health and rehabilitation practitioners that would acquaint them with the state of the art in working with the chronic mental patient. We did not buy into the general gloom and doom regarding treatment efforts with the chronically mentally ill. There were a number of studies, carried out by ourselves and others, that clearly signaled the responsiveness of chronic mental patients to behaviorally oriented interventions. The chronically mentally ill—individuals with schizophrenia and other severe mental disorders—could benefit from systematic and consistent programs that harnessed the best in thinking in the biomedical and psychosocial fields. Individuals with even the most chronic and unyielding symptoms of schizophrenia could learn or relearn skills enabling them to return to community life. The chronic mental patient was treatable and rehabilitatable!

What should a workshop include that was aimed at changing the knowledge and attitudes of professionals, many of whom were burned out and cynical in their help-giving with chronics? We decided to open the workshop with a challenge to unfounded prejudices. We selected seven programs that had empirical evidence of efficacy in working with the chronically mentally ill and presented them in a hard-hitting style that conveyed optimism and reality-based hope. We then followed this orientation with discussion of seven contemporary arenas of practice that when combined in a comprehensive program, could make a difference in the rehabilitation of the chronic mental patient. The arenas were psychiatric diagnosis, functional assessment, psychopharmacology, social skills training, behavioral family management, vocational rehabilitation, and community support programs.

Each section of a two-day workshop focused on these arenas of professional practice. We infused the syllabus for the workshop with the latest methods that were being reported as effective in the literature. We made a professional-quality videotape that depicted each of the arenas in action, a videotape that won first prize at the International Rehabilitation Film Festival. We also designed experiential learning exercises—such as modeling, role playing, and homework assignments—as intrinsic elements of the workshop. Each arena of rehabilitation practice had its own exercises because we wanted workshop participants to go through an active learning process. Workshops were led by three or four trainers who were selected for their knowledge, experience, and enthusiasm for the field.

To date, the workshop has been offered to more than 2,000 professionals in Georgia, Arizona, New Mexico, California, Pennsylvania, Idaho, Oregon, Florida, Alabama, North Dakota, Kansas, Iowa, Nebraska, and Nevada. Questionnaires and rating scales are administered to the participants before and after the workshop to test their acquisition of knowledge and changed attitudes. We have found that gains in knowledge did occur and attitudes toward working with the chronically mentally ill did become more favorable. The changes have been significant, both in absolute and statistical terms. Moreover, some participants responding to follow-up queries reported actually using the methods we introduced in the workshop.

The workshop and the seminars derived from it are still being offered. We hope to expand the potential audiences for this educational experience by training educators to take our syllabus and videotape into their own agencies, schools, and institutions and lead seminars, courses, and workshops on their own. And that is the reason for this book. To disseminate the educational experience and its materials, we needed to refine the materials we had assembled into a coherent text. Each chapter in this book summarizes one of the arenas of professional practice that are needed for effective treatment and rehabilitation of the chronic mental patient. Together with the videotape and an instructor's syllabus (available from The Training Director, Camarillo–UCLA Research Center, Box A, Camarillo, CA 93011), the text forms an educational package that we hope will continue to fuel the fires of change in mental health and rehabilitation practitioners' efforts with the chronically mentally ill.

Robert Paul Liberman, M.D.

INTRODUCTION

The National Conference on the Chronic Mental Patient, sponsored by the American Psychiatric Association in collaboration with the President's Commission on Mental Health, was held in Washington, D.C., in January 1978 and addressed the striking inadequacy of care, treatment, and rehabilitation of this group, estimated to number almost two million Americans. It was agreed at that conference that the chronically mentally ill were persons having major schizophrenic and organic psychoses and recurrent affective disorders, long-term disabilities, extreme dependency needs, high sensitivity to stress, and difficulty coping with the demands of everyday living. These characteristics summed to create difficulties in securing a job, steady income and self-support, and housing. As a result of their mental disorders and society's failure to compensate for their handicaps, the chronically mentally ill suffer from social isolation, lack of daily living skills, unemployment, poverty, and revolving-door hospitalizations, jailing, or homelessness. A second national conference on the chronically mentally ill convened six years later, in 1984, and underscored the continued public health problem posed by this population and delineated its unmet needs and societal challenges.

THE TERM "CHRONIC MENTAL PATIENT"
The authors of this book, together with most mental health and rehabilitation professionals, decry the use of the term "chronic mental patient." However, we view it as a necessary evil, because although it has many important drawbacks, it does have descriptive clarity and possesses

historical and current prevalence of usage. We agree with the framers of the Proposal for Public Policy on the Chronic Mental Patient, who point out that

> the term stigmatizes the person so designated and obscures their diversity and potential for improvement. It is not a desirable appellation because of its implication of hopelessness and progressive deterioration. While these people have a chronic illness that requires medical and psychiatric attention over a long period of time and are, therefore, appropriately called patients, it is equally important to recognize them as persons with continuing disability. (Talbott 1978, p. 57)

Various other terms have been proposed to define this population, such as "long-term mentally ill" or "severely psychiatrically disabled." We believe that the labels given to persons suffering from prolonged or intermittent symptoms and disabilities are not as influential in stigmatizing them as is the absence of adequate and effective treatment and rehabilitation programs. Other disorders that had been stigmatized in the past—tuberculosis and syphilis—were relieved of stigma when effective treatment measures became available. Therefore, in this book we have retained the term "chronic mental patient" and have placed high on our agenda the articulation of effective methods of evaluation, treatment planning, and rehabilitation.

The problems posed by the chronically mentally ill and their needs for medical and psychiatric treatment, housing, vocational rehabilitation, recreational programs, financial assistance, social rehabilitation, and crisis intervention are similar whether the afflicted individuals are living in the community or within institutions. The focus of supportive and rehabilitative intervention is necessarily broad and comprehensive regardless of the locus of services. But who are the chronically mentally ill, and how many are they?

WHO ARE THE CHRONICALLY MENTALLY ILL?

In former years, it was relatively simple to determine the chronically mentally ill population—they were the long-term residents of psychiatric hospitals. Today, these large custodial institutions are no longer host to the majority of chronic mental patients, who have been "trans-institutionalized" from the back wards and now live in a variety of community "back streets"—board and care homes, nursing homes, locked residential care facilities, foster homes, single-room-occupancy hotels, and substandard apartment rooming houses. To appreciate the shift in the locus of care for this population, consider the fact that in the mid-1950s state hospitals provided nearly 50 percent of all psychiatric care in the country, but by 1977 they provided only 9 percent (Sharfstein 1984). Many of

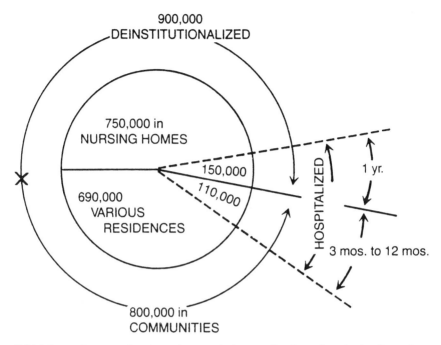

FIGURE 1. Residential locations of the nation's estimated 1.7 million chronically mentally ill persons. From Goldman HH, Gattozzi AA, Taube CA: Defining and counting the chronically mentally ill. Hosp Community Psychiatry 32:23, 1981. Reprinted with permission.

the chronically mentally ill are homeless, and they wander the skid rows of our nation living off scraps and handouts. Many return to live with their families, who continue to shoulder the major burden of caretaking for their disabled relatives. In Figure 1 is shown the location where the nation's estimated 1.7 million chronically mentally ill reside.

There are various ways to define the chronically mentally ill. Two criteria with validity are a) diagnosis of schizophrenia or major affective disorder and b) dependence on financial support from family and/or social security and welfare. In accordance with the *Diagnostic and Statistical Manual of Mental Disorders (Third Edition)* (American Psychiatric Association 1980), individuals who are diagnosed as suffering from schizophrenic, organic, or major affective disorders have almost always been impaired for six months or more, and since repeated episodes are the rule rather than the exception, chronicity is the usual pattern in these disorders. Chronic conditions may be marked by periods of remission or relative freedom from the active symptoms of the disorder, but there are usually residual disability and "negative" symptoms present even between periods of relapse or flare-ups of acute symptoms.

Another way to define the chronically mentally ill uses a three-dimensional grid delimiting those who are severely mentally ill (as measured by diagnosis), those who are psychosocially disabled (as measured by social and vocational level of function), and those who are chronically ill and disabled (as measured by duration of symptoms, disability, and hospitalization episodes). These three overlapping dimensions—diagnosis, disability, duration—are sufficiently accurate to provide a starting point for delimiting the chronic mental population in our society. Figure 2 displays these three dimensions with an estimate of 1.7 million as the size of the target population, as endorsed by the National Plan for the Chronically Mentally Ill, sponsored by the American Psychiatric Association and published by the federal government in 1980. A summary description, then, of the chronically mentally ill population is "persons who suffer severe and persistent mental disorders that interfere with their functional capacities in daily life such as self-care, interpersonal

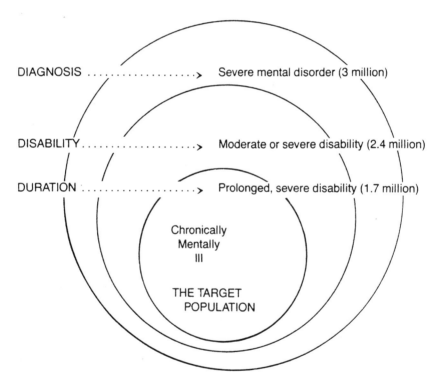

FIGURE 2. The three dimensions that together serve as the criteria for defining a person as chronically mentally ill. From Goldman HH, Gattozzi AA, Taube CA: Defining and counting the chronically mentally ill. Hosp Community Psychiatry 32:22, 1981. Reprinted with permission.

relationships, and work or schooling, and that often necessitate prolonged hospital care or psychiatric treatment" (Goldman et al. 1981,
p. 22).

The Community Support Program (CSP) of the National Institute
of Mental Health (NIMH) operationalized a somewhat different and
broader definition of the chronically mentally ill who are eligible for its
services: "Severe mental disability must satisfy at least one of the following: a single episode of hospitalization in the last five years of at least
six months' duration; or two or more hospitalizations within a 12-month
period" (Community Support Program Guidelines 1977). Treated prevalence rates for chronic psychiatric patients can be derived from statistics
collected by the NIMH Division of Biometry and Epidemiology on all
patients admitted to state, county, and private psychiatric hospitals as
well as to psychiatric units in general hospitals. The great majority of
patients have stays of less than 90 days in psychiatric facilities; however,
those who remain longer than 90 days have diminished likelihood of
release. It can be estimated that 110,000 patients were in psychiatric
facilities for 3 to 12 months in 1977 and an additional 150,000 remained
for longer than a year.

The following more specific definition of the chronically mentally
ill, offered by Goldman et al. (1981), has met with general acceptance.
It defines the chronically mentally ill as

> persons who suffer certain mental or emotional disorders (organic
> brain syndromes, schizophrenia, recurrent depressive and manic-
> depressive disorders, and paranoid and other psychoses), plus other
> disorders that may become chronic that erode or prevent the de-
> velopment of their functional capacities in relation to three or more
> primary aspects of daily life—personal hygiene and self-care, self-
> direction, interpersonal relationships, social transactions, learning
> and recreation—and that erode or prevent the development of their
> economic self-sufficiency. (Goldman et al. 1981, p. 23.)

The technical criteria for defining the chronically mentally ill are
described here to establish the objective boundaries of the target population, which are vital to the activities of planners and policy-makers.
But they do no more than hint at the clinical, socioeconomic, ethnic,
and cultural heterogeneity of this population. They cannot convey any
sense of the individual people involved, their families, or their hopes
and striving, however falteringly, for normalcy.

The chronically mentally ill population includes persons whose clinical conditions and functional disabilities vary widely at any point in time
and, moreover, change over time. Schizophrenia and other severe mental
disorders are multiply handicapping and lifelong. Only a minority of
patients have long periods of remission and normal levels of psycholog-

ical functioning. A majority have residual social and vocational disabilities even when the positive symptoms of the disorder are controlled by medications. Periodic relapse may be an expected part of their illness, and many are at least intermittently and partially dependent upon mental health and social services throughout their lives.

The variability inherent in severe, major mental disorders makes accurate determination of the size and nature of the population extremely difficult. At best we can provide an estimate to guide national policymakers in a more scientific assessment of needs. Suffice it to note here that although our definition encompasses persons with prolonged moderate-to-severe disability, a significant proportion possess the capacity to live in relative independence if adequate medical and psychiatric treatment, community-based services, social supports, and life opportunities are provided.

Throughout this book, we shall be describing assessment and treatment methods that have had their major impact and contribution on schizophrenic disorders. Most of the illustrative case material, for example, focuses on patients with schizophrenia. Similarly, the chapter on psychopharmacology presents the state of the art in the drug treatment of schizophrenia. However, it should be understood that most of what is presented as helpful in the diagnosis, treatment, and rehabilitation of individuals suffering from schizophrenic disorders is also of relevance to individuals with other severe and disabling mental disorders. Behavioral family management has been tested primarily with families containing a person with schizophrenia; however, just as the family emotional climate is as relevant a predictor of relapse in depression as it is in schizophrenia, we can expect that family management will eventually prove as helpful in affective disorders as it already is in schizophrenic disorders.

Robert Paul Liberman, M.D.

REFERENCES

American Psychiatric Association: Diagnostic and Statistical Manual of Mental Disorders (Third Edition). Washington, DC, American Psychiatric Association, 1980

Community Support Program Guidelines [mimeo]. Rockville, MD, National Institute of Mental Health, Community Support Program, 1977

Goldman HH, Gattozzi AA, Taube CA: Defining and counting the chronically mentally ill. Hosp Community Psychiatry 32:22, 1981

Menninger W, Hannah G (Eds): The Chronic Mental Patient/II. Washington, DC, American Psychiatric Press, 1987

Sharfstein SS: Sociopolitical issues affecting patients with chronic schizophrenia, in Schizophrenia: Treatment, Management, and Rehabilitation. Edited by Bellack AS. Orlando, FL: Grune and Stratton, 1984

Talbott JA: The Chronic Mental Patient: Problems, Solutions, and Recommendations for a Public Policy. Washington, DC, American Psychiatric Association, 1978

CHAPTER 1

COPING WITH CHRONIC MENTAL DISORDERS: A FRAMEWORK FOR HOPE

ROBERT PAUL LIBERMAN, M.D.

The heart bowed down by weight of woe
To weakest hope will cling.
A. Bunn
"Song from the Bohemian Girl"

Not enjoyment, and not sorrow,
Is our destined end or way;
But to act, that each tomorrow
brings us farther than today.
Longfellow
"A Psalm of Life"

The field of psychiatric rehabilitation is emerging as a coherent body of interdisciplinary theory and credible programs of intervention for the mentally ill. With the recognition that most psychiatric disorders are associated with persisting disability, acute treatment models are being supplemented by effective procedures for optimizing the long-term outcome of patients. Psychiatric rehabilitation—as practiced by clinicians representing psychiatry, psychology, social work, nursing, rehabilitation as well as self-help efforts by patients and relatives—aims to improve the long-term capabilities of persons with psychiatric disabilities for living, learning, working, socializing, and adapting in as normalized a fashion as possible (Anthony and Liberman 1986).

HISTORICAL DEVELOPMENT

The origins of the psychiatric rehabilitation field are rooted in several historical developments: a) the moral therapy era, b) the inclusion of the psychiatrically disabled into public-supported vocational rehabilitation programs, c) the development of community mental health ideology, d) the self-help and psychosocial rehabilitation movement, and e) the development of skills training techniques as an effective mental health intervention.

Moral Therapy Era

The nineteenth-century reformists for more humane care of the mentally ill aimed to "treat the patients as far as their condition would possibly admit, as if they were still in the enjoyment of the healthy exercise of their mental faculties . . . and to make their condition as comfortable as possible" (Bockoven 1963). Moral therapy stressed a comprehensive assessment of the psychiatrically disabled, examining the person's work, play, and social activities. For example, a chaplain at a British asylum recognized the importance of patients' reentry into social life "by obtaining for them a change of scene and air and assisting them to obtain suitable employment" (Hawkins 1871). Consistent with present-day rehabilitation practice, moral therapy recognized that structured activity can have therapeutic value. Today the goal of psychiatric rehabilitation practice is to have the person *do* something differently.

Vocational Rehabilitation Programs

Although initial governmental programs for employment of the disabled, sparked by the end of World War I, focused on the physically

Parts of this chapter are reprinted with permission from Anthony WA, Liberman RP: The practice of psychiatric rehabilitation. Schizophr Bull 12:542–559, 1986. In the public domain.

handicapped, they did demonstrate that rehabilitation principles could be effectively implemented and won public support for rehabilitation as a societal responsibility. It was the 1943 amendments to the United States Vocational Rehabilitation Act that provided financial support and vocational rehabilitation services to the psychiatrically disabled, with similar legislation appearing at the same time in England.

These governmental actions extended the social welfare umbrella over the mentally ill and provided legitimacy to the training and rehabilitation of persons with psychiatric disabilities. Moreover, these legislative advances, and others that have followed in the past 40 years, grounded the practice of psychiatric rehabilitation in the vocational arena (Beard et al. 1982; Grob 1983). The belief in work as a major ingredient of rehabilitation is exemplified by H. Richard Lamb, one of the major spokespersons of psychiatry's concern for the chronically mentally ill, who said, "Work therapy geared to the capability of the individual patient should be a cornerstone of community treatment of the long-term patient" (Lamb 1982).

Community Mental Health

National legislation in the United States and European countries enacted in the 1950s and 1960s established community-based treatment for the mentally ill and retarded. The community mental health movement introduced a new basic assumption, namely, that persons with major illness should be helped to maintain themselves in the community in as normal a manner as possible. Unfortunately, community mental health centers (CMHCs) failed to provide the comprehensive services needed by the severely psychiatrically disabled, who were not a high-priority population for the interdisciplinary staff of CMHCs, perhaps because the latter were ill equipped with techniques for effective work with chronic psychotics (Liberman et al. 1976).

The deinstitutionalization movement that accompanied the opening of the CMHCs fostered an appreciation of the value of work training in the preparation of patients for resettlement in the community. Psychiatrists were forced to match their view of a patient's abilities and disabilities against the realities of adaptation in the "real world." Studies were carried out in industrial therapy programs that showed the benefits and hazards of work for the mentally ill, changed the attitudes of citizens and professionals about the employability of mentally ill persons, and led to job placement programs (Bennett 1983).

Consistent with modern concepts of rehabilitation are those additional elements of community mental health ideology—accessibility to and comprehensiveness of services and continuity of care. The emphasis on treating patients in proximity to their natural families and work settings was extended by the 1977 National Institute of Mental Health

(NIMH) initiative for community support programs, which has encouraged state and local investments in a spectrum of services for the chronically mentally ill. In turn, this has meant an infusion of key operating principles for psychiatric rehabilitation, including case management, coordination, and advocacy with a variety of agencies capable of meeting the full range of needs of persons with severe psychiatric disabilities; involvement of patients and relatives in self-help; and assertive outreach.

Psychosocial Rehabilitation Centers

The realization that severely and chronically mentally ill persons rarely experience a full return of psychosocial functioning in the community led to a movement emphasizing accommodation to the needs of these persons in sustaining some semblance of normalization. With mental health professionals neglectful of the chronic mentally ill, nonprofessionals and the patients themselves initiated psychosocial self-help clubs, located in large cities where the mentally ill congregated in large numbers. The early clubs, such as Fountain House in New York and Horizon House in Philadelphia, were founded by groups of ex-patients for the purpose of mutual aid and support. These early social clubs gave birth to comprehensive, multiservice psychosocial rehabilitation centers such as Thresholds in Chicago, the Social Rehabilitation Center in Fairfax, Virginia, the Center Club in Boston, Fellowship House in Miami, Hill House in Cleveland, and Portals House in Los Angeles. The psychosocial centers assist patients in dealing with their "real-life" problems by providing opportunities for acceptable role performance and successful mutually interdependent relationships with others, by buffering stressors, and by making available a range of housing and employment options. From the very beginning, these centers have emphasized a) strategies to help people cope with the environment rather than succumb to it, b) health induction rather than symptom reduction, and c) improvement of the person's ability to do something in a specific environment, even in the presence of residual disability.

Skills Training

The most recent development shaping psychiatric rehabilitation has been the introduction of skills training methods derived from social learning principles, human resources development, and vocational rehabilitation. Effective coping with life stressors requires skills for problem-solving, successful affiliative and instrumental relationships, mobilizing supportive networks, and work. Rehabilitation techniques that utilize active-directive learning principles—behavioral practice and role playing, social and tangible reinforcement, shaping, coaching, prompting, and activities to promote generalization—strengthen an individual's problem-solving capacities and confer protection against exacerbations of psychiatric symptoms (Wallace and Liberman 1985).

REHABILITATION MODEL IN PSYCHIATRIC DISABILITY

Rehabilitation of persons with medical and psychiatric disorders proceeds from a four-stage framework for understanding the nature and consequences of disease: 1) pathology, 2) impairment, 3) disability, and 4) handicap. From the point of view of rehabilitation professionals, the psychobiological abnormalities in the nervous system that produce deficiencies in cognitive, attentional, and autonomic functions and in regulation of arousal and information processing represent the active pathology or disease state. Neurosciences are just beginning to develop instruments and techniques that can sensitively measure these abnormalities. High-technology, laboratory-based methods of detecting metabolic and structural defects in the brain are not yet validated that will differentiate one disorder from another; however, it is expected that specificity of assessment of underlying disease processes will emerge in the next decade. Future breakthroughs are promised by current studies using brain imaging via positron emission tomography, nuclear magnetic resonance, and computerized axial tomography; neuroendocrinological function tests such as the dexamethasone suppression test and the thyroid-stimulating hormone test; brain mapping through computerized electroencephalogram evoked potentials; component analysis of the electrodermal response; measurement of eye tracking and continuous attentional performance; and measurements of neurotransmitters through radioimmune and radioreceptor assays.

Neurosciences have not yet yielded the secrets of the brain sufficient to characterize a person's vulnerability or trait for a specific psychiatric disorder; however, specific psychiatric syndromes or diagnoses can be reliably inferred through assessment of impairments that presumably index the more basic disturbances in brain function.

While impairments in physical rehabilitation include vision or hearing loss, reduced range of motion in an extremity, and loss of strength in a muscle group, psychiatric impairments can include thought disorder and speech incoherence, delusions, hallucinations, anxiety, depression, loss of concentration or memory, distractibility, and apathy and anhedonia. Thus, psychiatric symptoms and cognitive-emotional deficits are both correlates of the course and outcome of psychiatric illnesses and of the pathological processes in the nervous system.

When functional limitations imposed by psychiatric impairments result in decrements in social role performance, the individual is said to have a disability. Disabilities are defined as inability or limitation to perform roles and tasks expected of an individual within a social environment (Frey 1984). Among patients with severe psychiatric disorders, such as schizophrenia, disabilities include poor self-care skills (cooking, cleaning, grooming, teeth care), social withdrawal and seclusiveness, abandonment of family responsibilities, and work incapacity. The *Diagnostic and Statistical Manual of Mental Disorders (Third Edition) (DSM-III)* has highlighted the importance of these disabilities by including them as criteria from many diagnosable psychiatric conditions. To be diagnosed as having schizophrenia, for example, it is not sufficient to experience the characteristic symptoms of thought disorder, delusions and hallucinations, but the person also must evince a "deterioration from a previous level of functioning in such areas as work, social relations, and self-care" (American Psychiatric Association 1980).

The disabilities shown by persons with psychiatric disorders are influenced by the same protective and risk factors that influence the appearance, exacerbation, and remission of symptoms or impairments. Thus, there are substantial correlations between symptoms and disabilities; however, not every impairment results in a disability. Furthermore, similar patterns of disability can result from different disorders that may have the same profile of disabilities as patients with schizophrenia. Social and vocational disabilities form a major cluster of behaviors that reflect the course and outcome of a psychiatric disorder.

A fourth element in the rehabilitation model is handicap, which occurs when a person's disabilities place him or her at a disadvantage relative to others in society. This can occur through stigma and discrimination, as when employers are reluctant to hire individuals with a mental illness. Handicap also occurs because society does not provide settings where mentally ill persons can find accommodation and compensation for their impairments and disabilities. Wheelchairs and ramps have enabled paraplegics to overcome their impairments and disabilities to find remunerative work and fulfilling recreation; hence, their handicaps are compensated. Because mentally ill persons require special social environments to compensate for their problems, overcoming handicaps is much more difficult. Long-term institutional care in state and county mental hospitals was formerly society's method for dealing with the impairments and disabilities of psychiatric patients; unfortunately, institutionalization also created its own set of secondary disabilities and handicaps.

In Table 1 is depicted the interrelationship among the four stages of a rehabilitation view of mental disorders. Each stage is associated with a particular emphasis by the rehabilitation practitioner; for example, syndromal diagnosis defines the boundaries of a person's mental impairments while functional assessment delineates a person's disabilities.

Given the intrusion of symptoms of major mental disorders—psychotic delusions and hallucination, depression, anxiety—on the cognitive and interpersonal capabilities of afflicted individuals, it is no surprise that such impairments lead to significant disability and handicap. For example, unemployment has been found to be as high as 70 percent in the chronic mentally disabled (Goldstrom and Manderscheid 1982). Unemployment is a prime index of handicap since the demands of work

TABLE 1: Stages in the Rehabilitation Model of Chronic Mental Disorders

Stage:	Pathology →	Impairment →	Disability →	Handicap
Definition:	Lesions or abnormalities in the central nervous system caused by agents or processes responsible for the etiology and maintenance of the bio-behavioral disorder	Any loss or abnormality of psychological, physiological, or anatomical structure or function, (resulting from underlying pathology)	Any restriction or lack (resulting from an impairment) of ability to perform an activity in the manner or within the range considered normal for a human being	A disadvantage for a given individual (resulting from an impairment or a disability) that limits or prevents the fulfillment of a role that is normal (depending on age, sex, social, cultural factors) for that individual
Example:	Brain tumors or infections etiologically linked to psychotic symptoms	Positive and negative symptoms of schizophrenia (delusions, anhedonia)	Deficient social skills	Unemployment; homelessness
Interventions:	Laboratory and radiographic tests	Syndromal diagnosis; pharmacotherapy; hospitalization	Functional assessment; skills training; social support	National and state vocational rehabilitation policies; Community Support Programs

Reprinted from Liberman RP (Ed): Psychiatric Rehabilitation [special issue]. Schizophr Bull 12(4), 1986. In the public domain.

in modern society accentuate the deficits, deviance, and stigma of mental patients. Employment rates following hospital discharge range between 10 percent and 30 percent, and only 10 to 15 percent sustain their employment one to five years following discharge, with more recent studies revealing lower rates (Anthony et al. 1972; Anthony et al. 1984). Difficulties in work tolerance, endurance, following instructions, cooperating with co-workers and supervisors, problem solving, task orientation, sustained concentration, and ability to accept criticism and ask for assistance are all examples of disabilities that are caused by symptomatic and cognitive impairments and that lead to significant handicap.

Thus the impairments, disabilities, and handicaps of individuals with psychiatric disorders are related to their psychiatric symptoms and their vocational and social deficits. Symptomatic and functional problems exist on a continuum. For example, the nature of illness can influence the severity and chronicity of the symptoms and social dysfunctions. Individuals with schizophrenia generally are more impaired and disabled than those with affective or anxiety disorders (Harrow et al. 1978). However, within any one type of disorder, symptomatic and social-vocational course and outcomes vary considerably, both for different individuals and for the same individual over time (Liberman 1982). Moreover, there are not always high correlations among the major dimensions of outcome of severe mental disorders: For example, social functioning may be good even in the face of poor vocational functioning and persisting symptoms (Anthony 1979). Alternatively, symptoms may be persistent but may still permit adequate job adjustment (Anthony and Jansen 1984; Strauss and Carpenter 1981). Variability in the manifestations of major mental disorders is one of the most salient features of these disorders and can be best understood and studied through the interplay of vulnerability, stress, coping, and competence factors.

While the symptoms and syndromal diagnosis of a patient clearly impair the afflicted individual's concurrent social and vocational performance, the remitting and exacerbating nature of most major mental disorders obscures the relationship between psychopathology at time A and behavioral functioning at time B. The changing character of the symptomatic impairments of psychiatric disorders with the passing of time accounts in part for the insubstantial correlations often found between psychopathology measured during an acute episode and index hospitalization and future work performance.

It also might be argued that modest correlations between impairments and disabilities reported by reviewers (Anthony 1979) were a result of the reviews' having been conducted in the era prior to the availability of objective and reliable instruments for eliciting and rating psychopathology. Research using the standardization in diagnosis brought about by the *DSM-III* have yielded studies that suggest a stronger relationship between syndromes and long-term outcome (Tsuang et al. 1979; Pfohl and Andreasen 1986).

STRESS-VULNERABILITY-COPING-COMPETENCE IN MENTAL DISORDERS

The overriding characteristic of mental illness is heterogeneity in the course and outcome of individuals with disorders. As shown in Figure 3, the impairments, disabilities, and handicaps that compose the course and outcome of psychiatric disorders can vary from minimal to maximal. One person with schizophrenia could have severely psychotic episodes but a very benign course with good recovery of social and vocational functioning and little in the way of psychopathology. Another person with the same number or severity of psychotic episodes might have considerable residual impairment and disability.

Variability also is the rule rather than the exception within any one person's course of disorder. Periods of relapse and incapacity may alternate with periods of remission and excellent social role functioning (Harding and Struass 1985). How, then, can one explain the tremendous interindividual and intraindividual variability in course and outcome of chronic and severe mental disorders? The multifactorial schema shown in Figure 3, including factors of vulnerability, stress, and protection, explains the sources for this heterogeneity.

The stress-vulnerability-coping-competence model of major mental disorders explains the onset, course, and outcome of symptoms and social functioning as a complex interaction among biological, environmental, and behavioral factors (Liberman 1982) and is congruent with the rehabilitation conceptualization. Psychobiological vulnerability may result in psychotic symptoms when stressful life events or ambient tensions in the family or work setting overwhelm coping skills.

Vulnerability and stressors are moderated in their impact on impairment, disability, and handicap by the presence and action of protective factors. Prime among protective factors are coping and competence exercised by individuals, families, natural support systems, and professional treatment. Examples of protective factors include rehabilitation programs that offer skill building, social support, or transitional employment. Coping and competence can be attributes of the individual or of the person's social environment. From this point of view, an exacerbation or relapse of schizophrenic symptoms that accompanied use of street drugs of abuse (for example, phencyclidine, amphetamines) would result from the stressful action of these drugs on an individual's underlying biological diathesis for schizophrenia. In like manner, stressful life events (for example, loss of a trusted therapist or discharge from long-term hospitalization) that overwhelm the protective effects of medication, personal coping, and social support can also lead to symptomatic

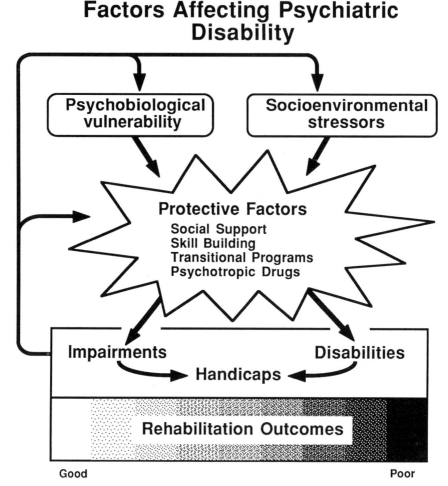

Factors Affecting Psychiatric Disability

FIGURE 3. A multifactorial model of chronic mental disorders and their disability that highlights the variables that contribute to variations in outcome. Protective factors of coping, competence, social support, and psychotropic medication can buffer or neutralize the deleterious effects of stress superimposed upon vulnerability. Reprinted from Liberman RP (Ed): Psychiatric Rehabilitation [special issue]. Schizophr Bull 12(4), 1986. In the public domain.

exacerbation. Even in the absence of a time-limited stressor, vulnerable individuals can succumb to ambient levels of challenge, tension, or conflict in their environment if they lack the protection conferred by medication, coping abilities, and social support.

CASE EXAMPLE _____

Joe lived all his growing-up years on his family's farm. The farm was far from neighbors and Joe had little contact with peers as a youth. He went to a small school but avoided contact with other children. Most of his time was spent on the slopes of his native mountains, tending sheep and cows. He had poorly developed social skills with peers. His parents were also socially withdrawn and did not provide opportunities to learn expressiveness or intimacy. There was, at the genetic level, a grandfather who spent many years in the state psychiatric hospital, presumably for a schizophrenic disorder.

At the age of 18, Joe entered military training. He lived in a barracks full of other young men, most of whom came from larger cities. They talked openly, fast, and loud. He was not used to this active and stimulating social intercourse and he experienced difficulty in processing the incoming information. He did not know how to make jokes with his fellow recruits. He did not know how to brag about his sexual exploits because he did not have any. After several stressful weeks of trying vainly to cope with the rigorous military discipline and peer pressure, he experienced confusion in his thinking and autonomic symptoms of anxiety. These prodromal symptoms of psychosis were quickly followed by ideas of reference and then delusions that thoughts were being put into his head by his officers. He showed lapses in attending his regular duty, was awake at night, and was brought to the military hospital with florid hallucinations and delusions, where the psychiatrist pronounced him as suffering from a schizophrenic disorder.

Joe then went into the hospital ward, which was supportive, nurturing, warm, and friendly. The staff were helpful to him and seemed to understand his needs for privacy and quiet. He did not have to polish his shoes or make his bed in the morning. He received antipsychotic medication and slowly but surely his symptoms subsided. He began to tentatively socialize, and his level of function returned to its premorbid level.

At this point, he was discharged from the military hospital and returned to his family home. Unfortunately, the protective factors provided by the military hospital did not get communicated to Joe's aftercare system. The psychiatrist in the military did not talk to the psychiatrist responsible for the rural clinic near Joe's parents. As a result, Joe returned home to family members who were baffled and confused about what had happened to him. He looked normal. There were no outward signs of illness. He was taking some pills, which his parents felt made him sleepy and were a sign of weakness. His parents told him that he did not really need to have those pills as long as he ate his ample farm meals and drank a lot of good milk. His parents urged him to again work on the farm. Their expectations for his work capacity were as high as before, if not higher, because they were frustrated and annoyed with him for having failed to complete his military service.

As the performance demands on the farm and pressures within the family mounted, Joe experienced the return of weird feelings. He felt unreal and became obsessed with concerns about bodily decay and dying. The long-acting antipsychotic medication was slowly metabolized and excreted, and Joe again developed the symptoms of schizophrenia.

Joe was hospitalized at a community mental health center located in a small city that was the county seat of the rural area in which his family's farm was located. There, Joe and his parents received education about schizophrenia and its management. A therapist who also functioned as a case manager was assigned to Joe and saw to it that he received continuity of care and social and vocational rehabilitation. Joe entered a social skills training group at the mental health center which met weekly and he joined a social club run by volunteers and ex-patients.

He decided to live apart from his parents in a supervised apartment that received consultation from mental health center staff. His medication was continued using a long-acting injectable form and he developed a trusting and collaborative relationship with his psychiatrist. Joe did well after this second episode of psychosis. He required monitoring over the years, and occasionally had exacerbations of his symptoms; however, his trajectory was upward toward recovery of function. Ultimately, he was able to find employment as a janitor and lived semi-independently.

COPING AND COMPETENCE CAN COMPENSATE FOR STRESS AND VULNERABILITY

Vulnerability factors that convey risk for major mental disorders are relatively enduring, pathological abnormalities of individuals that are present before, during, and after symptomatic episodes. Protective variables are environmental and personal factors that determine whether a given level of vulnerability to mental disorder leads to manifest symptomatology under a given current level of stress. Stressors are transient or ambient events that demand adaptive changes from the individual and that challenge the individual's current coping and competence.

The vulnerability/stress conception of psychiatric disorders also highlights the role of specific psychosocial interventions for developing personal and familial coping skills and interpersonal competence as protective factors. Psychosocial protective factors buffer the impact of stressors and thereby reduce the probability of psychotic relapse. Socially learned coping enables individuals to better obtain their instrumental and socio-emotional needs through meeting the challenges and solving the problems of everyday life. Coping and competence protect an individual with a given level of vulnerability to schizophrenia from stressful life events and ambient levels of environmental tension. At any level of psychopathology, coping can reduce the social, occupational, and self-care disabilities that are associated with the disorder.

The model also encourages investigators to design optimal psycho-pharmacological interventions to modify the effect of psychobiological vulnerability factors. For example, antipsychotic medication serves as a personal protective factor against biological vulnerability and thereby decreases relapse rates and improves the course of schizophrenic disorders. Antipsychotic medication also serves to raise the threshold at which environmental potentiators and stressors precipitate psychotic symptoms in an individual with a given level of vulnerability to schizophrenic episodes (Leff et al. 1973; Vaughn and Leff 1976). However, the modulation of biological vulnerability by antipsychotic medication cannot fully remediate a vulnerable individual's susceptibility to relapse when faced with severe stressors, loss of social support, or diminution in personal problem-solving skills. Even with reliable ingestion of neuroleptics, for example, upwards of 30 to 40 percent of schizophrenic patients relapse within a year (Liberman 1984).

In this vulnerability-stress-coping-competence model, the appearance or increase of characteristic schizophrenic symptoms and associated disabilities may occur in susceptible individuals when

1. underlying psychobiological vulnerability factors are triggered, which is more likely in the absence of optimal antipsychotic medication;
2. stressful life events intervene that exceed the individual's coping skills and competencies in social and instrumental roles;
3. the individual's social support network weakens or diminishes;
4. coping and problem-solving skills atrophy as a result of disuse, reinforcement of the sick role, or loss of motivation.

Coping refers to processes that may confer protection from relapse in major mental disorders when an individual with a given biological vulnerability is confronted with environmental stressors. Coping refers to the process of striving to master environmental stressors or challenges. Coping begins when an individual (or individual in concert with relatives or other social support elements) believes that his or her effectiveness is sufficient to engage in a course of action that aims at some desirable outcome. Termed "self-efficacy," the belief or conviction that one can successfully execute the behaviors required to produce a desired outcome is thought to be a precursor or at least a concomitant of the striving behavior itself. Previous performance accomplishments or success experiences are the main source of self-efficacy, but self-efficacy can also be influenced by vicarious experiences of seeing others cope with threats and succeed, by verbal persuasion, and by emotional arousal.

People fear and avoid threatening situations or environmental stressors and challenges if they believe that their coping abilities are not sufficient for mastery. Perceived self-efficacy also affects the persistence of coping efforts once a challenge is undertaken. The stronger the efficacy or mastery expectations, the more a person will persist in coping efforts. Those who persevere in coping, despite unpleasantness, and succeed in their goals will gain corrective experiences that further reinforce their sense of efficacy.

Coping behaviors may be carried out by the individual alone or in concert with others. A person who enlists the aid of friends or relatives in efforts to obtain a job or some personal need is using coping skills. The soliciting and recruiting of social and material resources in pursuit of a desired goal can be more important types of coping. Coping thus refers to the attempts and efforts to obtain some instrumental or social-emotional goal. Coping is linked, in temporal sequence, with competence, which is defined as the attainment of one's needs. Competence is an outcome measure while coping is a process.

In addition to perceived self-efficacy and already existing coping skills within one's repertoire, motivational factors also play a part in determining one's coping efforts. For example, an individual who is experiencing dysphoria from the side effects of a neuroleptic drug should be more motivated to use his or her coping skills (for example, conversational skills with doctor, ability to obtain transportation resources to get to doctor's appointment, ability to make a phone call or in-person appointment with doctor to negotiate changes in medication) than someone whose side effects are less dysphoric. Similarly, patients who are responsive to social reinforcement will be more motivated to attend treatment sessions than patients who find social contact aversive. Money and a host of other tangible reinforcers have been repeatedly shown to exert powerful effects on the coping activities of schizophrenic and other psychiatric patients (Liberman 1976; Liberman et al. 1974).

Contextual factors can also influence coping efforts. For example, some tasks require greater skills and more arduous performances and carry a higher risk of aversive consequences than do others. Despite high levels of self-efficacy and motivation, patients who do not have vocational skills or the social support to engage in a lengthy job search may fail to look for jobs. Failure in job seeking may also be compounded by fears of losing one's disability pension.

Coping efforts are dependent on the individual's social and living skills. The role of social and living skills as protective factors against the disabling effects of schizophrenia is highlighted by a study from Scotland in which 51 long-stay patients were followed for four years after they completed participation in a special rehabilitation unit. (Presly et al. 1982). The only factors that successfully distinguished the patients who made progress and were able to live in the community from their compatriots who remained unimproved were related to self-care skills (use of money, cooking, care of clothing, and so on). Similarly, a study of schizophrenic patients placed in homes after relatively brief hospitalizations found that relapse rates at one year after discharge were significantly higher among those patients who had prerelease deficiencies in social skills (Linn et al. 1980).

Measures of social competency during childhood, adolescence, and adulthood are related to and partially predictive of the severity and outcome of schizophrenic disorders within a population that has already become ill (Kokes et al. 1977; Strauss and Carpenter 1977, 1981). Many studies have shown that the higher the person's social level of adjustment prior to developing schizophrenic symptoms and requiring hospitalization, the better his or her posthospital outcome (Hersen and Bellack 1976; Kokes et al. 1977).

STRATEGIES OF PSYCHIATRIC REHABILITATION

The conceptual framework elucidated above, joined with the rehabilitation view of disability, provides a coherent set of strategies for rehabilitation interventions with the psychiatrically disabled. Psychiatric rehabilitation is the recovery of social and instrumental role functioning to the fullest extent possible through learning procedures and environmental supports. When restoration of functioning is limited by continuing deficits and symptoms, rehabilitation efforts aim at helping the individual a) acquire skills and living and working environments that are compensatory and b) adjust to the level of functioning that is realistically attainable. Rehabilitation begins immediately after the stabilization of an acute episode or exacerbation of psychiatric disorder, which usually results in the loss of social and role functioning. The goals of rehabilitation professionals are to sustain symptomatic improvement over the long haul, establish or reestablish interpersonal and independent living skills, and help the individual reach a satisfactory quality of life.

The practice of psychiatric rehabilitation is guided by the basic philosophy that disabled persons need skills and environmental supports to fulfill the role demands of various living, learning, and working environments. The assumption of clinical rehabilitation is that by changing psychiatrically disabled persons' skills and/or support in their immediate environment, they will be more able to perform those activities necessary to function in specific roles of their choice. In other words, interventions designed to lessen or compensate for the disability are assumed to lead to a decrease in the handicap.

Because the goals of rehabilitation center on adjustment to everyday life, it is vital that the individual himself or herself participate maximally in the choice of objectives and in the learning process. Comprehensive rehabilitation involves assessment, training, and modification of living environments in those areas relevant to personal and community life: self-care, including medication and symptom self-management; family relations; friendships; avocational and employment pursuits; money management and consumerism; residential living; recreational activities; transportation; food preparation; and choice and use of public agencies. Specific goal setting within these generic areas should be conducted with the active involvement of the patient and his or her family and significant others. This can help to keep the professionals' well-intentioned rescue fantasies and unrealistically ambitious goals of recovery from tipping a patient into a relapse.

Professionals contributing to psychiatric rehabilitation include psychologists, vocational rehabilitation counselors, occupational therapists, recreational therapists, nurses, social workers, psychiatrists, and mental health paraprofessionals. Professionals must be careful not to overlook the natural caregivers in the patient's living environment, namely, relatives and operators of board-and-care homes. Specific intervention programs, aimed at these natural caregivers as mediators of rehabilitation, are now available to magnify the impact of professionals.

Rehabilitation encompasses two major strategies: a) helping the patient to develop or reacquire social and instrumental skills and b) modifying the patient's social and physical environmental supports to compensate for continuing disabilities and handicaps. Usually, both strategies are employed to meet the individual needs and goals of the patient. Some patients, such as those who are reconstituting from an acute schizophreniform disorder or a major affective disorder, need assistance only in reestablishing their premorbid level of functioning, which may have been consistent with a good quality of life.

On the other hand, patients with more chronically disabling disorders, such as schizophrenia or organic brain disorders, may be unable to reestablish specific impaired or lost skills. Alternate compensatory skills and environments, such as learning to function in sheltered employment and residential settings, would be the focus of rehabilitative efforts. With chronic psychiatric disorders, some amount of continuing symptoms and residual impairment makes necessary the acceptance of disability and the identification of new, attainable goals. Learning how to cope with symptoms, manage medication, and use professional resources when necessary become important targets for rehabilitation. When deficits preclude gainful employment, the patient and family need assistance in generating alternative types of meaningful activity, social contacts, and daily structure. Although persisting symptoms may produce social and occupational disabilities, the reciprocal also holds; namely, the more that rehabilitation improves the patient's social and role performance, the more likely his or her symptoms will be held in check.

CASE EXAMPLE _____

In the most carefully controlled study of psychiatric rehabilitation (Paul and Lentz 1977), over 100 of the most residual, regressed, and dysfunctional chronic psychiatric patients in the Illinois state hospital system were randomly assigned to a skill-building social learning program, a milieu program based on therapeutic community principles, or a standard-care state hospital unit. Five years later, results showed marked superiority in all dimensions of outcome for the patients who received the skills training in a systematic token economy program (Paul and Lentz 1977). The data from this study are summarized in Figure 4. More than 98 percent of the patients enrolled in the social learning program achieved release from the hospital and at least 18 months of tenure in the community, compared with 71 percent and 46 percent for the milieu therapy and standard-care programs, respectively.

The costs for achieving these remarkably superior outcomes were less in the social learning program, and patients from that program required less neuroleptic medication to control their symptoms. Furthermore, the only program to produce significant improvement in daily functioning was the social learning ward, with almost 20 percent of the patients in that program attaining a near-normal level of functioning.

STEPS IN PSYCHIATRIC REHABILITATION

In the chapters of this book are detailed the steps for conducting psychiatric rehabilitation, from diagnosis and functional assessment through skills training, pharmacotherapy, and community support. Each chapter focuses on an area of psychiatric rehabilitation that has been validated through empirical studies. Here I will summarize briefly some of these functions of rehabilitation.

Psychiatric rehabilitation begins with a comprehensive medical-psychiatric diagnosis and functional assessment. This enables mental health and rehabilitation professionals to categorize individuals by diagnostic disorder and level of behavioral functioning, which are key to identifying their impairments and disabilities. Identification of impairments and disabilities permits the mental health and rehabilitation practitioner to prioritize problems, formulate specific goals, and organize and implement treatment and rehabilitation plans. Both medical-psychiatric diagnosis and behavioral assessment are necessary to match patients to effective drug and psychosocial treatment and rehabilitation programs (Taylor et al. 1982). Furthermore, knowing the patient's diagnosis aids the clinician in providing the patient and his or her family with a reasonable prognosis. The diagnosis also assists the clinician in making estimates of the ratio of environmental support to remedial skills training that will most likely assist the patient in minimizing disability and handicaps.

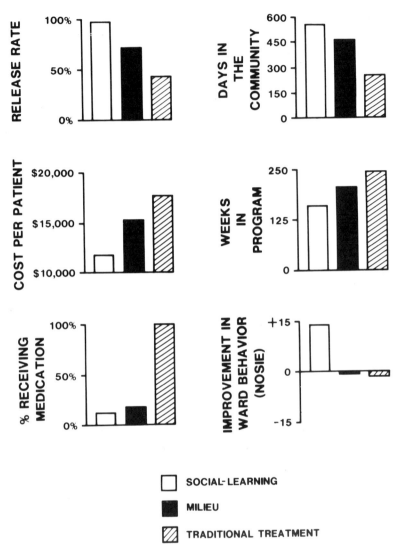

FIGURE 4. Multidimensional outcomes of a controlled study of three forms of psychosocial treatment for chronic mental patients. In each outcome dimension, social learning therapy was superior to milieu therapy or customary care. Reprinted from Liberman RP (Ed): Psychiatric Rehabilitation [special issue]. Schizophr Bull 12(4), 1986. In the public domain.

Reduction of Impairments

Rehabilitation interventions with psychiatric patients require reduction or elimination of the symptomatic and cognitive impairments that interfere with and intrude on social and vocational performance. Fortunately, interventions for reducing impairments are available from psychopharmacology. The past 20 years have seen major accomplishments in both treatment and prevention of morbidity from psychopathology through the use of antipsychotic, antidepressant, and anxiolytic drugs. It should be noted that these psychotropic drugs are not panaceas: They are frequently only able to partially reduce symptoms and delay rather than totally prevent relapse, even when taken regularly. Psychotropic drugs are also associated with unpleasant side effects that at times can interfere with skills training activities. However, they are usually helpful in reducing impairments to the point at which psychosocial strategies can be used with effectiveness to remediate disabilities and handicap.

As can be inferred from Figure 3, there are reciprocal relations among the various protective factors that mitigate stress and vulnerability. Thus, in the presence of effective skills-building rehabilitation programs, a patient's need for antipsychotic medication may be reduced. This was found in the Paul and Lentz (1977) study (described in the above case example), in which less than 18 percent of patients receiving social learning therapy required maintenance neuroleptic drugs after one or more years in the program.

CASE EXAMPLE ————————————————————————————

In a comparative, controlled study of behavioral family management versus supportive individual therapy for chronic schizophrenics (Falloon 1985), much better outcomes were accrued by the patients involved in family skills training. At the end of two years, 78 percent of the patients participating in the program that trained families in communication and problem-solving skills were in remission of their psychotic symptoms, compared with only 17 percent of their counterparts who had received supportive therapy. These vastly superior outcomes were reached with lower doses of maintenance neuroleptic drugs—on the average 100 mg per day less of chlorpromazine equivalents. These differences, highlighting the interactions between drug therapy and skills training in psychiatric rehabilitation, are shown in Figure 5.

Remediation of Disabilities Through Skills Training

Once a patient has benefited optimally from psychotropic drugs and the therapeutic effects of brief hospitalization, rehabilitation practitioners use skills training to remediate disabilities in social, family, and vocational

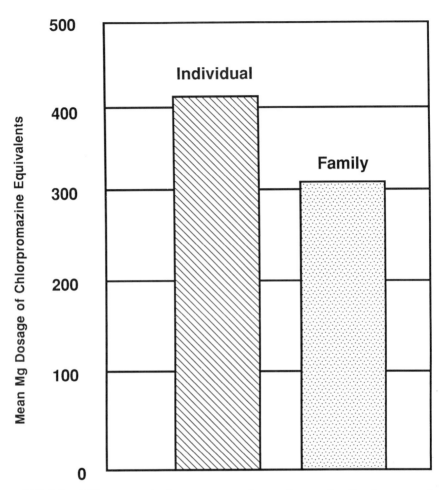

FIGURE 5.   Differences in the average dose of neuroleptic drugs used in the treatment of schizophrenic patients randomly assigned to either behavioral family management or individual supportive therapy over a two-year period. Despite vastly superior outcomes accruing to patients receiving behavioral family therapy, these patients required less neuroleptic maintenance medication than did their counterparts who received individual therapy.

functioning. Skills training as a principal strategy in psychiatric rehabilitation starts from the assumption that many patients will suffer persisting symptoms and residual impairments despite the best efforts at pharmacotherapy and hospitalization. A relatively new field, training of social and vocational skills, has relevance for a wide variety of psychiatric patients and for the professionals who serve them.

The psychiatric disorders with the greatest chronicity—schizophrenia, major depression, and organic syndromes—are those most in need of a skills-training focus. While appropriate drug treatment significantly reduces symptoms in most schizophrenics and depressives, many are refractory to drugs and others experience continuing social and vocational handicaps even with symptomatic improvement. The negative or deficit symptoms of schizophrenia, for example, pose a largely unanswered challenge to the pharmacopeia. Social withdrawal, apathy, anergy, slovenliness, and anhedonia do not respond as well to neuroleptic drugs as do hallucinations, delusions, and thought disorder. Neither do drugs teach life and coping skills, except indirectly through removal or reduction of symptoms. Most schizophrenic persons need to learn or relearn social and personal skills for surviving in the community.

Skills training can begin immediately after the stabilization of an acute episode or exacerbation of a psychiatric disorder which usually results in the loss of social and role functioning. Because of the pervasive disruption of daily living skills by chronic mental disorders, patients generally require training or retraining in a comprehensive array of functional domains relevant to personal and community life: self-care skills, including medication and symptom self-management; family relations; peer and friendship skills; avocational and employment pursuits; money management and consumerism; residential living; recreational and leisure skills; transportation; nutritional food preparation; and choice and use of public agencies.

CASE EXAMPLE _____

A comprehensive skills-training program for rehabilitating chronic mental patients was carried out in a day treatment center sponsored by a Veterans Administration hospital (Spiegler and Agigian 1977). The program was highly structured and emphasized teaching social and vocational skills in classes. Patients were assisted in transferring the knowledge and skills they acquired in the educational program into their community living. After one year, 90 percent of patients enrolled in the educational, skills-training program were still functioning in the community, while only 53 percent of patients assigned to a standard day program were able to sustain their community tenure.

Remediating Disabilities Through Supportive Interventions

When restoration of social and vocational functioning through skills training is limited by continuing deficits and refractory symptoms, rehabilitation strategies aim at helping the individual compensate for handicap by a) locating living, learning, and working environments that can accommodate to the residual deficits and symptoms; and b) adjusting the individual's and family's expectations to a level of functioning that is realistically attainable. Thus, environmental modification and supportive-prosthetic social and vocational environments are a complementary approach to skills training in the reconstitution of social roles for patients with severe and chronic psychiatric disorders.

Environmental interventions attempt to provide the patient with supportive persons, supportive settings, or both. A "support person" might reduce a person's disability and handicap through a number of different roles, that is, as an advocate, companion, counselor, and/or advisor. Attempts at making the setting more supportive focus more on the programs or resources within the environment rather than on support persons per se (for example, sheltered work and living settings, special discharge programs). The main identifying feature of both types of supportive interventions, as distinguished from skill development interventions, is that they do not attempt to systematically and directly change the patient's behavior. Rather, the attempt is simply to support and accommodate the patient's present level of functioning.

CASE EXAMPLE

Citizens from neighborhoods where psychiatric patients were discharged to live were recruited to function as "supportive case workers." They served as companions and "enablers" with the patients to ensure their community adaptation. Over a 12-month period, inpatient days were decreased by 92 percent, suggesting that the nonprofessional enablers were successful in buffering stress and easing transition into community life (Cannady 1982).

In another study of a support team for chronic mental patients (Witheridge et al. 1982), counselors were assigned to severely psychiatrically disabled persons who were at high risk for rehospitalization. They provided a variety of assistance to the patients in their homes and neighborhoods; after one year, the average days hospitalized for the patients dropped from 87 to 37.

Remediation of Handicaps

In addition to clinical rehabilitation interventions of skill and support development, psychiatrically disabled persons can be helped to overcome their handicaps through societal rehabilitation interventions (Anthony 1972). Societal rehabilitation is designed to change the system in which psychiatrically disabled persons must function. Unlike clinical rehabilitation, its focus is not on the skills of specific psychiatrically disabled individuals, nor on their unique environments. Rather, the focus is on system changes which can help many psychiatrically disabled persons overcome their handicaps. Examples of this type of system intervention are the Targeted Job Tax Credit legislation, changes in the length of the trial work period in the Social Security Disability program, and the development of a quota system for the employment of disabled workers. The importance of these system-type interventions cannot be overemphasized. Obstacles in overcoming a handicap may be more a function of a nonaccommodating and discriminating social and economic system than of the person's impairment and disability. Community support programs are another example of a system-wide response to the problems of persons who are severely psychiatrically disabled (Turner and TenHoor 1978).

CASE EXAMPLE

A 30-year-old male with a 15-year history of being in and out of private and state psychiatric hospitals decided he would like to get a job in the community after being in a psychosocial work adjustment program for one year. He did not have a good work history: For example, six months was the longest he had ever been able to hold a job. Using the Targeted Job Tax Credit legislation as an incentive to the employer, the psychiatric rehabilitation team was able to find the disabled person a job working in a video repair shop, a job consistent with the patient's interests and talents. In order to keep his job at the repair shop, the patient needed to learn the skills of taking orders from authority figures, such as showing understanding of what others said and expressing his own thoughts and feelings to others. The team also made the environment more supportive to the patient by educating the employer to the patient's needs and obtained employer agreement on reducing the initial work load/time until the disabled person became comfortable with the new environment.

SUMMARY

Given the pervasive impairments, disabilities, and handicaps of most persons with chronic mental disorders, a combined approach to psychiatric rehabilitation, employing skills training and environmental modification strategies, is most often required. Psychotropic medication, partial and full hospitalization, case management, skills training, social self-help clubs, environmental prostheses, and social change initiatives must be integrated to help patients achieve maximum feasible adaptation. The emphasis on each of the types of intervention will vary with the nature of the disorder, the premorbid level of competence of the patient, and the phase of the illness.

   With an emerging consensus that major psychiatric disorders are stress-linked, biomedical disorders, rehabilitation approaches have emerged from eclectic and empirical traditions emphasizing the development of patients' skills or supportive environments for coping with

---

LEARNING EXERCISE

A number of attributes of effective rehabilitation programs have been identified. While many exemplary psychiatric rehabilitation programs contain unique features that make them difficult to replicate, factors common to successful programs should be emulated by practitioners in any clinical facility or setting. A list of these attributes is given below; for each attribute, consider how your local psychiatric rehabilitation program stacks up in terms of staff, organization, and clinical techniques.

- Enthusiasm and commitment of staff
- Ability to set modest goals and be rewarded with limited progress
- Practice of setting concrete and specific goals with patients
- Administrative support and priority given to rehabilitation
- Comprehensiveness of services
- Networks established with other service providers
- Continuity of care
- Use of skills training and supportive interventions
- Assertive outreach and crisis services
- Emphasis on patients' assets and potential for responsible behavior

---

the enduring disabilities and handicaps of illnesses such as schizophrenia or affective disorders. The practice of psychiatric rehabilitation uses assessment and intervention techniques based on such orientations as social learning and behavior therapy (Liberman and Evans 1985; Paul and Lentz 1977; Liberman and Foy 1983), client-centered therapy and human resources development (Carkhuff and Berenson 1976), and life-span developmental psychology (Strauss and Carpenter 1981).

The psychiatrically disabled person must be involved as much as possible in the setting of rehabilitation goals—a process that necessitates the development of a trusting, mutually respectful and empathic relationship with service providers. The preferred mode of intervention combines judicious and rational psychopharmacology with an educational approach that employs training patients directly in the knowledge and skills they need to function in society.

The rehabilitation process encompasses three stages that are overlapping and recurring for as long as the patient requires professional services. Assessment at the symptomatic, functional, and resource levels guides the patient and professional through a collaborative planning phase. Through diagnostic and assessment interviews, inventories, informants, historical data, role plays, and direct behavioral observation, the evaluation yields information about the psychiatrically disabled person's current deficits, psychopathology, and skills and supports as well as the skill level demanded by the living, learning, and/or working environments in which he or she wishes to function.

The assessment information enables the rehabilitation practitioner to work with the patient and family members in the planning phase to develop a rehabilitation plan that specifies how the person and/or the person's environment must change to achieve the rehabilitation goals. With respect to changes in the person, the plan develops the skill steps that he or she needs to learn or use in order to move from the present level of functioning to the level required by his or her environment. With respect to changes in the person's environment, a sequential plan is designed that describes what and how the necessary coordination, advocacy, and modifications are to be made. The rehabilitation plan also identifies the persons (for example, practitioner, patient, agency, family member) responsible for implementing the various parts of the plan.

In the intervention phase, the rehabilitation plan is implemented to increase the person's skills and/or to make the environment more supportive of the person's functioning. These person- and environmentally focused interventions lead to the achievement of the person's rehabilitation goals, which were first identified during the assessment phase. Repeated and regular monitoring of the change process informs all concerned about goal attainment and enables clinical decisions to be made regarding continuation or change of interventions and goals.

There are many patients who, for the foreseeable future, will remain relatively refractory to skills training and environmental support programs aimed at independent living and full employment. Such individuals can still benefit, however, from rehabilitation. It is possible to improve social adjustment, role performance, and autonomy and quality of life even within the limited opportunities provided by a mental hospital or locked residential care facility in the community.

Research studies have been conducted by a large number of investigators in the United States and Europe that support the following conclusions:

1. Severely psychiatrically disabled persons can learn skills.
2. The psychiatrically disabled person's skills are positively related to measures of rehabilitation outcome.
3. Skill development interventions improve the psychiatrically disabled.
4. Environmental resource development improves the psychiatrically disabled person's rehabilitation outcome.

In conceptualizing psychiatric rehabilitation, the "key and lock" analogy is apt. While it is desirable to maximize an individual's social and instrumental role functioning through training and reeducative procedures, persistent deficits are likely to plague the patient, the family, and the rehabilitation team. Endeavors to upgrade the patient's repertoire of skills hone the "key," but it is often necessary to modify the "lock," the patient's environment. Recent interventions aimed at modification of the family environment have led to dramatic reductions in relapse, exacerbation, and rehospitalization of patients with schizophrenia (Strachan 1986). Other examples of environmental prostheses are sheltered workshops, transitional employment, halfway houses, and psychosocial clubs.

Guiding the rehabilitation professional is

1. the optimism that desirable change is possible, given the harnessing of principles of human learning to the needs of the patient;
2. the belief that motivation for change can come from special arrangements of the patient's rehabilitation and natural environments as well as from within the patient;
3. the confidence that building from the patient's assets and interests, including supportive treatment and family environments, even small improvements can lead to significant functional changes in and uplifting of the patient's quality of life.

The principles of rehabilitation have the potential to tie researchers and professionals engaged in psychiatric rehabilitation together into a cohesive, empirically based field. Rehabilitation practice has taken root in a variety of settings, including mental health centers and clinics, mental hospitals, general hospitals, psychosocial centers, and community support programs. More than ever before, psychiatric rehabilitation is perceived as a legitimate and credible field of practice, education, and research; as complementary to the existing fields of prevention and treatment; and as a necessary component of mental health system planning and policy-making.

REFERENCES

American Psychiatric Association: Diagnostic and Statistical Manual of Mental Disorders (Third Edition). Washington, DC, American Psychiatric Association, 1980

Anthony WA: Societal rehabilitation: changing society's attitudes toward the physical and mentally disabled. Rehabilitation Psychology 19:117–126, 1972

Anthony WA: Principles of Psychiatric Rehabilitation. Baltimore, MD, University Park Press, 1979

Anthony WA, Buell GJ, Sharratt S, et al: Efficacy of psychiatric rehabilitation. Psychol Bull 78:447–456, 1972

Anthony WA, Howell J, Danley K: The vocational rehabilitation of the psychiatrically disabled, in The Chronically Mentally Ill: Research and Services. Edited by Mirabi M. Jamaica, NY, SP Medical and Scientific Books, 1984

Anthony WA, Jansen M: Predicting the vocational capacity of the chronically mentally ill: research and policy implications. Am Psychol 39:537–544, 1984

Anthony WA, Liberman RP: The practice of psychiatric rehabilitation: historical, conceptual, and research base. Schizophr Bull 12:542–559, 1986

Beard JH, Propst RN, Malamud TJ: The Fountain House model of psychiatric rehabilitation. Psychosocial Rehabilitation Journal 5:47–59, 1982

Bennett DH: The historical development of rehabilitation services, in Theory and Practice of Psychiatric Rehabilitation. Edited by Watts FN, Bennett DH. New York, Wiley and Sons, 1983

Bockoven JS: Moral Treatment in American Psychiatry. New York, Springer, 1963

Cannady D: Chronics and cleaning ladies. Psychosocial Rehabilitation Journal 5:13–16, 1982

Carkhuff RR, Berenson BC: Teaching as Treatment. Amherst, MA, Human Resources Development Press, 1976

Falloon IRH: Family Management of Schizophrenia: A Study of Clinical, Social and Family and Economic Benefits. Baltimore, MD, Johns Hopkins University Press, 1985

Frey WD: Functional assessment in the 80s: a conceptual enigma, a technical challenge, in Functional Assessment in Rehabilitation. Edited by Halpern A, Fuhrer M. New York, Brooke Publishing, 1984

Goldstrom I, Manderscheid R: The chronically mentally ill: a descriptive analysis from the Uniform Client Data instrument. Community Support Services Journal 2:4–9, 1982

Grob S: Psychosocial rehabilitation centers: old wine in a new bottle, in The Chronic Psychiatric Patient in the Community. Edited by Barofsky I, Budson R. Jamaica, NY, SP Medical and Scientific Books, 1983

Harding CM, Strauss JS: The course of schizophrenia: an evolving concept, in Controversies in Schizophrenia. Edited by Alpert M. New York, Guilford, 1985

Harrow M, Grinker RR, Silverstein ML, et al: Is modern-day schizophrenic outcome still negative? Am J Psychiatry 135:1156–1162, 1978

Hawkins H: A plea for convalescent homes in connection with asylums for the insane poor. Journal of Mental Science 17:107–116, 1971

Hersen M, Bellack AS: Social skills training for chronic psychiatric patients: rationale, research findings, and future directions. Compr Psychiatry 17:559–580, 1976

Kokes RF, Strauss JS, Klorman R: Premorbid adjustment and schizophrenic heterogeneity: II. Measuring premorbid adjustment. Schizophr Bull 3:186–214, 1977

Lamb HR: Treating the Long-Term Mentally Ill. San Francisco, Jossey-Bass, 1982

Leff JP, Hirsch SR, Gaind R, et al: Life events and maintenance therapy in schizophrenic relapse. Br J Psychiatry 123:659–668, 1973

Liberman RP: Behavior therapy for schizophrenia, in Treatment of Schizophrenia. Edited by West LJ, Flinn D. New York, Grune and Stratton, 1976

Liberman RP: Social factors in schizophrenia, in American Psychiatric Association Annual Review (Volume 1). Edited by Grinspoon L. Washington, DC, American Psychiatric Press, 1982

Liberman RP: Psychosocial therapies for schizophrenia, in Comprehensive Textbook of Psychiatry (fourth edition). Baltimore, MD, Williams and Wilkins, 1984

Liberman RP, Evans CC: Behavioral rehabilitation for chronic mental patients. J Clin Psychopharmacol 5:8s–14s, 1985

Liberman RP, Foy DW: Psychiatric rehabilitation for chronic mental patients. Psychiatric Annals 13:539–545, 1983

Liberman RP, King LW, DeRisi WJ: Behavior analysis and therapy in community mental health, in Handbook of Behavior Analysis and Modification. Edited by Leitaiberg H. Englewood Cliffs, NJ, Prentice Hall, 1976

Liberman RP, Wallace C, Teigen J, et al: Interventions with psychotics, in Innovative Treatment Methods in Psychopathology. Edited by Calhoun KS, Adams HE, Mitchell EM. New York, Wiley, 1974

Linn MW, Klett CJ, Caffey EM: Foster home characteristics and psychiatric patient outcome. Arch Gen Psychiatry 41:157–161, 1980

Paul GP, Lentz R: Psychosocial Treatment of Chronic Mental Patients. Cambridge, MA, Harvard Universtiy Press, 1977

Pfohl B, Andreasen NC: Schizophrenia: diagnosis and classification, in American Psychiatric Association Annual Review (Volume 5). Edited by Frances AJ, Hales RF. Washington, DC, American Psychiatric Press, 1986

Presley AJ, Grubb AB, Semple D: Predictors of successful rehabilitation in long-stay patients. Acta Psychiatr Scand 66:83–88, 1982

Spiegler MD, Agigian H: The Community Training Center: An Educational-Behavioral-Social Systems Model for Rehabilitating Psychiatric Patients. New York, Brunner/Mazel, 1977

Strachan AM: Family intervention for the rehabilitation of schizophrenia: toward protection and coping. Schizophr Bull 12:678–698, 1986

Strauss JS, Carpenter WT: Prediction of outcome in schizophrenia: III. Five-year outcome and its predictors. Arch Gen Psychiatry 34:159–163, 1977

Strauss JS, Carpenter WT: Schizophrenia. New York, Plenum Press, 1981

Taylor CB, Liberman RP, Agras WS: Treatment evaluation and behavior therapy, in Treatment Planning in Psychiatry. Edited by Lewis J, Usdin G. Washington, DC, American Psychiatric Press, 1982

Tsuang MT, Woosen RF, Fleming JA: Long-term outcome of major psychoses. Arch Gen Psychiatry 36:1295–1301, 1979

Turner J, TenHoor W: The NIMH Community Support Program: pilot approach to a needed social reform. Schizophr Bull 4:319–348, 1978

Vaugh CE, Leff JP: The influences of family and social factors on the course of psychiatric illness. Br J Psychiatry 129:125–137, 1976

Wallace CJ, Liberman RP: Social skills training for patients with schizophrenia: a controlled clinical trial. Psychiatry Res 15:239–247, 1985

Witheridge TF, Dincin J, Appleby L: Working with the most frequent recidivists: a total team approach to assertive resource management. Psychosocial Rehabilitation Journal 5:9–11, 1982

CHAPTER 2

PSYCHIATRIC DIAGNOSIS

DAVID LUKOFF, PH.D
JOSEPH VENTURA, M.A.

A disease known is half cured.

Thomas Fuller, M.D.
Gnomologia

A reliable and carefully conducted diagnostic assessment of a chronic mental patient is the first step in treatment and rehabilitation. The very term "chronic mental patient" derives from a definition that owes much to diagnosis and monitoring of symptoms. It implies that the patient's diagnosis falls into certain categories, that symptoms must be severe enough to interfere with social functioning and community adaptation, and that symptoms of the illness have persisted for at least two years. (Goldman et al. 1981). Patients with chronic disabilities can be diagnosed as having schizophrenic disorders, affective disorders, other psychoses, organic mental disorders, and certain persisting anxiety, substance abuse, and somatoform disorders.

Because many chronic patients are likely to have a diagnostic label that was assigned to them years ago, before the advent of the *Diagnostic and Statistical Manual of Mental Disorders (Third Edition) (DSM-III*; American Psychiatric Association 1980), it is important to carry out reevaluations of their current diagnostic status. The earlier diagnosis may have been incorrect; the patient's diagnosis may have changed (for example, schizophrenia may evolve to schizoaffective disorder), the earlier diagnosis may have been based on faulty elicitation of symptoms, or a new additional diagnosis may need to be added (such as substance abuse disorder superimposed on an affective disorder).

Recent studies indicate that the assignment of a dual diagnosis— that is, the coexistence of more than one major mental disorder in a patient—is frequently missed in the chronic population. Approximately 46 percent of patients admitted to an inpatient unit at a Veterans Administration hospital for schizophrenia also met *DSM-III* criteria for alcoholism. Sixty to seventy percent had substance abuse problems. A significant minority, perhaps 10 to 15 percent, of chronic mental patients may also be mentally retarded (Menolascino and Stark 1984). Diagnosticians need to pay greater attention to maximizing the built-in potential of the *DSM-III* for recording multiple diagnoses for patients.

Why is it important to categorize patients into one or another of these disorders? Isn't it a fact that, unlike medical diagnosis, psychiatric diagnosis does not predict course or outcome? So why bother? Isn't assessment of functional disability more important than a diagnostic label for the person's symptoms and syndrome? What is the process of psychiatric diagnosis anyway? Since the true causes of mental disorder are unknown, how can a diagnosis help a patient, his or her therapist or case manager, or family? These are the questions that I will attempt to answer in this chapter. But first, let's understand how the symptoms and signs of a mental disorder fit into the stress-vulnerability-coping-competence model.

STRESS-VULNERABILITY-COPING-COMPETENCE MODEL

The onset and intensity of symptoms are the outcome of a complex interaction among genetic, vulnerability, stressor, protective, and potentiator factors that operate within an individual (biologically and behaviorally) as well as in the individual's environment. (These factors are described more fully in Chapter 1.) Monitoring the level of symptomatology present in a patient can help the therapist assess the impact of these factors, much as a thermometer reading of a person's temperature can help a physician gauge the status of an infectious process. Changes in any of these areas, such as the death of a patient's friend, an overstimulating work environment, or participation in a problem-solving training program that increases the patient's coping skills, can be expected to affect the occurrence and severity of symptoms.

Symptoms interact with social and occupational functioning in a reciprocal way; that is, psychopathology can affect and be affected by events in the social and work spheres. Symptoms, when severe, can also intrude on self-care. Symptoms themselves may become stressors, in that their emergence can frighten relatives, coworkers, and often the patients themselves. The interaction of stress, vulnerability, coping, and competence factors is a dynamic process, and therefore the symptom picture of patients varies over time. For example, an individual who is biologically vulnerable to frequent relapses may experience an episode of illness and hospitalization during a period of stress (for example, trying to succeed at college or working at a demanding job). The same vulnerable individual might have a better course of illness when involved in a vocational rehabilitation and community support program that confers protection against stress.

Both the development and intensity of symptoms are amenable to interventions of various types, which will be described in subsequent chapters of this book. However, the first step in the clinical management of chronic mental disorders is to use techniques that reliably permit symptoms to be measured. In addition to generating diagnostic information, the assessment of symptoms indirectly provides an index of the factors affecting the rehabilitation of the chronic mental patient.

IMPORTANCE OF DIAGNOSIS

Psychiatric diagnosis is the attempt to scientifically classify mental disorders into groups with similar characteristics of symptoms, signs, and associated behavioral disabilities. Although the majority of chronic mental patients carry the diagnosis of schizophrenic disorders, several diagnostic categories are contained within this population. Accurate diagnosis is a critical component of a comprehensive treatment package and should precede all other treatments. The choice of appropriate psychopharmacological and psychosocial treatments depends on accurate diagnosis. Neuroleptic medication for schizophrenia, developed in the 1950s, and the more recent antidepressant medication, antianxiety medication, and lithium for bipolar disorder have appeared as specific agents for these disorders. Thus, diagnosis is a critical determinant of pharmacological treatment.

The selection of psychoactive drugs on the basis of diagnosis is shown in Table 2. It should be made clear that drugs are not as specific to a diagnostic category or disorder as they are to the type of symptoms primarily experienced by patients having that disorder. For example, psychotic symptoms—whether related to a schizophrenic disorder or affective disorder or organic mental disorder—tend to respond to neuroleptic antipsychotic drugs. Antidepressants of both the tricyclic and monoamine oxidase inhibitor types tend to reduce symptoms of depression and block the experience of panic symptoms. The emerging combinations of drugs that are becoming useful in augmenting the effects of primary drugs, shown in Table 2, are also linked to the nature of a patient's psychiatric symptoms. For example, lithium has been found to be effective in combination with antidepressants in some primarily depressed patients who are refractory to antidepressants alone. Carbamazepine has been found effective in manic patients who don't respond satisfactorily to lithium.

At times, making a reliable primary diagnosis in a patient is key to selecting the preferred psychotropic drug. For example, a patient who sits in a chair without moving for hours at a time could be suffering from severe retardation secondary to depression or from catatonia as part of a schizophrenic disorder. In the first case, treatment with antidepressants is called for and would be likely to alleviate the motor retardation. In such a patient, use of a neuroleptic might not be effective. However, administration of a neuroleptic to a catatonic patient might alleviate the symptom. Moreover, if the patient's motor retardation was a result of developmental disability, psychosocial rather than drug treatment would be indicated.

Choice of psychosocial treatment also depends on diagnostic assessment. Extreme social withdrawal might be a result of depression, or it could be a symptom of schizophrenia. Cognitive therapy aimed at reducing the patient's negative thinking style and irrational beliefs would probably be helpful in reducing the withdrawal if it is secondary to depression, but it would not be effective if the withdrawal is a result of schizophrenia.

An important distinction in the diagnostic categorization of patients is between psychotic and nonpsychotic disorders. The *DSM-III* defines *psychotic* as

TABLE 2: Diagnosis of a Chronic Mentally Ill Person Often Leads to the Selection of a Diagnostically Specific Psychotropic Medication

Diagnosis	Primary Medication	Ancillary Augmenting or Adjunctive Medication
Schizophrenic disorders	Neuroleptic	Reserpine, carbamazepine
Schizoaffective disorder with depression	Neuroleptic	Antidepressant or lithium
Schizofffective disorder with mania	Neuroleptic	Lithium
Major depressive episode	Antidepressant	Lithium
1) with mood-congruent psychotic features	Antidepressant	
2) with mood-incongruent psychotic features	Neuroleptic	Lithium
Manic episode, with or without psychotic features	Neuroleptic and/or lithium	Carbamazepine
Bipolar disorder, depressed	Lithium	Antidepressant
Bipolar disorder, manic	Neuroleptic and/or lithium	Carbamazepine
Bipolar disorder, mixed	Neuroleptic, lithium	Antidepressant, carbamazepine
Bipolar disorder, mixed (with psychotic features)	Neuroleptic, lithium	Antidepressant, carbamazepine

gross impairment in reality testing. . . . When there is gross impairment in reality testing, the individual incorrectly evaluates the accuracy of his or her perceptions and thoughts and makes incorrect inferences about external reality, even in the face of contrary evidence. (American Psychiatric Association 1980, p. 367)

The following are psychotic disorders in the *DSM-III*: schizophrenic disorder, schizophreniform disorder, schizoaffective disorder, paranoid disorder, paraphrenia, major depressive episode with psychotic features, and bipolar disorder with psychotic features. Many patients with these disorders experience a chronic course of persisting or intermittent symptoms and social disability. Treatment personnel need to be aware if a psychotic disorder is present in a chronic mental patient. Medication is likely to play a greater role in the overall treatment approach, and medication compliance issues will often be a focus of the therapy. The family members of psychotic patients may play a greater role in providing diagnostic information, giving feedback on the patient's progress, and acting as adjunct supportive therapists. Relatives may need to be educated concerning the nature of the patient's disorder.

Many patients with psychotic disorders have persisting psychotic symptoms even when they are in their best clinical state. The determination of persisting symptoms, through structured and repeated ratings of the patient's psychopathology, is of importance in designing an optimal drug and psychosocial rehabilitation program. Drugs should be titrated down to the lowest level consistent with protection from exacerbation. Some patients are more refractory to the effects of neuroleptics than others and hence benefit less from them. In terms of psychotherapeutic approaches for patients with persisting psychotic symptoms, the therapy sessions should be shorter and the treatment more structured, behavioral, and focused on short-term goals.

RELIABILITY OF DIAGNOSIS

In the past, diagnosis of the major mental disorders has been plagued by problems with low reliability, that is, poor agreement between the diagnoses assigned by different professionals. In several studies conducted during the 1960s, agreement between psychiatrists on diagnoses was found to be only 50 percent. This impeded both the development of effective treatments and the delivery of appropriate services to psychiatric patients.

Diagnosis of the major mental disorders is hampered by the lack of any laboratory tests or known etiology, which aids in the diagnosis of most physical disorders. The primary sources of diagnostic information are 1) the patient's self-report of his or her inner experiences, termed "symptoms"; and 2) manifestations of pathological conditions that can be observed by the diagnostic examiner or significant others, termed "signs." The *DSM-III* does not recognize any single sign or symptom as pathognomonic, that is, as definitely indicating a diagnosis of schizophrenia. The signs and symptoms of schizophrenia are nonspecific and can be mimicked by many other conditions, including organic brain syndromes and affective disorders. The presence of signs such as memory impairment, clouding of consciousness, or disorientation especially warrant a neurological assessment to rule out these competing diagnoses. Frequently abused street drugs such as LSD, mushrooms, PCP, amphetamines, and cocaine, as well as prolonged abuse of alcohol, can also cause hallucinations and delusions that are similar to the symptoms of schizophrenia. In addition, the examiner must also determine whether any unusual beliefs (delusions) or perceptual alterations (hallucinations) reported by a patient occurred as part of a shared religious experience. Subculturally validated experiences should not be rated as diagnostically significant symptoms. Schizophrenia is a diagnosis of exclusion that should be assigned only after organic disorders, substance abuse disorders, and subcultural variables have been ruled out.

However, three major improvements in diagnostic procedures have occurred over the past 10 years. First, operational criteria that specify explicit requirements for classification have been developed. This reduces the incidence of diagnostic disagreement of professionals using different standards for diagnostic categories. The *DSM-III* includes operational criteria for almost all diagnostic categories. As a result, reliabilities of the major mental disorders are much higher in the *DSM-III* than in the *DSM-II* (American Psychiatric Association 1968), which lacked operational criteria.

Second, structured interviews have been developed that guide the interviewer in systematically covering all the relevant symptom areas. Interviews such as the Present State Examination (PSE), the Schedule for the Assessment of Affective Disorders and Schizophrenia, and the Diagnostic Interview Schedule reduce information variance between diagnosticians and also result in higher levels of agreement between professionals. An example from the PSE (Wing et al. 1974) of the questions for Thought Insertion is shown in Table 3. This chapter includes an abbreviated structured interview that covers the diagnostically significant symptoms of chronic mental patients.

Third, standard definitions have been prepared to accompany structured interviews. This ensures that all users mean the same thing by a symptom. The PSE includes a glossary with definitions for each of the 140 items in the interview. The definition for Thought Insertion contained in the PSE glossary is

The subject experienced thoughts which are not his own, intruding into his mind. The symptom is not that he has been caused to have

TABLE 3: Questions Used in the Present State Examination to Elicit and Rate the Symptoms of Thought Insertion

---

These symptoms are often recorded as false positives. The examiner must be satisfied that the subject is not simply assenting to a question he or she does not understand, but genuinely recognizes the experience and can describe it so that the examiner recognizes it.

Are thoughts put into your head which you know are not your own?
(How do you know they are not your own?)
(Where do they come from?)
RATE THOUGHT INSERTION: Include only thoughts recognized as alien. Do not include delusional elaboration, only basic experience. (Exclude hallucinations)

1 =   Symptom described clearly, but subject thinks it may be due to "own unconscious thoughts," etc. (that is, not certainly alien).
2 =   Symptom described clearly and thoughts described as alien, that is, inserted into mind from elsewhere (even if subject does not know from where). Not hallucinations.

---

unusual thoughts (for example, if he thinks the Devil is making him think evil thoughts the symptom should be rated as "delusion of control"), but that the thoughts themselves are not his. In the most typical case, the alien thoughts are said to have been inserted into the mind from outside, by means of radar or telepathy or some other means. Sometimes the subject may say that he does not know where the alien thoughts came from, although he is quite clear that they are not his own. (Wing et al. 1974, p. 160)

The *DSM-III* also includes a glossary with definitions and examples for many of the important symptoms and terms.

Chronic mental patients will usually have a diagnosis already assigned to them by the time you see them. Why then conduct another diagnostic assessment?

First, many, if not most, chronic mental patients are incompletely or incorrectly diagnosed. Second, there is a need to regularly reassess the diagnostic picture of psychiatric patients, particularly patients with major mental disorders. Most diagnoses are assigned during an acute episode. Often accurate historical information is not obtainable from the patient, and relatives may not be available to provide the necessary background data. Yet, by the time a patient is labeled as chronic (illness for a minimum of two years), information on course of the disorder should be available either from the patient or from case records. Many problematic cases become much easier to diagnose once accurate information on the past course of the illness is elicited.

CASE EXAMPLE

A consultation using structured interview methods often clarifies diagnostically confusing cases. At admission to a psychiatric unit of a state hospital, a 29-year-old single woman had been diagnosed as having major depression. After two weeks on the unit, her diagnosis was changed to schizophrenic disorder when it was discovered that she had been delusional in the past. During past admissions, she had received *DSM-II* diagnoses of schizoaffective disorder; manic-depression, depressed type; and depressive neurosis. At different times she had been treated with neuroleptics, antidepressants, and lithium.

The administration of a structured interview yielded responses indicating that she currently met the criteria for a *DSM-III* depressive episode. She had depressive mood and five depressive symptoms: insomnia, loss of interests, feelings of worthlessness, difficulty concentrating, and suicidal ideation. All of these symptoms had persisted for longer than the two-week period required for rating a depressive episode. However, further questioning about her past psychiatric history uncovered a manic episode two years previously that was not noted in her chart. During that episode, she reported feeling ecstatic as she developed the belief that she was the messiah and that God was sending her messages in the newspaper and signs on license plates. She believed she had been given the mission to save the world by giving people a leader they could look up to. She hitchhiked from California to New York City, planning to travel on from there to an Israeli kibbutz. She expected that she would be recognized as the messiah by the kibbutz and would redesign the Israeli flag. She stayed in New York for five weeks, supported by a succession of different men for short periods before the episode ended and she returned to California. She was not hospitalized during this period.

Her elevated mood, increased activity, inflated self-esteem, decreased need for sleep, and involvement with activities that might lead to painful consequences persisted for more than the one week required by the *DSM-III* for a manic episode. The psychotic features that were present during this episode, but not the manic symptoms, were noted in her chart and accounted for her diagnosis of schizophrenic disorder. However, with the full symptom picture available, it became clear that the psychotic symptoms were all congruent with her elated mood at the time of her manic episode. Therefore, her current diagnosis was readily clarified as bipolar disorder, depressed. The use of a structured interview along with careful elicitation of past history helped to resolve this diagnostic dilemma. Her condition could then be treated more rationally, with a change in medication from a neuroleptic to a combination of lithium and an antidepressant.

BENEFITS OF CAREFUL DIAGNOSTIC ASSESSMENT

A detailed interview of the chronic mental patient has therapeutic benefits beyond the assigning of an appropriate diagnosis. It greatly improves rapport with some patients as they share the details and depth of their experience, often for the first time. Following the structured diagnostic interview, the patient highlighted in the above vignette stated that it had been the most interesting day she had spent since coming to the hospital five weeks before. Thus it can be useful for all professionals who have sustained contact with the chronic mental patient—psychiatrists, psychologists, social workers, nurses, rehabilitation therapists—to conduct a diagnostic interview. In addition to contributing to the ongoing diagnostic evaluation, the information also helps the professional function as a therapist by making him or her better informed about the experiential world in which the patient lives. The therapist can better help the patient to sort out reality-based perceptions from delusional beliefs. Dynamically oriented and behaviorally oriented therapists can uncover a wealth of information for future therapy sessions. For example, one interviewer determined that a patient experienced auditory hallucinations when he stayed up late at night drinking coffee and listening to loud music. A contract with the patient was developed whereby no increase in medication would be prescribed if he agreed to drink only decaffeinated coffee after 6:00 pm.

A depressed patient reported hearing the voice of her dead mother making critical and hostile comments to her, such as, "You're no good. You'll never make it through college." The patient's mother had died suddenly in an automobile accident a year before the patient's depressive episode. Unresolved grief and guilt elicited during the structured interview became a major focus of the therapy sessions.

POINTERS FOR THE DIAGNOSTIC INTERVIEW

The following practical suggestions and guidelines may promote a more satisfactory and mutually valuable diagnostic interview between patient and professional.

Setting Up the Initial Appointment

Frequently, diagnostic interviews take place by appointment in the clinician's office. However, in institutional settings such as hospitals and board-and-care homes, a third party may arrange the time and place to meet with a patient. In other situations, you will need to make all the arrangements after being given only the patient's name and ward or board-and-care location. Regardless of whether the patient is well known or new to you, call ahead to ensure the patient's availability for a 45- to 90-minute block of uninterrupted time. It is usually possible to complete a diagnostic interview in one session; however, be prepared to make a second or more visits in difficult cases or where the patient's cognitive capacities have not reconstituted.

Interviews should be conducted in private. Most wards have a room available for such purposes. When the room is unavailable or when at facilities that do not have a private interviewing room, make the extra effort to find a location that maximizes privacy and minimizes the possibility of interruption. If you decide to use the patient's room, the patient should be requested to sit in a chair rather than lie in bed.

First Contact With the Patient

The interview begins the moment you meet the patient. Take note of the patient's general demeanor. Does he or she appear depressed? overly cheerful? preoccupied with inner thoughts? mumbling to himself or herself? highly distractable? or incoherent? These first few moments of careful observation of the patient can provide valuable diagnostic information.

In introducing yourself, be sure to give your name, professional title, and a brief rationale for the interview. For example,

Interviewer: Hello, I'm Mr. Smith, a psychologist here at the clinic. I'd like to ask you some questions about the types of problems you've been having recently. Would you come with me to the interview room so we can talk in private?

Avoid social pleasantries such as, "It's a pleasure to meet you." They interfere with the professional atmosphere required for disclosure of severe problems and embarrassing experiences. However, neutral comments or questions such as, "What have you been doing during the day?" can help break the ice.

With acutely ill and extremely thought disordered patients, it may be necessary to titrate the duration and focus of the interview depending on the patient's tolerance, cognitive status, and anxiety. Some diagnostic evaluations can be completed only over several sessions or must await the patient's clinical improvement.

Development of Rapport

Rapport develops as the interview proceeds. It results partly from the interviewer's nonjudgmental acceptance of the patient's beliefs and experiences, even when they seem bizarre. For example, a patient who claims that he sees UFOs and that they are stealing his thoughts could be responded to as follows:

Interviewer: You mentioned that UFOs were following you and stealing your thoughts. Could you tell me some more about that?

However, the basic function of the diagnostic interview can be contrasted with the therapy session that at a future date you may conduct with the same patient. During the diagnostic interview, your objective is to elicit and record pertinent symptomatology. This precludes engaging in reality testing, that is, trying to dissuade patients of their delusional beliefs. The interviewer also need not attempt to resolve the patient's anxiety associated with the symptoms. The interviewer should not continually reassure the patient that he is okay, although occasional empathic statements are helpful. For example, if the patient has persecutory delusions such as in the example above, the interviewer may offer a statement which conveys an understanding of that experience and patient.

Interviewer: That must have been frightening.
Patient: Yes, it was. In fact, I think that people at work have been programmed by the aliens and maybe even the nurses here at the hospital.

The diagnostician who communicates an understanding attitude toward the patient's unusual experiences will elicit a more accurate and complete picture of symptomatology.

Taking notes of the patient's verbatim statements provides an important record of the patient's symptoms. Most patients will not object to your recording examples. Occasionally, a suspicious patient will express concern about notes being taken, but you can usually allay this fear by explaining that you are trying to record his or her experiences as accurately as possible.

The verbatim description of symptoms should be written into the medical record so that clinicians meeting the patient in subsequent years can more readily document the diagnosis or changes in diagnosis.

LEARNING EXERCISE

To appreciate the problems attendant upon failures to record graphic examples of a patient's symptomatology in the medical record, locate the chart of a patient in your facility or practice setting. Go through the chart, including the reports of diagnostic interviews, and try to locate verbatim descriptions of symptoms and subjective experiences of the patient. If you cannot find verbatim descriptions of symptoms, are you able to find sufficient documentation of the symptoms to be certain that the symptoms were actually present? That the diagnostic criteria were satisfied?

Phrasing Questions

Using questions from a structured interview will help you get the interview underway. Once the initial question has been asked, you should continue to elicit more details of the patient's experiences. Useful probes include: "Can you tell me more?"; "What was that experience like?"; "When did that happen to you last?"; "What was it like?"; and "Can you give me an example?" The following vignette shows how the interviewer moves from the initial question for depression, listed in the structured interview reprinted later in this chapter, to probes of her own.

Interviewer: Have you felt depressed?
Patient: Yes, I have felt very depressed.
Interviewer: Could you describe what that was like.
Patient: It was awful.
Interviewer: How long have you been feeling depressed?
Patient: For the past month I have felt depressed constantly day and night.
Interviewer: Can you give me an example of how feeling depressed has affected you?
Patient: I stopped bowling and seeing friends. I even stopped watching my favorite shows on the TV.

Notice that the interviewer started with the standard introductory question contained in the structured interview. Then the interviewer followed up the patient's acknowledgment of depression with several questions designed to elicit more details of the severity of the depression. Close-ended questions, those which can be answered with a simple yes or no, are helpful in determining whether a given symptom is potentially present. However, to obtain examples, the interviewer then needs to switch to more open-ended questions, which provide the specifics. Non-verbal listening techniques such as head nodding, good eye contact, and vocalizing "uh-huhs" also contribute to the flow of material from the patient.

If the patient claims not to remember critical pieces of information, the interviewer should try to jog the patient's memory by helping her recreate the circumstances surrounding that experience. For example,

Interviewer: Were you hearing voices at that time?
Patient: I really don't remember.
Interviewer: Try to think back to sitting in your room at the Lost Pines board-and-care. Do you recall ever hearing voices there?
Patient: Oh yeah. I thought my roommate was using telepathy to transmit his voice into my mind.

Management of the Interview

Keeping the interview focused on diagnostically relevant topics is sometimes tricky. Actively symptomatic patients may try to direct the interview toward their areas of concern. In such cases, the interviewer needs to refocus the patient back to the pertinent areas. At times, you may have to ignore the topic the patient seems to want to discuss, a style you may not adopt for therapy sessions.

Patient: Yes, I have telepathy and I've been using it to read the minds of government leaders.
Interviewer: So that's a special power that you have. Now I'd like to ask you some different questions. Have you heard voices talking to you when no one was around?
Patient: Yes, it's the telepathy that they use on me. Sometimes I have the power and sometimes they do. I haven't figured it out yet, but I'm sure it's the government that's behind this.
Interviewer: What have you heard the voices say to you?
Patient: They tell me, "You'll be a world leader."

Similarly, some patients will ask many questions. If you respond to all of them, the interview will be impeded. Do not be afraid to defer the patient's questions to the end of the interview.

Patient: Do you think I'm crazy?
Interviewer: I'd like to collect as much information as possible before concluding this interview. We can discuss the results of my evaluation at the end of our session.

Conceptual disorganization is a core symptom of schizophrenia and also occurs frequently in bipolar disorder. Conceptually disorganized patients present special diagnostic problems because they may have difficulty providing the information required for making diagnoses. For example, blocking, circumstantiality, flight of ideas, illogicality, over- and under-inclusiveness, and loosening of associations can interfere with the comprehension of responses, even to structured interview questions. With such patients, the interviewer must be especially careful to repeat questions, define terms in very simple language, rephrase the patient's responses to verify the content, refocus the patient on the question, and sort out irrelevancies and illogicalities. Open-ended questions may tax the patient's already disorganized thought processes. In such cases, the interviewer needs to provide more structure in the questions, such as by providing a few choices of potential responses once a patient has acknowledged the presence of a symptom.

Interviewer: Do you hear voices when no one else is around?
Patient: I hear voices . . . not from temperature . . . around so new . . .
Interviewer: Are they male or female voices?
Patient: Male . . . I walk to the world over . . . .
Interviewer: Do they say nice things to you or do they criticize you?
Patient: Mean things or curse at me.

Duration of Interview

The duration and focus of an interview may need to be titrated on the basis of the patient's tolerance, cognitive status, and tension level. Diagnostic evaluations with conceptually disorganized patients and patients in the acute phase of a manic, depressive, or psychotic episode may need to be completed over several sessions.

In the first session with a 33-year-old male patient, the interviewer began by asking the patient's birth date and place of residence. The patient answered these questions coherently. Then the interviewer asked, "What problems led to your coming to the hospital?"

The patient responded, "I am the Creator . . . My cousin is a good guy . . . works as a plumber . . . the female part is always . . . I comprehensive the burden."

Since further questions also yielded similarly incoherent responses, the interviewer terminated the interview.

From this session, the only symptoms that could be confirmed were grandiose delusions and conceptual disorganization. Two days later, the interviewer returned. In response to a structured interview similar to the one delineated in the next section, the patient was able to provide information about his depressed mood and associated symptoms of depression. However, after 15 minutes, the responses again became conceptually disorganized and the interview had to be terminated during the questioning about elated mood. The interviewer could see that the patient's cognitive abilities were reconstituting under the influence of medication, and so waited two additional days and returned again. This time, the interviewer was able to complete the entire interview and elicit a complete picture of both psychotic and depressive symptoms, with the onset of the psychotic symptoms preceding the affective symptoms.

Neophyte diagnosticians often ask the following questions:

1. Should acutely ill patients be interviewed, or is it better to wait until symptoms remit?

The closer the patient is to the acute phase, the more accurate information you may be able to elicit. Many patients forget or "seal-over" diagnostically important symptoms. However, if the patient is severely incoherent (not just delusional), it may be necessary to wait until some degree of remission has occurred.

2. What if the patient becomes upset or agitated during the interview?

Although extreme agitation may require that the interview be terminated, often the interviewer can temporarily redirect the line of questioning to a more neutral area. Once the patient has calmed down, the previous line of questioning can be resumed at a less intense level.

3. What if the patient is suspicious or even accuses me of plotting against her?

This may happen. In fact, it is not unusual for patients to incorporate the staff into their delusional world. Calmly but firmly reassure the patient that you are there to help with her treatment. You can also inform her of confidentiality procedures which prohibit the information from being used by other agencies without her permission.

4. What if the patient provides contradictory information? Is it all right for the interviewer to confront the patient?

Yes, although the interviewer should not express irritation at the inconsistencies. The proper attitude to convey is that you would like to get as accurate information as possible. If done in a nonjudgmental manner, this sort of confrontation rarely elicits distress from patients. For example:

Interviewer: You mentioned earlier that you hear voices. What do they say to you?
Patient: I don't hear any voices.
Interviewer: Earlier you said that you heard God giving you instructions.
Patient: Oh yeah, I hear God talking to me, but not voices.

If the inconsistency is obviously due to delusional accounts of past events, such as claims to have been a marine, a priest, an undercover agent, and a student all simultaneously, there is no need to confront the patient to clarify the inconsistencies. The material should simply be noted as delusions.

5. What if you have completed asking all the relevant questions and are still not sure of the diagnosis?

In some studies, this diagnostic dilemma has been found to occur in 20 to 25 percent of cases. Although the interview is the heart of the diagnostic procedure, you are not constrained from obtaining information from any other sources. Relatives may often be able to fill in gaps in the patient's memory. They particularly can help with the sequence in which symptoms developed. Useful information is often available from nursing and other ancillary staff who interact and observe the patient over longer time periods under varying degrees of stress in naturalistic settings. Obtaining input from these staff can help clarify ambiguities in the patient's self-report of symptoms. Previous chart material is also a resource that can help resolve the diagnosis, although chart information may not always be acceptable unless a specific example of a symptom is recorded. Simple references to thought broadcast or auditory hallucinations without a confirming example are of dubious value. Diagnostic interviewers should be conservative, allowing data to accumulate over time and should err on the side of waiting for full documentation. A consensus diagnosis utilizing all sources of data (for example, structured interview, nursing staff observations, relatives' and friends' reports, historical documents from previous hospital or clinic treatment episodes, and current medical chart material) can maximize the validity of a diagnosis.

In a recent case, a patient presented with grandiose delusions but denied elevated mood. None was observed on admission. However some of the associated features of a manic episode were present, including inflated self-esteem, distractibility, increased activity, and talkativeness. The staff were undecided between a diagnosis of schizophrenic disorder and bipolar disorder. The resident contacted the relatives with whom the patient had been living, and found that for two weeks prior to admission, the patient had been talking constantly about "cosmic bliss" and feelings of being in "seventh heaven." With this additional information, it could be seen that the patient was admitted near the end of her manic episode.

In particularly questionable cases, medication may be cautiously withdrawn so that you can reexamine the patient while he or she is in a drug-free state. Many times, diagnostically significant symptoms will reappear or be identifiable more graphically, allowing a more accurate diagnosis to be made.

STRUCTURED DIAGNOSTIC INTERVIEW

A brief structured interview containing questions for making differential diagnoses of psychotic disorders is printed below. Using a structured interview will greatly improve your ability to elicit symptoms from patients. However, an equally important diagnostic task is rating the presence of symptoms. An interviewer may fully elicit a patient's auditory hallucinations and then misperceive the presence of voice commentary due to a misunderstanding of the definition of the symptom. Some definitions are available in the glossary of the *DSM-III*. The Description and Classification of Psychiatric Symptoms (Wing et al. 1974) contains an excellent glossary that gives guidelines and examples for rating psychotic symptoms.

A careful inquiry will often disconfirm the presence of a symptom that the patient seems to acknowledge. Such "false positives" are a major source of diagnostic error. Below is a vignette that illustrates that follow-up probes and obtaining an example are essential components of the diagnostic process.

Interviewer: Are thoughts put into your head which you know are not your own?
Patient: Yeah, the Devil makes me think some very evil things at times.
He makes me think about making love to women I've just met.
Interviewer: Could these possibly be your own thoughts?

Patient: Well, they could be my thoughts, but I wouldn't think them by myself. I'm a religious married man. It must be the Devil which makes me think about sex.

By probing further, the interview determined that the patient experienced unwanted thoughts which he believed were influenced by the Devil. This did not meet the criteria for thought insertion, which requires that the thought be experienced as inserted. While a cursory interview might rate this patient as having acknowledged thought insertion, his experience is probably not even rateable as a delusion. The full extent of the patient's beliefs in the powers of the Devil and his subcultural religious background would have to be explored further before making a final determination about the presence of delusional beliefs.

The interview below covers the major *DSM-III* diagnostic categories to which most chronic mental patients are assigned. These include schizophrenic disorder, schizoaffective disorder, bipolar disorder, major depression, atypical affective disorder, paranoid disorder, and atypical psychotic disorder. Although most chronic mental patients fit into one of these categories, some do not. Interviewers interested in a more comprehensive structured interview should consult the Diagnostic Interview Schedule (Robins et al. 1981), the Present State Examination (Wing et al. 1974), or the Structured Clinical Interview for *DSM-III* (Spitzer 1986).

Once the symptoms are elicited and rated and the interview is completed, the full criteria listed in the *DSM-III* should be consulted (pages 340–341 in the manual). The criteria for schizophrenic disorder are listed in Table 4 as an example of *DSM-III* operational criteria for all the major mental disorders.

BRIEF STRUCTURED DIAGNOSTIC INTERVIEW

Introduction
Could you tell me what kinds of problems you have been having recently?

Affective Symptoms

Depressed Mood: Have you felt depressed? sad? What was that like? How long has it lasted?
Irritable Mood: Have you felt irritable? Have you gotten into arguments or fights?
Weight Loss/Gain: Have you gained or lost any weight recently?
Insomnia/Hypersomnia: Have you had any difficulty sleeping? Have you been sleeping more than usual?
Agitation/Retardation: Have you been pacing or more restless than usual? Have you been slowed down in your movements? (not just subjective feeling of being slowed down)
Loss of Interest: Have your interests declined? Has your interest in sex changed?

TABLE 4: Diagnostic Criteria for a Schizophrenic Disorder (295.XX)

A. At least one of the following during a phase of the illness:
   1) bizarre delusions (content is patently absurd and has no possible basis in fact), such as delusions of being controlled, thought broadcasting, thought insertion, or thought withdrawal
   2) somatic, grandiose, religious, nihilistic, or other delusions without persecutory or jealous content
   3) delusions with persecutory or jealous content if accompanied by hallucinations of any type
   4) auditory hallucinations in which either a voice keeps up a running commentary on the individual's behavior or thoughts, or two or more voices converse with each other
   5) auditory hallucinations on several occasions with content of more than one or two words, having no apparent relation to depression or elation
   6) incoherence, marked loosening of associations, markedly illogical thinking, or marked poverty of content of speech if associated with at least one of the following:
      (a) blunted, flat, or inappropriate affect
      (b) delusions or hallucinations
      (c) catatonic or other grossly disorganized behavior.

B. Deterioration from a previous level of functioning in such areas as work, social relations, and self-care.
C. Duration: Continuous signs of the illness for at least six months at some time during the person's life, with some signs of the illness at present. The six-month period must include an active phase during which there were symptoms from A, with or without prodromal or residual phases.
D. The full depressive or manic syndrome (criteria A and B of major depressive or manic episode), if present, developed after any psychotic symptoms, or was brief in duration relative to the duration of the psychotic symptoms in A.
E. Onset of prodromal or active phase of the illness before age 45.
F. Not due to any organic mental disorder or mental retardation.

Loss of Energy: Have you felt exhausted or worn out?
Worthlessness/Guilt: Have you felt like you were worthless? no good? Have you felt guilty?
Inefficient Thinking: Have you had trouble thinking clearly? Have you had difficulty concentrating?
Suicidal Ideation/Attempts: Have you deliberately considered killing yourself?

Elevated Mood: Have you felt unusually cheerful? ecstatic? happier than you ever felt before?

Irritable Mood: Have you felt irritable? Have you gotten into arguments or fights?

Increased Activity: Have you been more active recently? developed new interests?

Pressured Speech: Have you been more talkative than usual?

Flight of Ideas: Have you noticed your thoughts racing?

Inflated Self-Esteem: Do you have any special abilities or talents?

Decreased Need for Sleep: Have you needed less sleep than usual?

Distractibility: Does your attention keep jumping to unimportant things around you?

Delusions

Reference: Does the TV or radio communicate messages specially meant for you? newspapers? magazines? license plates? Do people seem to say things which have a double meaning? drop hints about you? check up on your movements?

Persecution: Have you felt like anyone was trying to harm you or kill you?

Grandiose: Do you have any special abilities or powers? a mission? are you somebody rich or famous?

Religious: Do you communicate directly with God? get signs or omens?

Paranormal: Does telepathy, ESP, or hypnotism ever affect you?

Physical: Does anything like electricity, X rays, or laser beams ever affect you?

Delusion of Control: Do you ever feel under the control of some force or power? like a robot or zombie without a will of your own?

Somatic: Do you feel there is anything wrong with your body or your appearance?

Jealousy: Do you believe your spouse is cheating on you?

Guilt: Do you feel responsible for any crimes or catastrophes? or that you sinned greatly?

Nihilistic: Do you feel that you have died? part of your body has been removed? the world does not exist?

Thought Disturbance Symptoms

Thought Insertion: Do thoughts seem to be placed in your head that are not your own thoughts?

Thought Broadcast: Do your thoughts seem to be broadcast to others so that others seem to know what you're thinking?

Thought Withdrawal: Does it ever seem like thoughts are being removed from your mind?

Hallucinations

Nonverbal: Do you hear noises like bells or machinery when there is nothing around that could make that sound?

Auditory Hallucinations: Do you hear a voice or voices talking to you when no one is around?

Third Person Auditory Hallucinations: Do you hear voices talking about you or referring to you by name or as he or she?

Voice Commentary: Do you hear a voice commenting on your behavior or thoughts?

Visual: Do you ever see things (have visions) that other people don't see?

Olfactory: Do you ever smell things other people don't seem to notice?

Differential Diagnosis Questions

Duration of Episode: How long have you [specify symptoms]?

Impairment: Have these problems interfered with your ability to work? go to school? socialize? take care of yourself?

Mood Congruency of Symptoms: During the time you were hearing the voices (believing people were reading your mind, etc.), were you also depressed [elated]?

Sequence of Symptoms: Which came first, the [name a symptom] or the [name a symptom]? How long after did the [name a symptom] begin?

Signs of Psychosis

Incoherence: _____

Marked Loosening of Associations: _____

Poverty of Content of Thought: _____

Markedly Illogical Thinking: _____

Blunted Affect: _____

Inappropriate Affect: _____

Catatonic Behavior: _____

Grossly Disorganized Behavior: _____

LEARNING EXERCISE

1. Locate a patient who would be a good interview subject (that is, not conceptually disorganized or suspicious) and administer the structured interview presented in this chapter.
2. Insert a verbatim account of a symptom or group of symptoms into the chart of the patient or relay the description to the patient's primary caregiver or responsible psychiatrist.

RATING AND MONITORING SEVERITY OF SYMPTOMS

Rating scales of psychopathology are assessment tools that also aid work with chronic mental patients. The major mental disorders such as schizophrenia typically have a fluctuating course. Accurate monitoring of changes in symptomatology provides treatment personnel with highly useful information. In the typical outpatient clinic setting, patient visits may be separated by two weeks or more. Medication appointments are frequently very brief, for example, 5 to 10 minutes. The use of rating scales lets the prescribing psychiatrist and other treatment staff know in an objective manner whether symptoms are stabilizing, improving, or worsening. Thus, medication can be titrated more sensitively.

Markers of impending relapse can also be monitored to catch exacerbations in the prodromal phase. Research has found that relapse in schizophrenia is usually preceded by a prodromal period that the patient, relatives, and the therapist can learn to identify. When Herz and Melville (1980) retrospectively interviewed schizophrenic patients and their relatives about the period preceding a relapse, most were able to report a distinct prodromal period. The symptoms mentioned most frequently by patients and their relatives were nonpsychotic: symptoms of dysphoria that nonpsychotic individuals experience under stress, such as eating less, having trouble concentrating, having trouble sleeping, depression, and seeing friends less (Herz and Melville 1980). Preoccupation with previous hospitalizations, magical thinking, and visual illusions were also frequent precursors of relapse. Clearly, it would be desirable to be able to identify impending relapses during their formative prodromal stage. Increased medication and psychosocial treatment strategies could be employed in tandem with identification of prodromata to prevent a full-blown relapse.

The development of intermittent medication strategies (Carpenter and Heinrichs 1983; Herz et al. 1982), a promising innovation in psychopharmacological treatment, also requires the ability to reliably recognize the early signs of relapse to signal the reintroduction of medication. However, most chronic mental patients have persisting levels of such symptoms. Establishing the patient's baseline level allows the therapist to identify exacerbations and, perhaps, prevent their developing into full relapses.

Therapy can also be aided by the information generated from rating scales. The effectiveness of interventions can be evaluated on the basis of changes in ratings. For example, the therapist can determine whether the social skills training being provided is reducing the patient's anxiety at work and in the board-and-care home. The therapist can also determine whether changes in the patient's living situation are resulting in increased withdrawal and psychotic symptoms. Below is an example of how the use of the Brief Psychiatric Rating Scale (Overall and Gorham

1962) enabled a therapist to monitor a patient's condition and forestall an imminent relapse. Table 5 contains examples of the anchor points used for rating 3 of the 24 scales of the Brief Psychiatric Rating Scale (Lukoff et al. 1986).

CASE EXAMPLE ————————————————————————

A male patient at an outpatient clinic requested that the social worker help him move from a small board-and-care facility where he had been living for the past two years to a board-and-care closer to his parents. The social worker arranged a transfer to a much larger facility in the neighborhood where his parents lived. One month after the move, the social worker had a session with the patient and asked him how he was doing. He replied that he enjoyed being able to spend some evenings and weekends with his parents. If she had stopped the interview at that point, everything would have seemed fine. However, the social worker continued to ask questions from the Brief Psychiatric Rating Scale, a standardized rating scale. These questions uncovered a marked increase in anxiety, difficulty in sleeping, and the belief that others at the board-and-care were staring at him and talking about him. These prodromal symptoms concerned the social worker because they represented a definite exacerbation from the level of symptomatology present before the patient moved. Additional questioning revealed that the patient felt overwhelmed at the new larger placement and had not made any even casual friendships. However, he did not want to move further away from his parents. The social worker immediately scheduled an appointment that afternoon with his psychiatrist to determine if an increase in medication was warranted. With the patient's consent, the social worker notified the board-and-care manager and suggested that he pay some special attention to the patient. Then she contacted other board-and-care homes in the area to locate one that housed a smaller number of residents. Through the social worker's careful monitoring of the patient's symptomatology and her efforts to alter the stressful situation, a potential relapse was averted.

When symptom levels are graphed, the resulting picture of the covariance of symptoms and medication can be used to prescribe medications and titrate drug therapy.

CASE EXAMPLE ————————————————————————

When Joan was first seen in the hospital, she was totally preoccupied with messages from the TV, radio, and computers. On the Brief Psychiatric Rating Scale she was rated a 7 on Unusual Thought Content, the highest possible rating. She also reported hallucinations several times

TABLE 5: Operational Descriptions for Anchoring the Ratings of Three Categories of Psychotic Symptoms for the Brief Psychiatric Rating Scale

---

Unusual thought content: Unusual, odd, strange, or bizarre thought content. Rate the degree of unusualness, not the degree of disorganization of speech. Delusions are illogical or clearly impossible ideas verbally expressed. Include thought insertion, withdrawal, and broadcasting. Include grandiose, somatic, and persecutory delusions even if rated elsewhere.

2	Very mild	Ideas of reference (people stare/laugh at him/her). Ideas of persecution (people mistreat him/her). Unusual beliefs in psychic powers, spirits, UFO's. Not strongly held. Some doubt.
3	Mild	Same as 2 but with full conviction.
4	Moderate	Delusion present but not strongly held—functioning not disrupted; or encapsulated delusion with full conviction—functioning not disrupted.
5	Moderately severe	Full delusion(s) present with some preoccupation or some areas of functioning disrupted by delusional thinking.
6	Severe	Full delusion(s) present with much preoccupation, or many areas of functioning are disrupted by delusional thinking.
7	Extremely severe	Full delusion(s) present with almost total preoccupation, or most areas of functioning are disrupted by delusional thinking.

Have you felt that you were under the control of another person?

Have things or events had special meanings for you?

Did you see any references to yourself on TV or in the newspapers?

Has anything strange been going on?

How do you explain the things that have been happening (specify)?

Hallucinations: Reports of perceptual experiences in the absence of external stimuli. When rating degree to which functioning is disrupted by hallucinations, do not include preoccupation with the content of the hallucinations. Consider only disruption due to the hallucinatory experience. Include thoughts aloud—*gedankenlautwerten.*

2	Very mild	While resting or going to sleep, sees visions, hears voices, sounds, or whispers in absence of external stimulation, but no impairment in functioning.
3	Mild	While in a clear state of consciousness, hears nonverbal auditory hallucinations (e.g., sounds or whispers) or sees

illusions (e.g., faces in shadows) on no more than two occasions and with no impairment in functioning.

4	Moderate	Occasional verbal, visual, olfactory, tactile, or gustatory hallucinations (1–3 times) but no impairment in functioning.
5	Moderately severe	Occurs daily or some areas of functioning are disrupted by hallucinations.
6	Severe	Occurs several times a day or many areas of functioning are disrupted by hallucinations.
7	Extremely severe	Persistent throughout the day or most areas of functioning are disrupted by hallucinations.

Have you heard any sounds or people talking to you or about you when there has been nobody around?

Have you seen any visions or smelled any smells others don't seem to notice?

Have these experiences interfered with your ability to perform your usual activities/work?

Conceptual disorganization: Degree to which speech is confused, disconnected, or disorganized. Rate tangentiality, circumstantiality, sudden topic shifts, incoherence, derailment, blocking, neologisms, and other speech disorders. Do not rate *content* of speech. Consider the first 15 minutes of the interview.

2	Very mild	Peculiar use of words, rambling.
3	Mild	Speech a bit hard to understand or make sense of due to sudden topic shifts.
4	Moderate	Speech difficult to understand due to tangentiality, circumstantiality, or topic shifts on many occasions or 1–2 instances of severe impairment, e.g., incoherence, derailment, neologisms, blocking.
5	Moderately severe	Speech difficult to understand due to circumstantiality, tangentiality, or topic shifts most of the time or 3–5 instances of severe impairment.
6	Severe	Speech is incomprehensible due to severe impairments most of the time.
7	Extremely severe	Speech is incomprehensible throughout interview.

Note. The questions keyed to each symptom group are excerpted from the Present State Examination (Wing, Cooper and Sartorius, 1974). The operational definitions for the anchor points on the rating scale were developed by the Diagnostic and Psychopathology Unit of the Clinical Research Center for Schizophrenia and Psychiatric Rehabilitation at the University of California at Los Angeles (Lukoff, Liberman, and Nuechterlein, 1986).

a day, thereby warranting a 6 on that item. She was taking oral flu-phenazine (Prolixin) 20 mg daily. By hospital discharge, her hallucina-tions had remitted totally. When she came to the outpatient clinic for her visit two days after discharge from the hospital, Joan told her case manager that she still was getting messages, but only from the radio. She did not think about them and they did not interfere with her func-tioning (this warrants a 4 on the Unusual Thought Content item of the Brief Psychiatric Rating Scale). After Joan had been seen for four weeks as an outpatient, the case manager was concerned about the persistence of Joan's delusions of reference about messages from the radio, even though they were at a low level of intensity. The finding of persisting delusional thinking was discussed with the clinic's psychiatrist, and a decision was reached to increase Joan's daily Prolixin dosage to 30 mg. Six weeks later, another administration of the Brief Psychiatric Rating Scale revealed no change in Joan's ratings; however her motor retar-dation had increased to a moderately severe level. With her agreement, she was switched to biweekly 20 mg IM Prolixin to rule out compliance as a factor in her persisting symptomatology. When Joan came in for her third injection, she announced that she would not take her shot. She stated that the shots were painful and that she wanted pills. Review of the Brief Psychiatric Rating Scale ratings revealed no additional thera-peutic impact from the increased dosage or from IM administration; indeed, the only change was an increase in motor retardation and ak-athisia, both likely side effects of the neuroleptic drug (see Figure 6). On the basis of this reevaluation, the case manager and the psychiatrist agreed to place Joan back on oral Prolixin at the original discharge dosage. Two weeks later, Joan's unusual thoughts were no longer of delusional proportions, and her extrapyramidal side effects had begun to lessen. Her maintenance Prolixin dose was further decreased to 10 mg daily with continued improvement in her thinking and functioning. The serial ratings using the Brief Psychiatric Rating Scale enabled Joan's psychiatrist to titrate her neuroleptic therapy to the lowest effective dose compatible with the least side effects.

Clinicians and researchers have paid most attention to the so-called positive symptoms of schizophrenia: hallucinations, delusions, and thought disorder. Negative symptoms are deficiencies in qualities such as acti-vation and effort (amotivation), ability to experience enjoyment (anhe-donia), need for socialization (asociality), flow of thought processes (alogia), affective expression and experience (blunted affect), and energy (aner-gia). Early theorists such as Bleuler considered negative symptoms to be a primary feature of schizophrenia. In the past 50 years they have been largely ignored because they are difficult to rate reliably and they do

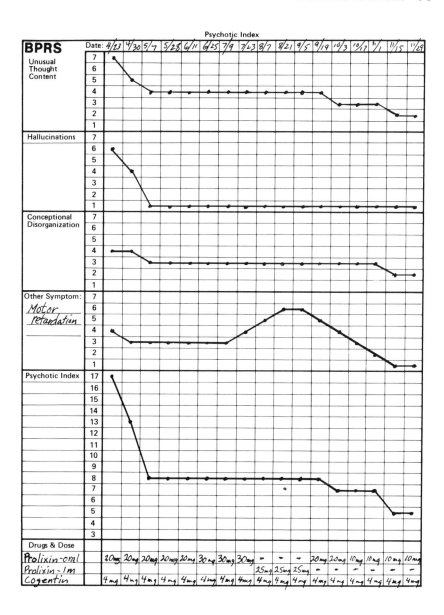

FIGURE 6: Use of serial ratings graphed from the Brief Psychiatric Rating Scale (BPRS) in making drug treatment decisions in the case of Joan. The Psychotic Index is the sum of ratings made in the core psychotic scales of the BPRS: Conceptual Disorganization, Hallucinations, and Unusual Thought Content. This graphic monitoring of a patient's psychopathology and side effects can assist the prescribing clinician in making benefit/ risk decisions on choice and dose of psychotropic drugs.

LEARNING EXERCISE

Rate the following three cases for specific symptoms and signs and make a tentative *DSM-III* diagnosis.

Case 1. The patient is a 47-year-old male. He was admitted to psychiatric hospitals on three previous occasions and currently lives on SSI. For the past year, he has lived by himself in an apartment. Two months ago, he began to believe that the Mafia had moved into the apartment next door. He claims to hear laughing and screaming through the adjoining wall. He reports that they have put him on "mind control," which is a drug they have placed in his drinking water. He can tell because the water tastes very bitter. Using the mind control, he believes they have been projecting thoughts of theirs into his mind telepathically. They put thoughts of racial hatred and the end of the world into his mind. These thoughts interfere with his own thoughts. He thinks they want to use his brain to plan crimes and send him to jail. He refused to leave his apartment for the past two weeks because he was sure they arranged for a warrant for his arrest for crimes he did not commit.

Symptoms?   Diagnosis?

Case 2. The patient is a 37-year-old married woman. For the past eight months, she has suspected that her husband can read her mind. Two months ago, she became convinced this was happening and that her thoughts were being broadcast so that everybody nearby could hear what she was thinking. She believed that her husband was in control of her thoughts and that she was like a robot. At times, she would believe that she was being forced to say and do things that were not her own thoughts and ideas. She suspected there was some telepathic process controlled by her husband. She felt he was trying to help her and did not find this particularly distressing.

Symptoms?   Diagnosis?

Case 3. The patient is a 28-year-old man who was brought in by his parents because they were afraid he might kill himself. He has been up for the past seven nights and still shows high energy. He reports that he has a special mission to save the world. He hears the voice of God giving him special instructions. He admits to wanting to jump from the top of the Bonaventure Hotel. He has chosen this spot because a nearby sign says "Jesus Saves" and he believes that means he and the world will be saved if he jumps. He believes the hospital staff are CIA agents and he can and must outwit them.

Symptoms?   Diagnosis?

not contribute to making diagnoses. Recently, negative symptoms have again attracted the attention of clinicians and researchers. Rating scales have been developed that permit negative symptoms to be rated reliably, for example, the Schedule for the Assessment of Negative Symptoms (Andreasen 1982). Studies have found that negative symptoms have a major impact on social and occupational functioning during the post-psychotic phase of schizophrenia and in other disorders as well. Since negative symptoms mainly concern functioning in the activities of daily living, they are discussed in more detail in Chapter 3, "A Framework for Functional Assessment."

SUMMARY

Although most chronic mental patients already carry a diagnosis, careful diagnostic assessments can contribute significantly to the quality of care they receive. Patients' diagnoses may change over time, or additional diagnoses may need to be assigned. Treatments, both pharmacological and psychosocial, are greatly aided when the patient is accurately di-agnosed. Careful monitoring of symptoms can help the therapist pre-scribe the appropriate type and dosage of medication, make choices regarding treatment and residential placements and therapeutic activi-ties, and improve the patient's strategies for coping with and mastering psychopathology.

REFERENCES

American Psychiatric Association: Diagnostic and Statistical Manual of Mental Disorders (Third Edition). Washington, DC, American Psychiatric Association, 1980

Andreasen N: Negative symptoms in schizophrenia: definition and reliability. Arch Gen Psychiatry 39:784–788 1982

Carpenter W, Heinrichs D: Early intervention, time-limited, targeted pharmacotherapy of schizophrenia. Schizophr Bull 9:533–542 1983

Goldman HH, Gattozzi AA, Taube CA: Defining and counting the chronically mentally ill. Hosp Community Psychiatry 32:22, 1981

Hertz M, Melville C: Relapse in schizophrenia. Am J Psychiatry 137:801–805, 1980

Herz M, Szymanski H, Simon J: Intermittent medication for stable schizophrenic outpa-tients. Am J Psychiatry 139:918–922 1982

Kohler K: First rank symptoms of schizophrenia: questions concerning clinical boundaries. Br J Psychiatry 134:236–248 1979

Lukoff D, Liberman R, Nuechterlein K: Symptom monitoring in the rehabilitation of schizophrenic patients. Schizophr Bull, in press 1986

Menolascino F, Stark J: Handbook of Mental Illness in the Mentally Retarded. New York, Plenum Press, 1984

Overall J, Gorham D: The Brief Psychiatric Rating Scale. Psychol Rep 10:799–812 1962

Robins L, Helzer J, Croughan J: National Institute of Mental Health Diagnostic Interview Schedule. Arch Gen Psychiatry 38:381–392 1981

Spitzer R, Endicott J, Robins E: Research diagnostic criteria: rationale and reliability. Arch Gen Psychiatry 35:773–782 1978

Spitzer R, Williams J: The Structured Clinical Interviews for DSM-III, 1986. Available from Robert Spitzer, New York State Psychiatric Institute, Biometrics Research Department, 722 West 168th Street, New York, NY 10032

Strauss J, Carpenter W: The prediction of outcome in schizophrenia II: Relationships between predictor and outcome variables. Arch Gen Psychiatry 31:37–42 1974

Wing J, Cooper J, Sartorius N: The Description and Classification of Psychiatric Symptoms: An Instruction Manual for PSE and CATEGO System. London, Cambridge University Press, 1974

CHAPTER 3

FUNCTIONAL ASSESSMENT

TIMOTHY G. KUEHNEL, PH.D.
ROBERT PAUL LIBERMAN, M.D.

Do all the good you can,
In all the ways you can,
In all the places you can,
At all the times you can,
To all the people you can,
As long as ever you can.
John Wesley
"Rules of Conduct"

While the assessment of the symptoms or impairment of a person with a major mental disorder is a necessary first step in diagnosis and choice of drug treatment, the functional assessment of a person's behavioral assets and deficits is a prerequisite for the provision of psychosocial services. The psychiatric diagnosis, with its focus on a patient's impairments, must be accompanied by a comprehensive and multimodal behavioral assessment of a patient's disabilities and potentialities for rehabilitation. Only with both types of evaluation can rehabilitation goals and plans be formulated.

The vulnerability-stress-coping-competence view of chronic mental disorders highlights the importance of both of these assessment approaches. Symptomatic diagnosis and assessment provide information on the prescription and monitoring of optimal psychopharmacological interventions to protect against psychobiological vulnerability. In contrast, functional assessment provides the rehabilitation professional with information on

1. stressors that may overwhelm the individual's coping skills and competencies in social and instrumental roles, thereby evoking an exacerbation or relapse of symptoms;
2. the presence or absence of premorbid and current coping skills and competencies that may serve as buffers against stress; and
3. the reasons for deficits in an individual's coping and problem-solving skills, such as disuse, reinforcement of the sick role, or loss of motivation.

In short, functional assessment assists in the identification of behavioral assets, excesses, and deficits that help or hinder a patient's performance in social and occupational roles. While the social, personal, and occupational disabilities of an individual tend to capture the attention of clinicians, treatment and rehabilitation of the chronic mental patient should begin with an accurate inventory of a patient's capacities, namely, what a person has been and is able to do in everyday life.

The importance of functional assessment in rehabilitation practice is illustrated by findings from long-term follow-up studies of persons diagnosed as suffering from schizophrenia. These studies document that social recoveries are possible in many individuals, given a reasonable amount, quality, and continuity of treatment services. For example, in one longitudinal study of 79 schizophrenic patients from Chicago, good social functioning was found in 45 percent and good vocational functioning in 36 percent on the average of 2.7 years after discharge from a psychiatric hospital (Harrow et al. 1978). Even more striking are the findings from a 30-year follow-up of severely impaired, chronically hospitalized schizophrenic patients from the Vermont State Hospital. In this study, approximately ⅔ of the patients were functioning within normal limits, had few symptoms, and were constructively involved in work or domestic life (Harding and Strauss 1985; Harding et al. 1987). These and a host of other studies suggest that even in the face of recurrent psychotic episodes, individuals with chronic mental disorders can use social and vocational skills to their advantage.

As highlighted by the multiaxial framework of the *Diagnostic and Statistical Manual of Mental Disorders (Third Edition)* (*DSM-III*; American Psychiatric Association 1980) criteria for mental disorders, symptomatic and functional assessments each make a complementary contribution to the evaluation of impairment, disability, and handicap. For example, before a diagnosis of schizophrenia can be made, the individual in question must be documented as having at least six months of disability in vocational, self-care, or interpersonal spheres of functioning as well as the characteristic symptom impairments of the disorder.

Psychiatric symptoms and other psychological deficits (for example, attention, concentration, memory) represent a patient's impairment. Disability in the domains of self-care, social relations, family relations, work, and learning refers to activities that the individual is impeded from doing as a result of symptomatic impairments. A handicap represents the degree to which an impaired person with disabilities is disadvantaged in particular environments and social roles. For example, an individual with schizophrenia may suffer a disability in socialization because of the impairment of incoherent or impoverished speech. In purchasing food in the modern supermarket environment, this would not pose a large handicap since the majority of items are available on a self-serve basis. This same disability, however, would have posed a real handicap in the mercantile environments of yesteryear where consumers had to verbally interact with a clerk who retrieved items from inaccessible locations and measured out desired quantities of foodstuffs.

Antipsychotic medications can improve positive symptoms of chronic mental illness, thereby reducing the patient's impairment; psychosocial treatment of behavioral excesses, deficits, and assets is necessary to reduce negative symptoms, disability, and handicap. While symptomatic and diagnostic assessments provide direction to the prescribing physician and treatment team, functional assessment provides direction for 1) setting short- and long-term goals, 2) monitoring progress, and 3) determining optimal rehabilitation outcomes.

FRAMEWORK FOR FUNCTIONAL ASSESSMENT

The general framework for functional assessment presented in Table 6 can guide the clinician in carrying out a systematic and comprehensive evaluation prior to selecting appropriate psychosocial interventions. It is important to involve the patient and significant others—parents, sib-

TABLE 6:   Outline of Functional and Behavioral Approach to History Taking, Assessment, and Therapy

I. Problem identification and goal setting

   A. Define and translate problems and goals into behavioral terms, using as dimensions the frequency, the intensity, the duration, form or quality, and the appropriateness of the context.

   B. Goals should be
—specific and clear
—chosen or endorsed by patient and significant others
—short-term linked to long-term
—frequently occurring
—salient and functional
—attainable

   C. Engage patient actively in goal setting:
—offer rationales
—solicit options and pros/cons
—provide visual displays
—check for acceptance and understanding

   D. Develop a multimodal inventory of the problems and goals in which all levels of human behavioral expression and experience are covered:
—social affiliative behavior
—instrumental behavior
—activities of daily living
—affects
—cognitions

   E. Determine behavioral deficits: Which behaviors need to be initiated, increased in frequency, or strengthened in form?

   F. Determine behavioral excesses: Which behaviors need to be terminated, decreased in frequency, or altered in form?

   G. Determine behavioral assets: Consider strengths in multimodal terms.

   H. Determine if interfering symptoms or side effects can be better controlled through pharmacotherapy.

II. Functional (behavioral) analysis of conditions maintaining the problems in living

   A. Antecedents of problems:

—Where, when, with whom?

—What life events and stressors, both episodic and ambient, may be triggering or influencing problems and relapse?

—Are symptoms side effects of drugs or cognitive impairments interfering with function?

B. Consequences of problem behaviors:

—What would happen if the problems were ignored? Consider the roles of sympathy, nurturance, attention, anger, coercion by others.

—What reinforcers or benefits would the patient gain or lose if the problems were diminished?

C. Self-motivation:

—Does the patient acknowledge problems and desire change?

—Does verbal behavior match follow-through in participation in treatment and homework?

III. Sources of assessment

A. Self-report questionnaires and inventories (for example, Fear Survey, Target Complaint Scale, Beck Depression Inventory, Independent Living Skills Survey)

B. Interviews (for example, Social Behavior Assessment Schedule, Reinforcement Survey)

C. Self-monitoring (for example, diaries, logs)

D. Behavioral observation (for example, naturalistic and role plays)

E. Permanent products of behavioral outcomes

F. Biological measures (for example, heart rate, biofeedback, physical disabilities, drug-behavior interactions)

G. Sociocultural measures (for example, recent changes in milieu or relationships, values and norms, social network and social support)

IV. Resource management

A. What resources are available or mobilizable to assist patient in

—learning skills

—using skills

TABLE 6: *(continued)*

    —compensating for skill deficits
    —managing symptoms or preventing relapse

  B. What are the socioenvironmental strengths and deficits in terms of achieving rehabilitation goals?

  C. What resources can be developed to motivate and maintain progress toward rehabilitation goals?
    —People
    —Transportation
    —Places
    —Activities
    —Telephone and Mail
    —Money
    —Reinforcement Survey

V. Planning rehabilitation

  A. Delineate overall and specific goals (for example, monthly, yearly)

  B. Establish longer term (for example, monthly, yearly) and short-term (for example, daily, weekly) goals

  C. Prioritize skills to be acquired and resources to be mobilized

  D. Set time lines

  E. Coordinate agency and natural supports and interventions (for example, pharmacotherapy, case management)

  F. Identify personnel responsible for interventions and liaison

VI. Monitoring progress

  A. Track progress toward goals rather than persistence of problems

  B. Measures should be practical, relevant, and convenient

  C. Involve patient and significant others in recording and acknowledging progress

  D. Methods of ongoing assessment:
    —Goal attainment
    —Frequency counts
    —Interval ratings

—Intensity ratings
—Permanent products

VII. Behavior therapy tactics

A. Develop trusting, caring, warm, and mutually respectful therapeutic alliance to serve as the foundation and lever for many of the behavioral techniques.

B. Develop time-limited treatment program.

C. Use behavioral rehearsal or role-playing to simulate "real world" problem situations.

D. Prompt, cue, signal, and coach patient to make improvements.

E. Give "homework assignments."

F. Reinforce small, discrete steps in adaptive directions.

G. Use therapeutic instructions and promote favorable expectations of outcome.

H. Have patient repeatedly practice the desired behavior.

I. Give feedback information on behavioral changes to patient and periodically reevaluate progress and reset goals.

J. Reinforce progress, underplay reversals.

K. Generalize gains to natural environment by involving family members and other aspects of the "real world."

---

lings, residential supervisors, agency staff—in as many of the steps of functional assessment as is realistically possible. Involvement of the patient provides quick and verifiable information as to the acceptability of the proposed rehabilitation program. It also provides a convenient method to assess the patient's comprehension of each of the goals and proposed interventions. The patient's input is also very helpful in selecting the initial goals of rehabilitation. Involving the patient in this manner increases motivation to participate in the rehabilitation program and helps to counter the "amotivational syndrome." The involvement of significant others provides reliability checks on the information gathered by the clinician and provided by the patient. Significant others may also be called upon to help prioritize goals and to actively participate in selected elements of the rehabilitation program.

Judicious doses of psychoactive drugs, appropriate to the patient's diagnosis and stage of illness, may be a necessary prerequisite to conducting and completing a comprehensive functional evaluation or assessment. This is because reconstitution of symptoms of the illness, through pharmacotherapy, may bring about large-scale improvements in social behavior and permit a more accurate assessment of a patient's true baseline functional state.

It is also important to note that functional assessment procedures are not implemented in a sequentially linear fashion. Rather, they are overlapping, and should be recurrently administered during the course of treatment and rehabilitation. Assessment and treatment are inextricably linked in clinical decision making; thus intervention proceeds from data obtained from evaluation and should be redirected by regular infusions of assessment data. In Figure 7 is depicted the way in which assessment and treatment interlock in a continuing fashion over time. If a high-priority goal has been attained, the clinician and patient together can decide whether enough progress has been made or whether new goals can be pinpointed for rehabilitation. If progress toward a goal is not being made, then it is important to consider whether the problem was initially identified incorrectly, the rehabilitation goals were improperly selected or set too high, or the treatment methods are inappropriate for this patient. As Figure 7 depicts, errors at any of these steps could contribute to a lack of progress.

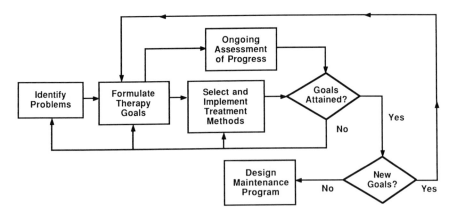

FIGURE 7: Flow chart of the empirical approach to treatment of the chronic mental patient. Both drug and psychosocial therapies can be guided by this goal-oriented sequence of clinical operations. The key element is the monitoring of progress using operationalized goals and instruments that can reliably rate psychopathology and social functioning. When clinincal goals are achieved, the rehabilitation practitioner or team—in concert with the patient, relatives and other caregivers—consider whether to work on new goals or to switch into a maintenance program to consolidate and reinforce treatment gains.

The following case example illustrates the interplay between symptomatic assessment and functional assessment. It also serves as a vehicle to clarify the steps or stages of functional assessment and the kinds of data that may be gathered to pinpoint areas of intervention.

CASE EXAMPLE

Al graduated from high school as a straight-A student, intending to pursue a career in science, which was his special area of interest. His father, an engineer, and his mother, a lawyer, both encouraged him to develop his intellectual skills. They were concerned, though, that Al didn't pay enough attention to his social life. While he had a few casual friends, he didn't chum around and had never gone out on a date. He enrolled at a nearby state university and for two semesters commuted daily from home to class. Although he passed his courses, he found it increasingly difficult to concentrate and complete homework assignments. He and his parents were puzzled by his decline in academic performance but they did not think of seeking medical or psychiatric consultation.

Instead of returning to college the next fall, Al decided to work. He tried a succession of jobs from file clerk to bus boy. He withdrew from his few acquaintances and family, preferring to spend long hours listening to music in his room. He told his parents that he was tense and fearful, but they thought it was because of pressures at work and suggested that he quit his job. Now spending all of his time at home, Al became more isolated and fatigued. He had trouble falling asleep and had several frightening nightmares. His mind wandered to strange thoughts, such as a belief that he had leprosy and might be dying. Frequently, while lying in bed alone he heard two male voices commenting on his indolence and referring to him as a "failure" and a "loser."

He refused to eat, stayed in bed, and stopped caring for his personal appearance. He told his father one night that he thought his actions were being controlled by a force from outer space. He went on to say that by remaining perfectly still, he could prevent this external control. His father shrugged off these fantastic ideas and reassured Al that no one was controlling him. The next day, Al fretfully told his mother that he discovered that he could broadcast his thoughts and was afraid that the neighbors would hear what he was thinking.

After several weeks of increasing indolence, Al stopped talking. He stared into space, urinated in his pants, sat immobile, and failed to respond to questions. He could be physically prompted to change positions, but it was as though he had no volition, and he was as passive as a lump of clay. Finally, Al's parents, weary of waiting for him to "snap out of his daze," brought him to a mental health center, where he was admitted for inpatient treatment.

Al was treated with a neuroleptic drug and showed gradual improvement in his appearance and behavior. He resumed speaking, first in a whisper and only in response to questions. His confusion and disorientation cleared. He took a shower and brushed his hair, albeit with some prompting. His eating improved, and, after five days of hospitalization, he began smiling and looking at people. However, he avoided interacting with fellow patients or staff and secluded himself in his room or in remote corners of the ward whenever possible. The medication appeared to improve his self-care skills and cognitive abilities, but he remained socially withdrawn and passive. He appeared to be returning to his premorbid personality—a shy, quiet loner.

Problem Identification

As is the case with many schizophrenic patients, Al presents with severe and disabling problems in almost every sphere of functioning. The decision to use neuroleptic medication at the time of his hospital admission was prompted by the diagnosis of schizophrenia made on the basis of initial clinical observations of his catatonic immobility, mutism, and incontinence, and by the specific history of characteristic delusions and hallucinations provided by his parents. The first problem to attack was his symptoms.

With an acutely and floridly psychotic patient such as Al, intervention is initially aimed at cognitive and behavioral reconstitution so that more definitive comprehensive assessment and treatment planning can be carried out with a reasonably attentive and socially responsive patient. The therapeutic environment, with proper programming, can facilitate the benefits of pharmacotherapy in improving the florid symptoms of schizophrenia. Along with neuroleptic medication, the treatment team responsible for reducing Al's level of symptomatology also arranged for him to

1. be removed, at least temporarily, from a possibly stressful family environment;
2. receive clear and concise messages from the staff regarding daily needs;
3. spend time in a quiet, unstimulating part of the ward;
4. receive prompts and positive feedback for any signs of self-awareness, social communication, and self-care.

After the acute and floridly psychotic or positive symptoms of schizophrenia subsided, the staff could then more clearly define Al's problems and appropriate rehabilitation goals.

Defining Problems in Functional, Behavioral Terms

In reviewing Al's problems, the staff operationalized or translated them into behavioral terms, using as dimensions the frequency, intensity, duration, latency, and form or quality of his actions and verbalizations. In addition, assessment was made of the appropriateness of Al's behaviors in their social context. These modes of monitoring progress toward treatment goals are listed in Table 6.

Frequency refers to how often a behavior occurs. The number of times each day that Al engaged in verbal interaction with staff or peers on the ward would be an example of how his problem of social withdrawal could be assessed.

Intensity of a problem refers to its magnitude or severity. To measure his subjective dysphoria, Al was asked to rate the magnitude of his tensions, fear, and discomfort on a 12-point Target Complaint Scale. Intensity levels on this scale ranged from "Couldn't be worse" (12 points) to "A little" (3 points) to "None" (zero points). Figure 8 depicts the successive ratings made by Al on this scale.

Duration refers to the amount of time spent behaving in a specific way. Al's history indicated that he spent "long hours listening to music." Listening to music for no more than 3 hours per day was operationalized as an appropriate initial goal of treatment. Alternatively, staff could have measured the duration of his self-initiated seclusiveness. Number of seconds, minutes, or hours can all be used as measures of the duration of problem behaviors such as social isolation, agitation, and excessive time engaged in stereotypies or self-stimulation.

Response latency also uses the passage of time to measure some behavioral function of the individual patient interacting with the environment. Here the focus is on the amount of time required for the patient to respond or act after a cue or signal has been given. You'll note below, when further examples of Al's problem list are presented, that the psychiatrist used response latency during weekly interviews, measuring the elapsed time between his questions and Al's response. Initially, when catatonia was present, there were pauses of up to 30 seconds, but as Al's cognitive capacities reconstituted, the latency was reduced to 5 seconds or less.

The form or quality of behavior can be measured reliably if the behavior in question is well specified. For example, in evaluating Al's overall social skill, each nursing staff made consensus ratings that included the quality of his eye contact, tone of voice, facial expression, and body language. Al was initially lethargic, avoidant, and sluggish, which was reflected in low ratings of overall social skill. As he became more comfortable interacting with staff and patients on the ward, his social skills became more demonstrative. Much later in his hospital course, he displayed even higher levels of vitality and enthusiasm.

Behaviors can be problematic because they occur under inappropriate conditions or at inappropriate times; that is, the patient has adequate skills, but they are not used in an adaptive manner, at a suitable time, or in the proper context. Inappropriate affect, a frequent sign of

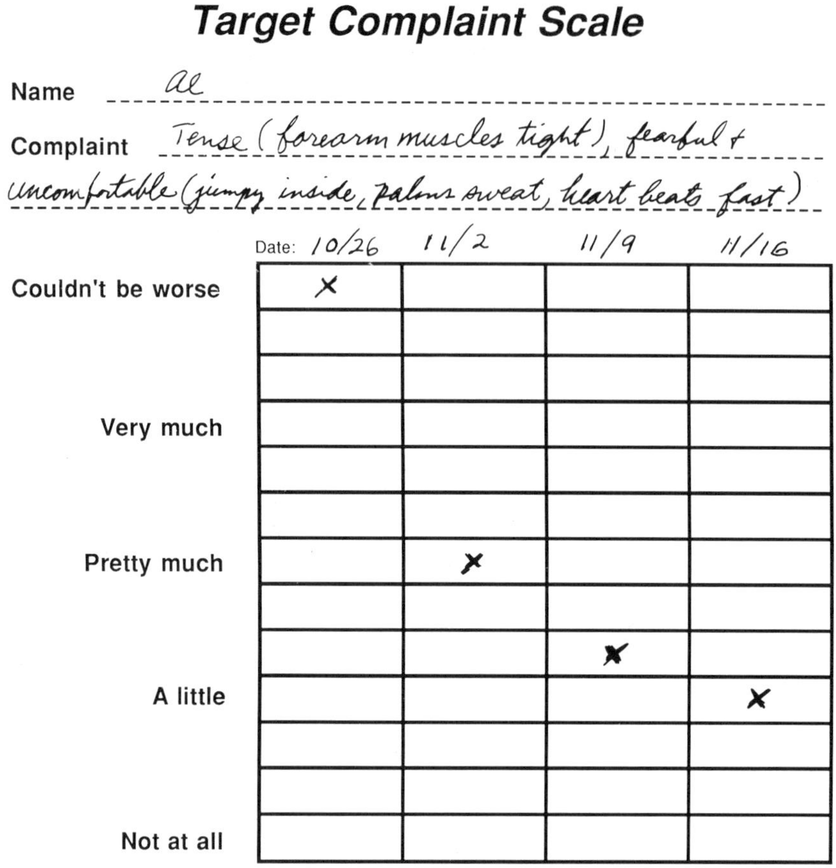

Target Complaint Scale

Name _al_

Complaint _Tense (forearm muscles tight), fearful + uncomfortable (jumpy inside, palms sweat, heart beats fast)_

	Date: 10/26	11/2	11/9	11/16
Couldn't be worse	✗			
Very much				
Pretty much		✗		
			✗	
A little				✗
Not at all				

FIGURE 8: Target Complaint Scale used to monitor tension and anxiety in the treatment of Al. The complaints were elicited from Al, in his own words, and then were repeatedly rated in terms of their severity by the patient on a weekly basis.

psychosis, is an example of a behavioral problem that can be assessed by its context. A patient who falls in love with his or her therapist is also revealing a problem that can be defined by the appropriateness of its context.

Once Al's catatonic symptoms subsided, efforts were made to pinpoint persisting behavioral problems in operational terms. For each of the identified problem behaviors, pinpointing involved translation or operationalization of general and vague problems into specific behaviors. For example, "socially withdrawn" was translated into "does not initiate conversation; does not eat meals with others; spends more than 80 percent

---

LEARNING EXERCISE

Now that you have seen some examples of how Al's general problems were operationalized into specific behaviors, take a few minutes to operationalize the following clinical terms into specific behavioral descriptions. A helpful tip for writing clear behavioral descriptions is to ask yourself, "Will someone else be able to observe the same behavior in the patient and agree with my assessment?"

Hostile
Poor self-concept
Angry, belligerent
Suicidal
Self-injurious, apathetic
Disheveled
Autistic, resistive
Withdrawn
Depressed, sad
Aggressive
Manipulative

---

of time alone." Further examples of pinpointing and operationalizing Al's problems are provided in Table 7. The concrete behavioral descriptions of Al's problems permit staff to assess their severity as well as their responsiveness to treatment.

Multimodal Inventory Of Problems And Goals

All levels of human behavioral expression and subjective experience should be examined in a truly comprehensive functional assessment of the chronic mental patient. Given the constraints imposed by time, resources, and settings, however, compromises and abbreviations are usually necessary. In the case of Al, psychiatric and functional assessment proceeded along multiple dimensions, as outlined in Table 8. The corollary of a multimodal problem list is an assessment strategy that uses a variety of methods for collecting information and monitoring clinical progress.

At first glance, it appears that a tremendous amount of assessment data is required to conduct a multimodal assessment of a chronic mental patient. Although it is crucial to define problems, set goals, and monitor progress on a variety of dimensions, it is often difficult to collect data of sufficient reliability and usefulness in inpatient or community settings. However, simple clinical judgment of improvement in global terms is nearly always unreliable and insensitive to actual change. The challenge

TABLE 7: Operationalization of Al's General Problems Into Specific Behaviors

Vague Problem	Behavioral Translation
Auditory hallucination	Believes two males are commenting about his laziness and referring to him as a "failure" and a "loser." Is noted when he yells, "I am not a failure, you SOB"; "I hate you Bob!!"; "I'm going to kick your butt, Fred!"; and similar kinds of combative statements made about Bob or Fred. Typically, verbal statements are followed by shadow boxing.
Low self-esteem	Feels no one likes to talk to him; uses critical and negative descriptions about himself, such as "I'm a jerk, no wonder nobody likes me."
Withdrawn; isolation	Does not initiate conversation; does not eat meals with others; spends more than 80 percent of time alone.
Anxiety, tension, fear	Palpitations; sweating; apprehensive that something catastrophic may occur; muscles tense; fearful of losing control of self.
Poor self-care	Incontinent; fails to eat without prompting; unable to dress and groom self.
Poor social skills	Does not speak with audible volume; has poor eye contact; unable to ask open-ended questions; does not vary pitch, rate, and tone of speech (sounds bored).

is to develop an assessment and data collection system that balances the need for accurate, consistent information with the time, training, and expert attention available for collecting it. Acceptable functional assessment systems should be reliable, valid, and useful. The assessment system should also collect data at an appropriate frequency and use environmental cueing to ensure that data will be collected.

Reliability. Steps should be taken to ensure that different staff collect assessment data in similar ways across time and settings. In the clinical setting, reliability can be assessed by occasionally comparing the data kept by two staff members who are recording independently at the same time and place. In the example below, the psychiatrist and another member of the professional staff might both interview Al and independently

TABLE 8: Problems of a Schizophrenic and Methods for Assessment—
The Case of Al

Level of Behavior	Specification of Problem	Methods of Assessment
Cognitive	Delusions of hypochondriasis; delusions of control; thought broadcast; reduced span of attention and concentration	Mental status interview of patient (for example, Present State Examination or Schedule For Affective Diseases and Schizophrenia); family interview; on-ward observations
Affective	Tension, fear	Interviews; on-ward observations; checklists; questionnaires (for example, Fear Survey Schedule)
Social	Isolation; withdrawal; poverty of speech; and mutism	Inteviews; on-ward observations; family interviews; questionnaires
Instrumental behavior including self-care	Immobile; requires prompting and manual guidance; incontinent; failure to eat; does not respond to instructions; unable to work, groom, and dress self	On-ward observations (for example, Behavioral Performance Tests); family interviews
Sensory	Auditory hallucinations with depreciatory content—voices talking about him	Patient interview
Imagery	Fantasies of body being distorted with leprosy	Patient interview; drawings by patient

rate him on the 12 dimensions of psychopathology assessed by the Brief Psychiatric Rating Scale (BPRS; Overall and Gorham 1962).

Validity. Assessment data must measure what they are supposed to measure. In general, a direct measure of a behavior will be more valid than an indirect measure. For example, Al's self-care skills could be globally rated and recorded by care providers on a monthly basis. However, a more valid measure of self-care skills would be to specify the skill area that Al is particularly deficit in, such as grooming, and to develop a scale for this area that clearly specifies and differentiates between good and poor performance. A valid measure distinguishes accurately between patients who show the behavior and those who do not.

Appropriate Frequency of Collection. Since it is impossible to carry along a chart or data sheets for each patient, decide on the longest interval between recordings that will allow fairly clear memory of the target behavior. Depending upon the level of behavior being assessed, this may be every 15 minutes or once a week. Alternatively, decide whether sampling the variables of interest during particular intervals (say, once a month) will yield data that reflect occurrence adequately. In the case example below, you will note that Al's social-interpersonal problems were measured by nursing staff using a Social Interaction Schedule four times daily. This Schedule requires only one to two minutes to complete. The intensity of Al's hallucinatory experiences was rated by the psychiatrist weekly on the BPRS.

A problem with too frequently collecting assessment information is not seeing the forest for the trees. Clinicians who daily measure discrete and frequently occurring behaviors (such as number of appropriate conversations with staff members for a socially withdrawn patient) may miss less frequent but more functional indications of behavioral change (such as the establishment of a new friendship outside the treatment setting). Thus, the frequency of behavioral assessment must be focused on activities, interactions, and performances that are also located in the patient's "real world" and that may be more important for long-term adaptation (Liberman et al. 1976).

Environmental Cueing. Assessments will more likely be carried out if they employ logical and clear data sheets that are located in a convenient place, are integrated into staff schedules, and are monitored by a supervisor.

Utility. A consideration important to an assessment system is the degree to which the data are useful in helping the care providers make decisions about the appropriateness of the treatment procedures being used. It is better if the sensitivity of the data to actual change in the patient's behavior is high, so that indications of both positive and negative changes appear quickly in the measures.

Please keep these dimensions or characteristics in mind as you read the following case example. How would you measure these dimensions? If time and personnel resources are scarce, which of these measures of multimodal assessment would you collect to help you define treatment goals and to monitor progress? Which measures would you omit? How would you decide if a particular assessment device was useful to your treatment program? Functional assessment of the illustrative case example of Al is presented below in a format organized around the key domains of Al's psychosocial functioning. The assessment begins with a description of Al's cognitive and psychopathological impairments to highlight the necessary integration of all dimensions of a patient's mental, clinical, and social status in an effort to evaluate the "whole person."

COGNITIVE PROBLEMS AND PSYCHOPATHOLOGY

On a weekly basis Al was interviewed by the unit psychiatrist, who rated him on 12 dimensions of psychopathology using the Brief Psychiatric Rating Scale (BPRS; Overall and Gorham 1962). As David Lukoff and Joseph Ventura described in Chapter 2, through measures of frequency and intensity, the BPRS enables a clinician to evaluate each dimension of psychopathology. (The BPRS and a host of other convenient and valid rating scales of psychopathology can be found in the *Assessment Manual for Psychopharmacology* [Guy 1976].) To supplement the BPRS ratings of delusions and hallucinations, Al's psychiatrist also used response latency to measure cognitive capacity during weekly interviews with his patient, measuring the elapsed time between his question and Al's response. Initially there were pauses of up to 30 seconds, but as Al's cognitive functioning reconstituted, the latency was reduced to 5 seconds or less.

During daily sessions of social skills training, therapists kept a record of the frequency of correct and incorrect responses Al made to questions probing his ability to solve interpersonal problems. For example, after family or peer interaction situations were role-played, Al was asked such questions as, "Who were you talking with?"; "What did the other person want?"; "How was the other person feeling?"; "What was your short-term goal in the situation?"; and "What alternatives could you have used to deal with the situation?" Al's ability to accurately perceive and process the information inherent in the role-playing gradually improved, with his error rate eventually declining to zero, which reflected his growth in attentional and cognitive abilities.

The intensity of Al's hallucinatory experiences was rated by the psychiatrist weekly on the BPRS. When he became more insightful about his illness, he self-monitored the frequency of auditory hallucinations by activating a wrist counter for each occurrence during the day. By the time of discharge, hallucinations were no longer occurring.

Al's fantasies and hypochondriacal delusions were followed during weekly recreational therapy sessions by his drawing pictures of himself. The first few drawings revealed distorted body shapes and numerous sores placed on the figure's hands and face. Subsequently, the drawings showed a figure isolated from others, but having coherent outlines and no sign of lesions. It was felt that these changes reflected positive improvements in the quality of his self-perception.

AFFECTIVE PROBLEMS

Each week, Al checked on a Target Complaint Scale the intensity or magnitude of his tension, fear, and discomfort. His self-ratings enabled the treatment team to remain sensitive to his subjective dysphoria, complementing functional assessments made by observing clinicians. Al's Target Complaint Scale graph for a three-week period revealed a decrease from "couldn't be worse" to levels between "a little" and "pretty much." It is of interest that a similar type of global rating of dysphoria, after "test doses" of neuroleptics, has been shown to accurately predict a schizophrenic patient's ultimate clinical response and adherence to neuroleptic drugs (VanPutten et al. 1981). Thus early and systematic assessment of the affective domain not only may reflect stress levels but also may enable clinicians to predict effectiveness of neuroleptic treatment.

SOCIAL-INTERPERSONAL PROBLEMS

Four times daily, the nursing staff unobtrusively observed Al on the ward, following a Social Interaction Schedule, and recorded indices of his engagement in unit activity, his interaction with other patients, and the occurrence of a variety of inappropriate behavior. All of these measures were frequency counts of specific appropriate or inappropriate behaviors. During his first week, Al was noted to be isolated and inactive for 90 percent of the nursing staff's observations. He showed 18 instances of inappropriate behaviors such as posturing, rocking, and grimacing. When initially approached for a 2- to 3-minute pleasant conversation at these four daily Social Interaction Schedule sessions, Al would actively move away and close his eyes. As time went on, observations revealed his more active engagement with the environment, although still isolated from others. By the third week of hospitalization, Al was interacting with other patients and staff about 40 percent of the time and was responsive in conversations with staff 60 percent of the time.

During the social-skills training sessions, which began after a week of hospitalization and positive response to drug treatment, Al was rated on the adequacy of his performance in role-played scenes. He was rated as satisfactory on eye contact and voice volume but as needing improvement in voice tone, fluency, and facial expression, which reflected his blunted affect. He also filled out an assertiveness inventory prior to starting the training and again at the end of training. The inventory showed an increase of 15 points, moving Al close to the normal range by the time his one-month hospitalization was over.

INDEPENDENT LIVING SKILLS

Al's self-care and work skills were evaluated by the nursing staff numerous times a day within the context of a credit incentive system, a type of token economy. The number of prompts that were required to get Al to satisfactorily wash himself, shower, brush his teeth, comb his hair, and dress himself in appropriate attire were recorded as a frequency measure. Full credits were given for satisfactory completion of these tasks without prompts; half credits were given for satisfactory completion after one prompt. Varying amounts of credits were also given for room maintenance and ward chores, depending on the quality of the performance and the number of prompts required to instigate their completion. Frequency ratings of appropriate self-care behaviors and quality ratings of his performance of ward chores translated into the total number of credits earned each day. Thus, Al's credit earnings reflected his role performance on the unit and served as an ongoing quantitative assessment of Al's progress.

In addition, an Independent Living Skills Survey (Wallace 1986) was filled out during Al's initial evaluation to pinpoint the areas of community functioning that needed intervention and training. The Independent Living Skills Survey contains 112 items concerning how much a person is able to do for himself or herself in self-care activities such as eating and grooming, domestic activities, health care, money management, transportation, leisure activities, and work. Each item is rated in terms of how often a particular behavior has occurred (frequency) in the past month and how much of a problem the behavior (or lack of it) has been for the patient, the family, or the facility in which the person lives during the past month. The Independent Living Skills Survey was completed by Al's parents. Both the Grooming and the Leisure subscales indicated that Al was having substantial difficulties in these areas. Grooming behaviors such as "bathes or showers using soap at least twice a week without prompting" and "uses deodorant daily without prompting" were rated on the frequency scale as "never." These behaviors were viewed

---

LEARNING EXERCISE

Using the multimodal framework for functional assessment, review a patient with a severe psychiatric disorder with whom you are familiar. On a piece of paper, list the different assessment modalities that apply to that patient. Then write, in behaviorally descriptive terms, the problems experienced by the patient in each modality of functioning.

After formulating the problems in this manner, consider whether you could use measures or instruments to assess the frequency, intensity or severity, latency, duration, or context in each problem domain. Use your ingenuity to design a method of measurement that would yield reliable and clinically relevant data in a feasible and practical way.

by Al's parents as being severely dysfunctional since they rated these items as "always a problem" during the past month.

BEHAVIORAL EXCESSES, DEFICITS, AND ASSETS

In conducting a functional assessment with a chronic patient like Al, where a plethora of problems can easily overwhelm the responsible clinician, it is also usually helpful to define targets for intervention in terms of behavioral excesses and deficits. Behavioral assets should also be defined since these can serve as building blocks for priorities in the treatment process. While it may not be necessary to develop interventions for all of the problem areas, segmenting them in this way often helps to clarify and prioritize the selection of problems for treatment. By working with the patient's positive assets, rehabilitation can strengthen a patient's adaptive behavior, thereby displacing problematic deficits and excesses.

Behavioral Excesses. Behaviors may be problematic because they are maladaptive in and of themselves or they occur at a frequency, intensity, or duration that is judged to be too high for a particular environment.

Some of Al's initially identified behavioral excesses included the following:

spends too much time alone—is withdrawn, isolated
urinates in pants
has difficulty in falling asleep
has nightmares
spends too much time listening to music
is fatigued all the time
fantasizes strange thoughts
has auditory hallucinations with depreciatory content

Behavioral Deficits. Often, adaptive and desirable behaviors may present problems because they occur at an insufficient frequency, inadequate intensity, or inappropriate form. These are termed "negative symptoms" of mental disorder.

Examples of some of Al's initially identified behavioral deficits included the following:

poorly sustained concentration
not completing tasks
unable to make or maintain friendships
not eating
diminished self-care skills
lack of social or instrumental activities
unresponsive to questions; poverty of speech
lack of affect
mute

Behavioral Assets. Assets or strengths include social competence, coping efforts, and social supports that the patient brings to the treatment setting. Chronic patients with "poor" premorbid histories usually possess few of these assets; however, it is important to identify whatever level or type of skills, interests, and abilities a patient has had in the past. It is expedient to build treatment goals on the individual's assets, since these give both the clinician and patient a running start with already-existing behavioral repertoires. In many clinical cases, the therapist is well advised to give priority to goals that are not directly linked to symptoms but are based upon the patient's strengths.

A paranoid schizophrenic's delusions may be impenetrable through direct treatment efforts but might less interfere with daily living if social interaction and work performance are improved. An obese individual may be extremely resistant to efforts aimed at changing eating habits directly, but might eat less if alternative social and recreational activities are engaged in, especially at times of peak hunger. A person with a somatoform disorder might respond better clinically to interventions aimed at the goal of improving communication in marriage rather than at the symptoms per se, particularly if the symptoms serve the function of gaining concern and reinforcement from the spouse. In other words, goals that strengthen the assets or strengths of the individual can often indirectly displace and reduce psychopathology and symptomatology.

Development of an inventory of assets is of use, of course, in determining Axis Five of *DSM-III*, the patient's highest level of adaptive psychosocial functioning in the past year. The clinician should obtain from the patient and significant others, as well as from historical records, answers to questions such as

1. What are the areas in which the patient functions well, now or in the past?
2. What are the patient's interpersonal resources and social support network?
3. What agencies and helping professionals can be mobilized for participation in a treatment plan?
4. How aversive are the patient's current impairments to himself or herself and his or her family, and can this serve as a source of motivation for change?
5. How responsive is the patient to the therapeutic alliance and setting?

As in identifying problems and formulating goals, assets should be inventoried from a multimodal perspective. While levels of functioning vary from one patient to another, each patient does have a unique set of assets in areas of affect, cognition, instrumental role behavior, interpersonal relations, and biological endowment. These assets can be matched against those skills and changes needed for the patient to attain chosen goals. Steps toward reaching long-term goals can build on patients' resources in a way that facilitates gradual and comfortable change, taking advantage of already-existing and developing assets.

Examples of Al's behavioral assets are listed below:

good academic skills
conscientious and reliable in meeting commitments
concerned family members willing to be involved in treatment

The need to identify and consider behavioral assets in the development of a treatment plan for Al can be illustrated in two ways. First, the frequency of an undesirable behavior is often maintained by well-meaning but inadvertently reinforcing attention. Al's delusional preoccupation with his health prior to and in the first few days of his hospitalization was inevitably reinforced with concern and sympathy by his family and by the hospital staff. Rather than helping Al, this attention may have actually enhanced this delusional preoccupation. Of course, enough attention must be devoted to eliciting and examining psychopathology to make a diagnosis and monitor improvements in mental status. Striking a balance between too much or too little focus on symptoms requires clinical acumen. Family and professional caregivers can redress psychopathology by attending to and reinforcing the positive strengths or progress of the patient.

A second reason for attending to behavioral assets is their importance as vehicles for developing new adaptive behaviors. Treatment programs are more likely to be successful if they build on existing talents, skills, and resources.

Al's conscientiousness and reliability were capitalized upon by having him self-monitor with a wrist counter the decreasing frequency of his hallucinating experiences. His having completed a year of college and having held (although briefly) jobs in the competitive marketplace were also viewed as assets to be built upon for after-care goals.

FUNCTIONAL ANALYSIS OF CONDITIONS MAINTAINING THE PROBLEMS

Once the presenting problems are clearly defined, the assessment process moves to the identification of biological and environmental influences on the problems. Since most major mental disorders have a biological substrate that confers vulnerability to the characteristic symptoms and psychopathology, a functional analysis must be preceded by the diagnostic evaluation process (described in Chapter 2). The delineation of the *DSM-III* diagnosis leads naturally to the choice of a rational plan for psychopharmacotherapy for the disorder, as outlined in Chapter 4. There is clear agreement that biomedical variables are foremost in the etiology of the psychopathology that characterizes the major mental disorders.

LEARNING EXERCISE

Read the following case history and identify the patient's behavioral deficits, excesses, and assets by responding to the questions that follow.

Eve presented as a pleasant but agitated and tense 56-year-old woman who typically answered in a monosyllabic manner. She was hospitalized briefly in Iowa approximately 25 years previously following a brief extramarital affair that was followed by extreme guilt, remorse, and an unremitting delusion that people, whom she didn't know, were "saying evil things about her." She had been twice hospitalized for brief periods of 5 to 7 days since this initial hospitalization, but managed to raise two children and maintain a job as a bookkeeper.

According to her husband she had continued to function poorly and had not "snapped out of it" since her last hospitalization, two years earlier. Upon probing, Eve revealed that she had felt "down in the dumps" for the last six or seven years, lacking energy and not having the courage to "face the world."

During the initial evaluation, Eve was administered a Brief Psychiatric Rating Scale and Beck Depression Inventory. Results indicated a moderate degree of depression with extremely high ratings of guilt and tension.

A functional assessment revealed that Eve had not ventured out of the house by herself in the last 15 months. She occasionally ventured out on weekends if her husband accompanied her and if they were going someplace where no one knew her. Her isolation was so complete that she would not even walk down their driveway to pick up the mail or into the backyard to maintain the vegetable garden that used to be her pride and joy. Eve often spent her nights pacing the floor. During the interview she was observed continually wringing her hands, tapping her feet, and moving her lips and jaw in an odd manner. Presently, she engages in no leisure or recreational activities, although she used to enjoy going for long walks, traveling, shopping, planning dinner parties, volunteering at the botanical center, and playing bridge. Her speech content was also noted to be predominately self-depreciating and concerned with her misfortune, and when pressed to describe something that she formerly enjoyed, she rarely displayed any affect.

Eve was diagnosed as suffering from "double depression"— a psychotic depressive disorder superimposed on an underlying chronic dysthymia (Keller and Shapiro 1982). An antidepressant

continued

Learning Exercise *continued*

was prescribed that helped to decrease the depression after six weeks. Perhaps most difficult for Eve and her husband to handle, in spite of the gains from medication, was her extreme reluctance to leave the house by herself to attend to routine tasks such as grocery shopping, banking, and going to the post office. Both Eve and her husband also desired to socialize with friends and travel in their motor home once again.

1. Behavioral Deficits: Which of Eve's adaptive behaviors need to be initiated, increased in frequency, or strengthened in form?
2. Behavioral Excesses: Which of Eve's maladaptive behaviors need to be terminated, decreased in frequency, or altered in form?
3. Behavioral Assets: Consider Eve's strengths in multimodal terms. Which interests and skills does Eve have either in overt or latent form? What material and interpersonal resources does the patient have?
4. How could you determine if the patient's self-description of her problems is congruent with that of other observers? Who, besides the patient, can be relied upon to monitor Eve's progress and response to treatment?

Beyond still poorly delineated biological causes, environmental factors that are implicated in the onset, exacerbation, relapse, or chronic course of a disorder must also be teased out so that effective psychosocial treatment and rehabilitation can be designed and implemented. The task here is to gather information on the environmental conditions that typically occur before the problematic behavior and the consequences that tend to follow it. Antecedents and consequences of problem behaviors in the patient's present and past environments contribute to the initiation and maintenance of the problems. A delineation of environmental antecedents of clinical disorders enables the practitioner to rate Axis Four of *DSM-III*, the severity of psychosocial stressors.

A common first step in the functional or behavioral analysis is to have the patient, family member, or friend describe a typical day of the patient in detail. Active questioning of the patient often yields a description of his or her daily activities from awakening to retiring. A review of the typical day indicates antecedents and consequences that may function to maintain or motivate behavior. The following questions illustrate the specificity needed to ascertain person-and-environment relationships that can influence the multimodal pattern of behavioral problems.

1. Setting—"In what situations does the problem behavior occur? At home? At work? In public places or when you're alone?" "Who is usually with you when the problem is present or maximal? How does the person respond to you?" "At what times of day does this happen?" "What else are you likely to be doing at the time?"
2. Antecedents—"What usually has happened right before the problem occurs? Does anything in particular seem to start this behavior?"
3. Consequences—"What usually happens right afterward?" "How do you feel when that happens?" "Does anyone respond or interact with you at that time?"

The following examples of antecedents and consequences highlight the importance of these variables in a functional analysis of patients' behavioral problems. As you read these sections, think about how you would use interviews and observations to link possible antecedents and consequences to the problem behaviors of interest.

Antecedents

Events, situations, and other people, as well as physical stimuli, can all serve to evoke human behavioral responses. Cues, prompts, signals, or instructions can influence a person to behave in a certain way. Examples of antecedent events in obsessive-compulsive disorders are words, colors, furniture, dirt, stove knobs, door locks, and light switches that serve as cues to elicit unwanted thoughts and rituals. Similarly, phobic patients generally avoid certain situations that are anxiety-provoking, for example, driving on busy streets or visiting crowded stores and theaters. These situational antecedents of anxiety and avoidance should be identified in specific detail so they can be used in developing behavioral treatment procedures.

Antecedents usually occur in combination across multimodal levels of behavioral experience. As an example, various antecedents may contribute to a depressed person's withdrawing from a social event: 1) He anticipates awkwardness and rejection (cognitive), 2) he feels especially low that day (affect), 3) he observes a person in the setting who previously had been critical and rude (interpersonal), 4) he fantasizes humiliation (imagery), 5) he enters a room which had been the scene of an unpleasant experience (situational), and/or 6) he did not sleep well the night before (biological).

Some situations spontaneously elicit maladaptive behavior because in the past the behavior has been reinforced in that situation. For example, a child's crying and tantrums when put to bed might be prompted by contact with the bed, which in turn has been associated with parental nurturance, reassurance, and attentiveness. Similarly, agitation in a patient about to receive a PRN dose of an antipsychotic drug may be heightened by the past experiences of physical contact and attention with staff associated with administration of PRNs. Other situations can affect physiological responses, such as when stressors in work settings increase the secretion of gastric acid or muscle tension in the neck and head. Major life events and interpersonal losses are also important precipitants to many psychiatric disorders, given an individual with the biological predisposition and vulnerability to stressors.

Modeling, or being influenced by observing the behavior of others, is a particularly powerful antecedent in determining behavioral responses. Models include parents and relatives, entertainment and television figures, and subjects in advertisements. The process of acquiring attributes through identification occurs essentially through modeling. Most complex skills and symptoms are learned on a vicarious basis, by observing other persons' behavior and its consequences for them. Thus, for example, a patient with hypochondriasis may have initially acquired the sick role and somatic complaints through observing another person with similar complaints. Similarly, epidemics of hysterical symptoms quickly spread among individuals who are in proximity to each other through seeing or hearing graphic accounts of those afflicted.

Cognitive responses are a special class of antecedents that can function as mediating steps in maintaining or exacerbating clinical problems. The labeling given to emotional states, self-perceptions, and self-instructions can perpetuate maladaptive behavior. For example, a person with

---

LEARNING EXERCISE

Using a case that you are familiar with, describe the antecedents that appear to be eliciting or maintaining maladaptive behavior by answering the following questions.

1. What typically happens right before the problem behavior occurs?
2. Does anything in particular seem to start this behavior?
3. Is there a particular place or situation that is associated with the onset of the problem behavior?
4. What combination of multimodal levels of behavioral experience appear to contribute to the maladaptive behavior?
5. Might the maladaptive behavior be prevented by blocking the occurrence of one or more of the multimodal levels of behavior?
6. What cognitive response or labeling appears to be functioning as a mediating step in maintaining the clinical problem?
7. Does modeling influence the form or occurrence of the problem behavior?

a chronic schizophrenic disorder who says to herself, "I am a loser and can't work," may increase anticipatory anxiety to the degree that her work performance and interest in job seeking may decline.

CONSEQUENCES

Most mental health professionals are sensitive to the antecedents or precipitants of emotional problems; they give less attention to the consequences or reinforcers of the problems. Consequences can either strengthen and increase or weaken and decrease the frequency, duration, and intensity of the behaviors that precede them.

Reinforcers are environmental consequences that increase the probability that a preceding behavior will occur in the future or be learned. When consequences of a behavior decrease the likelihood of future occurrences of that behavior, the unlearning process of punishment or extinction is in play.

The contingency, which defines the temporal relationship between the occurrence of a behavior and the environmental consequence, is very important in determining whether a particular consequence will affect preceding behavior. For example, consequences that occur immediately after a problem behavior are more likely to influence the future status of the problem than are delayed consequences.

How does the clinician evaluate the pertinent antecedents and consequences of the patient's problems to determine their salience and potential contribution to treatment planning? Information on the environmental antecedents and consequences can be obtained from the patient through careful and systematic interviewing and questionnaires. The Fear Survey Schedule (Wolpe and Lang 1964) can be filled out by the patient, indicating how much fear or discomfort each of 120 items or situations produces. A variety of reinforcement surveys elicit reports by the patient of things, people, events, and activities that are viewed as desirable and pleasant and thus are presumed to be reinforcing. However, the clinician is not limited to the patient as a source of information. In fact, because behavioral assessment requires our knowing the antecedents and consequences of behaviors, it may be necessary to interview significant others or directly observe the patient in the situations in which the troublesome behaviors take place.

Significant discrepancies may exist between what the patient reports as being antecedents and consequences and what is actually observed. Reasons for discrepancies include retrospective distortion, social anxiety, and poor self-observation. When such discrepancies occur, the behavioral clinician gives greater credence to what the patient does than to what the patient says he does. Although not always convenient or possible, direct observations of the patient are the most reliable means of determining the factors in the environment that are maintaining the

---

LEARNING EXERCISE

Read the following case history and identify the consequences that are maintaining this patient's maladaptive behavior by responding to the questions that follow.

Miss Jones is a 47-year-old patient at a state mental hospital. She has been hospitalized for the past 15 years. For the past 7 years, Miss Jones has been eating cigarette butts (including the filters) that she finds on the unit or grounds. She has been known to occasionally barge into the nursing station to grab a handful of cigarette butts, which she then stuffs into her mouth. By the time staff intervene and attempt to remove the butts from her mouth, she has already swallowed some. She also grabs food from other patients' plates at meals and stuffs the food into her mouth. Since she often doesn't chew the food she steals, she frequently chokes and gags as she tries to swallow and has consequently required resuscitation on three occasions in the past year.

She has been lectured and counseled on numerous occasions, deprived of meals, and put in seclusion, but all to no avail. After several episodes of gagging, Miss Jones was provided one-to-one supervision to prevent her insertion of cigarettes. She has also required medical attention on six occasions because of other patients striking out at her following her theft of cigarettes butts or food.

1. What are Miss Jones's behavioral problem(s)? Be specific.
2. What are the staff doing that might be contributing to Miss Jones's problem behavior?
3. How might the staff deal more effectively with the problem behavior(s)? Develop two or three suggestions.

---

problems. The behavioral-environmental interrelationships observed on an inpatient unit, in a day hospital, and even during an outpatient therapy session provide useful information in making a functional analysis. Home visits and community outings, perhaps conducted by a nurse or paraprofessional, can also improve the scope and quality of the behavioral assessment.

CASE EXAMPLE ————————————————————————

Without minimizing the critical role of biological causes of schizophrenic symptoms, let's examine what environmental antecedents and consequences were influential in the development and sustaining of Al's clinical problems. Al's earlier life events were likely formative in determining his premorbid personality, assets, and limitations), it appears that his increasing social isolation, lack of a peer network, and parental criticism all contributed to his symptomatic impairments. Many who have studied schizophrenia believe that either understimulating or overstimulating social environments can lead to symptoms and their worsening. Al was exposed to both types of stressors, alternating between total isolation and family criticism and overconcern.

It is also likely that his parents' cajolery may have served as a reinforcer of his growing self-negativism and isolation; that is, their emotional responses to his attempts to reduce intolerable levels of arousal may have inadvertently increased his withdrawal. Al's lack of peer relationships deprived him of age-appropriate models from which he could have learned social skills to acquire friends. In attempting to reduce external pressure on Al, his parents may have gone too far by excusing him from reasonable work responsibilities. Instead of receiving recognition and acknowledgement for chores and continuing in a remunerative job, Al received his parents' concern and solicitude for being increasingly helpless and dependent.

A functional analysis of antecedents and consequences influences on behavior problems, such as the above analysis of Al's, despite its reliance on retrospective guesswork, can be helpful in the goal-setting process. In Al's case, it seemed important to alter the contingencies of reinforcement and communication patterns in the family, to find a reasonable work role for Al to develop, and to start him on the path toward social relationships with peers.

LEARNING EXERCISE

The following case example illustrates some of the potential effects of antecedents and consequences on the behavior of a chronic schizophrenic patient.

Mr. West is a 37-year-old patient on a chronic ward of a state hospital. He spends most of the time sleeping on the floor or sofa in the day room and watching TV. His two friends, Bill and Bob, also spend most of their days in this manner. When the three of them watch TV together they seem to delight in playing a one-upmanship game to see who can make the most

continued

bizarre statements about themselves relative to the TV program. In addition, Mr. West is usually at the front of the line at meal time and never misses an opportunity to bum cigarettes or spare change.

Mr. West is an Army veteran who completed two years of college. Treatment staff find it almost impossible to get him to attend rehabilitation groups or to start making any vocational or discharge plans. He seems to vanish or become unresponsive whenever anyone approaches him for an interview or prompts him to attend a treatment session. He's been heard to say "just leave me alone." The staff refer to him as a "good patient"— he never becomes aggressive, doesn't pester the staff, and is on time for medication. He has been hospitalized for nearly two years, but no one has been able to engage him in a constructive discussion about his illness, plans, or treatment program. Staff describe him as "not being ready yet" and needing to develop some "motivation" before he can be helped.

Evaluate the role of the staff's efforts with Mr. West in terms of antecedent and consequent conditions that might be maintaining his clinical problems.

1. What are the behavioral problems shown by Mr. West? Be specific and descriptive in a multimodal assessment.
2. What is it about the ward setting and his pals, Bill and Bob, that might be contributing to Mr. West's present problems? Identify at least two possible antecedents to his apathetic, bumming, and bizarre behavior. (Note that the lack of activities or structured programs can be a corollary of deviant behavior and expression of symptoms.) Identify at least two consequences of Mr. West's behavioral problems that appear to be maintaining these problems. (Note that reinforcing consequences can be positive or negative. Positive reinforcers are operating when the behavior of interest triggers the desired consequence in the environment; negative reinforcers operate when the targeted behavior permits the individual to escape from or avoid some unpleasant or undesired environmental consequence.)
3. What might the staff do differently as they interact with Mr. West?

INSTRUMENTS AND METHODS FOR FUNCTIONAL ASSESSMENT

Behavior is multidimensional; thus, behavioral assessment must encompass all of the levels of human functioning that contribute to clinical symptoms, role impairments, and treatment outcome. Instrumental role performance, social interaction, imagery, sensory experiences, cognition, affect, and psychobiological processes need to be assessed during both the initial evaluation and the course of therapy and rehabilitation. In short, functional assessment includes all modalities of human expression and experience. The key, however, is to understand how problem behaviors interfere with the functional domains necessary for maximum independence and life satisfaction. From this vantage point, the most critical areas of everyday function needing assessment are

relationships with family members
social relationships with peers
vocational skills
leisure activities

A variety of methods and instruments are available to assist the clinician in obtaining information relevant to these functional domains. Behavioral interviewing provides one method of assessment. The interview may consist of questions that cover the areas listed above or the use of structured interview guides. A second method for functional assessment is direct observation of behavior. Although direct observation methods can be time consuming and require staff expertise to ensure reliability, they are particularly useful in inpatient or day treatment settings where patients are unable to articulate their problems. Behavioral coding systems can yield highly sensitive standardized assessment for program evaluation, quality assurance, treatment and discharge planning, and careful monitoring of patient response to particular interventions.

Self-observation approaches provide a third method of obtaining a reliable picture of the frequency and context of the patient's problems. A fourth method of functional assessment involves the use of paper-and-pencil checklists, questionnaires, and rating forms that are related to specific skills.

These four methods are described below and examples are given for some of the instruments in use. These multimethod approaches to functional assessment are desirable because they permit the astute care provider to gather information relevant to the rehabilitation needs of the patient from a variety of sources and in a variety of ways. For example, if the patient is able to actively assist the professional in the assessment process, behavioral interviewing, self-monitoring, and paper-and-pencil measures may be used. If the functional level of the patient precludes active participation, then direct observation methods can be used. Optimally, a combination of these methods may be selected in line with the resources and time constraints of the treatment setting.

Behavioral Interviewing

In functional assessment through behavioral interviewing, the practitioner begins by asking the patient to describe the nature and context of behavioral deficits, excesses, and assets. Questions such as, "What's causing you difficulty? When or how often does it happen? Where are you when it occurs? How does it impact on you?" can yield useful assessment data. It is preferable to have the patient give recent examples of behavioral functioning in their environmental contexts, rather than a general summary or overview of his or her difficulties. It is essential to help the patient translate vague and general problem descriptions into more specific or concrete terms. If the patient is unable to translate his or her vague complaints into behavioral terms, the assessment task becomes the identification of events and behaviors associated with the ambiguously phrased feelings or problems. For example, a depressed patient's complaints of "depression" and "worthlessness" may lead to a clearer assessment if interviewing can associate such complaints with excessive free time, a lack of social interaction, negative cognitions or self-deprecating thoughts, and criticism from family members or friends. An example of questions used in an assessment interview to elicit information about the patient's functioning relative to family, social contacts, work, and leisure activities is provided in Table 9.

Sometimes the patient may be reticent to disclose a specific undesirable behavior, for example, exhibitionism or paranoid thoughts. In this case, the assessment task is to help the patient feel comfortable enough to talk about the problem. More often, the patient finds difficulty in associating general dysphoria with any specific behavior or environmental context. In such cases, it is useful to consider whether a deficiency of desirable adaptive behavior is reducing the amount of positive reinforcement received from the environment and thus is responsible for malaise and dysphoria.

During the initial evaluation interviews, it is important for the clinician to understand the problems from the patient's point of view, adopting a "consumer" approach in which the patient describes his or her concerns and reasons for seeking help. After discussing the patient's view of the problems, the clinician encourages the patient to translate the feelings and problems into operational terms, focusing on what the patient is doing, feeling, and thinking. The goal is to determine which behaviors in the multimodal spectrum need to be modified, that is, which specific behavior patterns require change in their frequency of occurrence, intensity, duration, or the conditions under which they occur. At this point of behavioral assessment, the clinician should determine if the

TABLE 9: Sample Questions for Eliciting Functional Needs in a
Behavioral Interview

Family:

How have you been getting along with relatives?

Are there things your relatives do that annoy you?

Is there anyone in the family you avoid because you're uncomfortable
with that person?

Social contacts and comfort:

Have you had a chance to do anything socially with your friends or
family?

Do you generally make plans for social activities or does someone else
usually ask you to go along?

Do you enjoy being with people?

Do you feel anxious or want to get away or be alone when with
people?

Work:

Have you had any trouble keeping a job?

Do you get to work on time?

Do you perform any household tasks?

Leisure activities:

What kinds of things do you do in your free time?

Could you tell me about these?

Do you have any trouble keeping yourself busy in your spare time?

---

problems consist of an excess of maladaptive behaviors and/or a deficit
of adaptive behaviors.

During an initial evaluation, patients often overestimate the frequency or severity of self-reported problems. Depressed persons might
spontaneously report that they feel miserable, hopeless, and pessimistic
"all of the time," when in fact they may be able to elaborate periods of
feeling okay when questioned more specifically. Direct, clear questions
about the frequency of the occurrence of a problem help to elicit more
reliable information. Structured interview guides are available to assist
the clinician in the task of obtaining reliable information on the scope
and impact of problems on social functioning (Platt et al. 1980; Hersen
and Belleck 1981; Harris 1975; Cautela 1977). One such guide, the Social
Attainment Scale (Goldstein 1970), has proved useful in quickly evaluating the level of social adjustment of patients. An excerpt of this scale
is shown below in Table 10.

TABLE 10: Excerpt from the UCLA Social Attainment Survey (Adapted from Harris 1975)

The following ratings are based upon the social adjustment of male and female patients for the preceding 3 months. Ratings should be based on best information available.

Same-sex peer relationships
Number and closeness of relationships with like-sexed youngsters his own age. Do not include in this rating transient relationships, those with younger or older individuals, or relationships with relatives.
1. No friends his own age.
2. One or two casual friends only.
3. Several casual friends or close relationship with one individual only.
4. Several casual friends, with one or two close relationships.
5. Several casual friends, with three or more close relationships.

Leadership in same-sex peer relations
Frequency with which patient assumed a leadership role with like-sexed youngsters his own age. How often did he seek out others, or make plans or decisions for his group?
1. Never assumed leadership. Almost always waited for others.
2. Rarely assumed leadership.
3. Sometimes assumed leadership.
4. Often assumed leadership.
5. Usually assumed leadership role. Actively showed initiative in making plans and decisions with others every day.

Opposite-sex peer relations
Involvement with, and emotional commitment, to a member of the opposite sex. The extent to which the patient extended himself for another, showed concern for their needs and interests.
1. No emotional involvement with an opposite-sexed peer.
2. Mild emotional involvement.
3. Moderate emotional involvement.
4. Strong but intermittent emotional involvement.
5. Strong continuous involvement and commitment to an opposite-sexed peer.

TABLE 10: (continued)

Dating history
1. Never dated.
2. Dated a few times.
3. Occasionally went out on dates.
4. Dated often but never had a lasting steady association.
5. Dated regularly and went steady.

Sexual experience
1. No interest in sex.
2. Interested but no sexual play or intercourse.
3. Sexual play only on one or two occasions.
4. Sexual play or intercourse on one or two occasions.
5. Sexual intercourse and sexual play on several occasions.

Outside activities
Number of activities outside the home the patient initiated on his own, e.g., movies, dances, parties, shopping, picnics, hobbies, camping, riding, hiking.
1. Initiated no activities outside the home.
2. One or two outside activities.
3. Several outside activities.
4. Moderate number of outside activities.
5. Initiated many outside activities.

Participation in organizations
Attendance and participation in activities of organizations or social clubs on his own initiative, e.g., church, scouts, YMCA, school sports, or social club.
1. Did not attend any of these activities.
2. Belonged to none but occasionally attended.
3. Belonged to at least one organization and sometimes attended, but rarely participated.
4. Belonged to at least one organization and sometimes participated.
5. Belonged to at least one organization, attended regularly, and participated actively.

Direct Observation of Behavior

Direct observation methods can be used for assessment of individual patients and to evaluate the effects of programs on groups of psychiatric patients in an efficient and economical manner. Multidimensional or multicategory behavioral measures are used to target specific skill deficits and behavioral excesses in need of treatment and rehabilitation. Whereas intensive individualized measures of behavior of large numbers of patients are prohibitively expensive, multicategory behavioral observations based on time-sampling procedures and administered by nonprofessionals can be conducted in a less expensive manner, while maintaining the specificity necessary for rigorous assessment and evaluation. Behavioral observation instruments must have psychometric qualities of reliability and validity. They must also be a) sufficiently inclusive of general classes of behavior to be relevant to assessment questions of interest, b) simple enough to be used by nonprofessional observers, and c) sensitive enough to be responsive to changes in the patient.

One system that has proved to be exceptionally reliable and useful for assessment and ongoing monitoring of patient functioning in any residential setting is the Time-Sample Behavioral Checklist (Paul and Lentz 1977; Power 1979). The Time-Sample Behavioral Checklist (TSBC) is an observational assessment system designed to measure the level of functioning of patients in residential treatment facilities. The TSBC is designed to assess behavior in enough detail to allow situation-specific problem identification and ongoing clinical monitoring, while concurrently yielding higher-level adaptive and maladaptive scores to allow absolute and comparative evaluation of individual and group differences in treatment programs. The TSBC is based on random, two-second observations made throughout the patient's waking hours. The presence or absence of 69 behavioral codes at each observational interval are recorded on a TSBC response sheet. The patient's "appropriate" or "inappropriate" behavior can thus be identified through the occurrence or nonoccurrence of the relevant behavioral codes. A single observation has relatively little meaning, but with a minimum of 10 or more observations daily, an accurate picture of the patient's level of functioning can be obtained. Table 11 provides a listing of the TSBC observational categories, and Table 12 shows the discrete components entering into the Inappropriate and the Appropriate Higher Order Scores of the TSBC.

Figure 9 provides an example of changes in two of the TSBC category codes—chattering or talking to self; and pacing—that were observed in a patient, "Ralph," over a two-month period on the University of California at Los Angeles Clinical Research Unit at Camarillo State Hospital. Talking to self and incoherent speech were clearly reduced by the introduction of neuroleptic drug therapy. Pacing behavior increased somewhat, probably a result of the akathisia induced as a side effect of the medication.

To give a sense of the degree of specificity required in observational codes, chattering or talking to self is defined by the TSBC as "talks, makes meaningless vocalizations, moves lips at any time during 2-second observation in absence of recipient of communication." Pacing is defined as "walks alone without apparent destination throughout the 2 second

TABLE 11: Time Sample Behavior Checklist Categories and Codes for Observer Notation

I. LOCATION (Record 1)
1. classroom lounge
2. T.V. Room
3. corridor lounge
4. own bedroom
5. other bedroom
6. activity area
7. living room/day room
8. office
9. hallway
10. dining area
11. kitchen
12. restroom
13. bathing area
14. laundry room
15. sitting room
16. seclusion room
17. off unit (specify)
18. unauthorized absence—no observation
19. sick—no observation (specify)
20. authorized absence—no observation (specify)

II. POSITION (Record 1)
21. sitting
22. standing
23. lying down
24. walking
25. running
26. dancing

III. AWAKE-ASLEEP (Record 1)
27. eyes open
28. eyes closed

IV. FACIAL EXPRESSION (Record 1)
31. smiling, laughing with apparent stimulus
32. grimacing, frowning with apparent stimulus
33. neutral with apparent stimulus
34. smiling, laughing with NO apparent stimulus
35. grimacing, frowning with NO apparent stimulus
36. neutral with NO apparent stimulus

V. SOCIAL ORIENTATION (Record All)
37. alone
38. with residents ("patients")
39. with staff
40. with others

VI. CONCURRENT ACTIVITIES (Record All)
1. watching others
2. talking to others
3. listening to others
4. singing
5. reading
6. writing
7. hobby or handicraft
8. smoking

TABLE 11: (continued)

VI. CONCURRENT ACTIVITIES (continued)

9. eating	13. watching T.V.
10. drinking	14. group activity
11. playing a game	15. personal grooming
12. listening to radio, phonograph	16. working
	17. other (specify)

VII. CRAZY BEHAVIORS (Record All)

1. chattering, talking to self	9. repetitive and stereotypic movements
2. screaming	
3. swearing, cursing	10. posturing
4. verbal intrusion	11. shaking, tremoring
5. verbalized delusions, hallucinations, suicidal threats	12. pacing
	13. blank staring
	14. destroying property
6. incoherent speech	15. injuring self
7. crying	16. physical intrusion
8. rocking	17. other (specify)

Reprinted from Power CT: Journal of Behavioral Assessment 1:199–210, 1979.

observation and period immediately before observation." Lack of destination is further specified by "1) walking directly toward a blank wall and 2) walking in an identifiable pattern—such as circles." The specificity of these definitions of observable behaviors may seem overly precise, but it is only through such detailed articulation of observable behaviors that the reliability of the ratings may be maintained.

In the assessment of the behavioral problems and functional needs of chronic mental patients, direct observational methods like the TSBC may provide less biased and more detailed descriptions of behavior than retrospective ratings or questionnaires alone. However, as an indicator of the range, distribution, and frequency of symptomatic behaviors, such observational instruments as the TSBC may provide a necessary but not singularly sufficient assessment measure. Optimally, self-report and rating scales should be empirically combined with direct observations of behavior to provide a multidimensional assessment.

Self-Observation

Another approach to obtaining a reliable picture of the frequency and context of the patient's problems is to assign the patient homework to count the episodes when the problem occurs. This can be done through a daily diary or log, along with wearing a wrist counter such as those

TABLE 12: Discrete Components Entered into the Inappropriate and Appropriate Higher Order Score Categories on the Time Sample Behavior Check-List (TSBC). Higher order scores are obtained by summing the incidence of discrete components in each category.

Appropriate Higher Order Scores

Interpersonal Interaction

(All require a concurrent "with" social orientation)
Smiling—laughing with stimulus
Grimacing—frowning with stimulus
Watching others
Talking to others
Listening to others
Playing a game
Group activity

Self-Maintenance

Eating
Drinking
Personal Grooming

Instrumental Activity

Reading
Writing
Hobby or handicraft
Working

Individual Entertainment

Singing
Smoking
Listening to radio, phonograph
Watching TV
Playing a game (alone)

Total Appropriate Behavior

All of the above regardless of social orientation, plus
Sitting
Standing
Walking
Running
Dancing
Neutral with no stimulus
Other concurrent activity

Inappropriate Higher Order Scores

Bizarre Motoric Behavior

Lying down
Eyes closed
Neutral with stimulus
Rocking
Repetitive stereotypic movement
Posturing
Shaking—tremoring
Pacing
Blank staring

Hostile—Belligerent

Screaming
Swearing—cursing
Verbal intrusion
Destroying property
Injuring self
Physical intrusion

Bizarre Facial and Verbals

Smiling—laughing—no stimulus
Grimacing—frowning—no stimulus
Chattering—talking to self
Verbalized delusions, hallucinations, suicidal threats
Incoherent speech
Crying

Total Inappropriate Behavior

All inappropriate behavior, plus:
Seclusion room
Unauthorized absence
Other crazy behavior

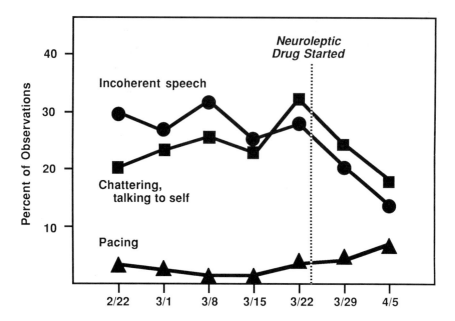

FIGURE 9:   Changes graphed in three of Ralph's behavioral problems, as monitored by the Time Sample Behavioral Checklist. Measurement of multimodal domains of behavioral functioning permits evaluation of therapeutic and side effects of treatment—in this case, the introduction of a neuroleptic drug.

used by golfers, carrying the inexpensive plastic counters used to tabulate grocery prices, or making checkmarks on a piece of paper. Self-observation and recording promotes commitment by the patient to the evaluation and treatment effort and provides further detailed information to either substantiate or qualify initial complaints. The use of self-observation techniques is illustrated by the following case example.

CASE EXAMPLE
According to his parents, Matt had been unable to "fit in" since his early teenage years. Now 35 years old, Matt's daily routine consisted of eating at fast food restaurants, working as a stock boy at a local retailer, and spending most of his time alone in his apartment with the exception of family gatherings that he was invited to attend. He complained that people "looked at him funny" when he tried to converse with them and laughed at him when they thought he could not hear them. He had previously been diagnosed as schizophrenic, but this diagnosis had been recently changed to schizotypal personality disorder and avoidant personality disorder. Matt had no friends, attended no social gatherings,

and talked in a circuitous and tangential manner. His parents complained during the initial interview that Matt failed to groom himself regularly and was being threatened with eviction from his apartment due to his hoarding of plastic trash bags filled with old newspapers and junk mail in his bedroom, which had resulted in a roach and silverfish problem. They also felt it would be beneficial if Matt could learn to manage his affairs independently without having to check with them constantly. Although he had received psychotherapy for these problems for the past 15 years and was able to express some insight into the nature of his difficulties, he was unable to make changes he felt were desirable to improve the quality of his life.

Initial treatment goals focused on increasing his social skills and improving his self care. In addition to social skills training to increase his ability to interact appropriately, a variety of self-observation techniques were used to help further define the parameters of Matt's problems and to help him monitor his progress. For example, Matt was initially given a homework assignment to count the number of opportunities he had in each work day to briefly interact with someone. It became clear to Matt rather quickly that he had 15 to 25 opportunities each day to say "Hello" to other employees or residents at the apartment building. After learning some brief conversation skills and when to apply them, Matt was next assigned to count the number of times each day that he actually engaged people in brief conversations, as well as the percentage of these engagement attempts that were successful. Similar self-observation techniques were used to monitor Matt's engagement in self-initiated social gatherings and his feelings of comfort/anxiety in these situations using the Target Complaint Scale. Self-observation checklists for appearance, hygiene, and apartment maintenance were also devised and assigned as homework. At the start of each treatment session the self-observation measures were reviewed by his therapist to ensure completion and to assess Matt's progress. The checklists were revised or new ones were added in accord with his progress.

Checklists, Questionnaires, and Rating Forms

While observational methods and interview strategies can elicit useful information about the treatment and rehabilitation needs of a particular patient, functional assessment can also proceed through the use of paper-and-pencil instruments. Most functional assessment instruments are skill related and behavioral in nature, focusing on the interaction between the individual and his or her surrounding environment. Examples of some of these instruments are provided in Table 13 (Wallace 1986). Checklists and questionnaires can be administered through an interview, a necessary method of obtaining assessment information from patients

TABLE 13: Major Characteristics of Instruments Used to Measure Functional Living Skills of Chronically Mentally Ill Individuals

Name, Author Source	Areas Assessed	Time Frame of Assessment	Data Collection Method
Katz Adjustment Scale (Katz and Lyerly 1963)	Symptoms, expected activities, rec/leisure activities	Past "few" weeks	Form R, 205-item questionnaire completed by significant other; Form S, 138-item questionnaire completed by patient
Personal Adjustment and Role Skills Scale (Ellsworth et al. 1968)	Symptoms, substance abuse, general community functioning	Past month	5 versions, all questionnaires, of 29 to 79 items— completed by significant other
Social Behaviour and Adjustment Scale (Platt et al. 1980)	Symptoms, role performance, objective burden, household distress	Past month	Semistructured interview conducted with significant other that covers 329 items
Psychiatric Status Schedule (Spitzer et al. 1970)	Symptoms, instrumental role performance	Past week (symptoms); past month (role performance)	Patient version, 321 items rated during structured interview; informant version, items rated during structured interview
Psychiatric Evaluation Form (PEF) (Endicott and Spitzer 1972a)	Symptoms, instrumental role performance	Past week (symptoms); past month (role performance)	28 items completed by experienced clinician using all sources of information
Current and Past Psychopathology Scale (Endicott and Spitzer 1972b)	PEF plus past adjustment, symptoms, and personality	PEF plus from age 12 to one month prior to evaluation	PEF plus 13 items of current symptoms plus 130 items of Psychiatric History Scale completed by experienced rater
Social Adjust Scale (SAS) (Weissman et al 1971)	General and interpersonal performance and satisfaction in 6 instrumental roles	Past 2 months for SAS and SAS-II; past 2 weeks for SAS-SR	SAS: 42 items rated during interview with patient; SAS-SR: 42-item questionnaire completed by patient; SAS-II: 52 items for chronic patients rated in interview
Social Stress and Functioning Inventory (Serban 1978)	Performance and stress in 21 areas of community living	Not reported	174 performance items and 130 stress items rated during interview with patient

Denver Community Mental Health Questionnaire (Ciarlo and Riehman 1977)	Distress, isolation, drug and alcohol abuse, productivity, use of agencies, satisfaction with service	Past 24 hours to past month	61 items rated during interview with patient
Community Adaptation Schedule (Burnes and Roen 1967)	Behavior, affect, desire for change in 34 areas of functioning	Current	Questionnaire of 212 items completed by patient
Rehabilitation Evaluation of Hall and Baker (Baker and Hall 1983)	"Deviant" behavior and "general" behaviors (Speech, interaction, etc.)	Past week	7 deviant behavior items and 15 general behavior items completed by trained institutional staff

who cannot be relied upon to give reliable responses without clear prompting and verbal encouragement.

Attributes of Functional Assessment Tools. Some of the dimensions of functional assessment tools that need to be considered in selecting one that fits the specific needs of potential users include the instrument's relevance, feasibility, utility, and reliability/validity (Brown et al. 1983).

Relevant instruments will generate information of the type that fits a user's given need for information. Functional assessment instruments vary widely in terms of the content and structure of the data that emerge, in at least the following ways:

1. Sensitivity to change in functioning.
2. Breadth of content of functioning that is described.
3. Relative emphasis on detailed profiles versus measures of overall amounts of impaired functioning.
4. Focus of assessment on the micro level versus focus on the macro functioning of the person in a community context.
5. Emphasis upon specific elements or components of behavior (for example, eye contact) versus characteristics of functioning (for example, social appropriateness).
6. Emphasis on production of behavior versus competency of functioning.
7. Emphasis on unobservable versus observable aspects of functioning.
8. Emphasis on descriptive measurement (for example, frequency counts of behaviors) versus evaluative measurement (for example, judgmental ratings).
9. Emphasis on developmental markers of progress versus adult-level (societal norms) markers.

Each of these parameters needs to be considered from the vantage point of the need for information on patients' functional status.

The amount of resources necessary to use an assessment tool can vary greatly. Resource limitations can determine the feasibility of an instrument. One constraint is the amount of time required for data gathering, for example, a few minutes to several hours or a month. Another constraint is one's access to the necessary informants to collect the information for functional assessment. Sources include self-report, informant interviewing, direct observation, or situational assessment. Specialized resources, such as computers and highly trained data collectors, can reduce the benefit/cost of using a particular instrument for functional assessment. Prior to using checklists, questionnaires, and/or rating forms, the practitioner should weigh their pros and cons relative to some other method of functional assessment. For example, a well-done behavioral interview may quickly identify behavioral deficits, excesses, and assets, which can be readily translated into appropriate rehabilitation goals. The behavioral interview may also be preferable for patients who are illiterate or who have difficulty in reading and writing.

The utility of functional assessment information can be diverse or limited. Tools that are insensitive to measuring change cannot be used for outcome measurement, but they may provide a global picture of functional characteristics that may assist in goal setting or other aspects of treatment planning. Instruments that are sensitive to change may also be used to state goals, track progress, and describe outcomes.

How is the precision of data gathering maximized? Selectors of instruments need to know the limits to precision and also the conditions associated with reliable data collection. Reliable data collection means that multiple users of an instrument will obtain the same results. Validity refers to what the measure tells us relevant to the patient's daily life. If A scores better than B on socialization, does A socialize more than B? Can A socialize appropriately on the job, with friends, in the community? Many of the "standardized" functional assessment tools fail to report reliability or validity data.

One functional assessment instrument that appears to meet the above criteria in an acceptable manner is the Independent Living Skills Survey (Wallace 1986). This 112-item survey of social adjustment covers the independent living domains of self-care skills, eating and grooming, domestic activities, health care, money management, transportation, leisure activities, and work. The survey is completed by a relative or care provider who rates each item in terms of how often the particular behavior has occurred in the past month and how much of a problem the behavior (or lack of it) has been for rater, the family, or the facility in which the person lives during the past month. In other words, each behavior in the eight functional domains covered by the survey is rated for its frequency of occurrence and on its severity. Excerpts from the survey are shown in Table 14. Once the survey is completed, it is a

TABLE 14: Excerpts From the Independent Living Skills Survey
(Wallace 1986)

For each item on this questionnaire the following scales are used.

Scale 1: Frequency of occurrence of behavior

0	1	2	3	4
Never	Sometimes	Often	Usually	Always

Scale 2: Degree of behavioral problem

0	1	2	3	4
Never a problem	Occasionally a problem	Sometimes a problem	Frequently a problem	Always a problem

[Selected items from each of the ILLS domains]

Please score each item in terms of the <u>previous month</u>	1 Occurrence during past	2 Degree of problem
I. <u>Eating</u>		
4. Chews food with mouth closed (without prompting)	_____	_____
II. <u>Grooming</u>		
3. Uses deodorant daily (without prompting)	_____	_____
III. <u>Domestic Activities</u>		
2. Keeps room clean (without prompting)	_____	_____
IV. <u>Health</u>		
10. Can reliably self-administer medication (times and dosages)	_____	_____
V. <u>Money Management</u>		
8. Cashes a pay check or SSI check (without prompting)	_____	_____
VI. <u>Transportation</u>		
9. Acts appropriately on buses, trains, or airplanes (without prompting)	_____	_____
VII. <u>Leisure</u>		
1. Works regularly on a hobby (without prompting)	_____	_____
VIII. <u>Job-seeking</u> or job related skills		
5. Has realistic job aspirations	_____	_____

relatively straightforward process to identify behavioral assets, deficits, and excesses. These may then be prioritized according to their severity (degree of problem) and frequency of occurrence as rehabilitation goals.

Reinforcement Surveys

One type of functional assessment strategy is the reinforcement survey. Identification of reinforcers that can provide motivation for treatment and for maintaining the improved behaviors in the community is an essential step in behavioral assessment. One of the characteristic negative symptoms of schizophrenia is amotivation. To the extent that a patient has few reinforcers or incentives to motivate progress in a program, responsiveness to therapy will be diminished. Psychotropic medications, rationally selected to fit the syndromal diagnosis (for example, neuro-leptic antipsychotic drugs for persons with schizophrenia; lithium or carbamazepine for persons with bipolar disorder) can help to restore the patient's responsivity to the spectrum of reinforcers that were effective in motivating the individual prior to the illness or relapse.

It may be necessary to use tangible reinforcers initially, particularly in a hospital, residential care, or day treatment setting. More naturally occurring reinforcers, such as praise and attention, should be used whenever possible. Reinforcement surveys can be done through interviews, questionnaires, direct behavioral observation, or a combination of all three methods. An excerpt from a reinforcement survey developed by Clement et al. (1971) is shown in Table 15. It can be administered to the patient and/or his or her significant others in questionnaire or interview formats.

Reinforcers can be considered to fall on a hierarchy, depending upon the level of functioning and sophistication of the patient. The hierarchy ranges from primary biological reinforcers to symbolic reinforcers (see Table 16). It is important to note that reinforcers can be found in the patient (such as preferred activities, relief from dysphoric symptoms), in the therapeutic relationship (such as positive feedback from the therapist), in tangible items (such as food, money, tokens), and in the natural environment (such as attention and recognition from family members and friends). Often one must search for effective reinforcers using trial and error over time, since a reinforcer is determined only by virtue of its impact on the behavior of concern. For example, food items would not serve as tangible reinforcers for an anorectic patient, nor would cigarettes for a nonsmoker.

One can identify reinforcers through a variety of methods:

1. Observe the patient's behavior. You may discover behaviors that occur frequently that can be used to reinforce low-frequency behaviors (for example, access to bedroom time can be made contingent upon par-

TABLE 15: Excerpts From the Reinforcement Survey for Adults (Clement et al. 1971)

A. PEOPLE

List below the 10 people with whom you spend the most time each week. Put them in order beginning with the person with whom you spend the most time. In making the list, consider family, relatives, work associates, etc.

1. _____   6. _____

2. _____   7. _____

There may be other people with whom you would like to spend more time each week, but don't get to. List below any such persons with whom you feel you would like to spend more time than you presently get to.

1. _____   4. _____

C. THINGS

List in order the 10 things with which you spend the most time each week. In making the list consider such things as books, hobbies (be specific), projects, musical instruments, etc.

1. _____   6. _____

2. _____   7. _____

List below the things you do not own or to which you do not have ready access which you would most like to have.

1. _____   4. _____

2. _____   5. _____

3. _____   6. _____

List below the 10 foods and drinks which you like best. Include candy, desserts, and other treats in the list. Record the items according to preference beginning with the most preferred. Include items which you may not allow yourself to have or be allowed to have very often, but which fall high on your list of preferences.

TABLE 16:   Reinforcement Hierarchy

Type of Reinforcer	Examples
Primary/biological	Candy, food, cigarettes
Immediate, tangible	Money, tokens
High-frequency behavior	Physical activity, conversation, TV watching
Immediate symbolic or informational feedback	Checkmarks, points, biofeedback
Delayed symbolic	Academic grades, prizes
Social	Approval, attention, sympathy
Self-reinforcement	Positive self-statements
Cognitive	Mastering a challenge

ticipating in occupational therapy, or for a patient who loves to watch television, access to the television might be permitted only after the patient attended a specified number of social and independent living skills training groups each day). The use of high-frequency behaviors to reinforce low-frequency behaviors enables a high degree of individualization in using reinforcers to promote therapeutic change.

2. Ask the patient. Patients' own reports of what foods they consume, which people they spend time with, and which activities they engage in can identify useful reinforcers. Reinforcement surveys or questionnaires can also be administered to identify useful positive reinforcers. The Pleasant Events Schedule (MacPhillamy and Lewinsohn 1982), for example, contains 302 activities, situations, and events about which the patient reports the frequency and pleasure of his or her involvement. It is important to validate any reinforcers identified by patient's self-report by observing their impact on the behavior of concern.

3. Reports by significant others. Relatives can usually identify potentially useful reinforcers in the patient's natural environment.

4. States of deprivation of the patient. Patients who are socially isolated may find interaction with others (including the therapist) highly reinforcing.

Social interaction as a reinforcer nicely illustrates the temporal specificity of positive activities, situations, and events. Many schizophrenic patients shun social interaction initially but come to enjoy and look forward to social interaction with the acquisition of appropriate social skills. Another caution regarding reinforcers concerns the effects of satiation. Eating a small amount of a favorite food item may be reinforcing; however, with increasing amounts of the food item, the patient may become satiated and may no longer respond to its reinforcing properties.

CASE EXAMPLE _____

Reinforcers that could be utilized in Al's treatment program came from two general sources: social and symbolic rewards and more tangible rewards. Once neuroleptic medication had restored Al's responsiveness to reinforcers, nursing staff, the psychiatrist, therapists, and family members were able to use social attention, recognition, and praise to reinforce Al's progress in attaining his treatment goals. For example, therapists liberally praised Al for giving correct answers and responding assertively in the social skills training scenes. Praise was paired with credits to reinforce Al's improvements in self-care and work. Tangible reinforcers, such as Al's favorite beverages and candy, were effective in backing up the value of the credits he received for grooming, showering, dressing, and interacting.

As time went on, Al experienced reinforcement from higher level rewards, such as the feeling of mastery at having successfully engaged a stranger in a 10-minute conversation on the hospital grounds. A high-probability behavior of Al's, his preference for social isolation, was identified as a reinforcer and was used contingently to increase his social involvement. Al was given access to his room for privacy after he first engaged in brief conversations with three different staff members or patients on the unit. This was part of a "contract" which Al negotiated with the unit treatment team as a prerequisite to being promoted to the highest level of autonomy and privileges in the credit system.

The information required for a comprehensive functional assessment of a chronic mental patient comes from interviews of the patient and family; from checklists, questionnaires, and rating forms filled out by the patient, family, and/or service providers; and from direct observations by professional and nursing staff of the patient's problematic and adaptive behavior on the ward, in the home, or in community settings. Using these assessment modes, the clinician can generate relevant information to set treatment and rehabilitation goals, assess progress, and measure outcome.

RESOURCE MANAGEMENT

Once functional and behavioral problems and goals are evaluated and identified, and prior to the formulation of a rehabilitation plan, resources must be organized and inventoried that will enable the patient

---

LEARNING EXERCISE

1. For each of the following types of reinforcers, give two concrete examples that are relevant and appropriate for you. Be specific in your examples and remember that items, people, places, and activities are reinforcers only if they increase, maintain, or strengthen the behavior upon which they are contingent.

   Primary or biological
   Immediate tangible items
   High-frequency behaviors or preferred activities
   Symbolic or informational feedback
   Social rewards
   Self-reinforcement
   Cognitive mastery

2. What is the difference between positive reinforcement and bribery? (Hint—check your dictionary.)

3. Think of a patient whom you know fairly well and describe the types of reinforcers you use or could use to motivate improvements in his or her behavior. Give at least three examples.

4. How might you use high-frequency or preferred activities that you engage in to increase one of your own low-frequency behaviors?

---

and his or her caregivers to achieve the desired rehabilitation outcomes. Resources are time, money, people, places, agencies, materials, transportation, communication media, and other tangible provisions within a community and family that permit goals to be attained. For example, in achieving recreational goals, transportation and money might be required resources to enable an individual to reach and participate in desired leisure time activities. Similarly, achieving well-conceived vocational goals might require the active involvement of a state vocational rehabilitation agency as a resource for funding the costs of a uniform, tools, and transportation to a job training site.

Patients, in collaboration with their treatment and rehabilitation caregivers and their relatives, need to generate resources useful in implementing a rehabilitation plan. Patients may need to be prompted to consider available or required resources. Questions such as, "What are some of the materials you may need to cook for yourself in your own apartment?"; "Which friends or relatives could assist you with transportation to the sheltered workshop until you have earned enough money for bus transport?"; and "Whose telephone could you borrow to make needed appointments at the Recreation Center?" are useful. In Table 6, under Section IV, constructive questions are listed that practitioners must be prepared to answer as part of the process of designing a rehabilitation plan.

CASE EXAMPLE _____

One functional skill that most chronic mental patients must learn is how to effectively negotiate medication issues with psychiatrists and other health-care providers. Once communication skills are learned through role playing, coaching, and reinforcement, resources must be organized to enable the patient to put into practice the acquired negotiation skills. The following procedure is excerpted from a training program on medication self-management. The procedure guides the practitioner serving as group leader through the steps of teaching patients how to manage the resources required to bring their medication side effects and other concerns to the attention of their doctors.

The leader reads the following statement to the patients: "Let's think about what resources we may need to negotiate medication issues with physicians and other health-care professionals. When you think about resources here, I want you to remember that we are talking about people, skills, information, or anything else that will facilitate calling or visiting your physician, and effectively communicating your needs and questions."

The leader then asks the patients two more questions: "What is your goal in this situation?" and "What is the goal of the entire module?". The leader asks the patients to think about what would happen if they wanted to ask their doctor about a problem they were having with their medication. What kinds of things would they need to have in order to negotiate with the doctor? After generating resources needed, the patients identify methods for obtaining each resource. The therapist writes down these resources and methods. The patients are then asked to identify the advantages and disadvantages of each method identified for obtaining the resources.

PLANNING REHABILITATION

Functional assessment procedures are not implemented in a sequentially linear fashion; rather, they are overlapping and should be recurrently administered throughout the course of treatment and rehabilitation. However, many service settings do have formal and regularly scheduled meetings to integrate functional assessment information from all members of the treatment team, and the patient and family as well. Different professional disciplines use this opportunity to provide their input, leading the treatment team to reach a consensus for a rehabilitation plan. The following steps are required in developing a rehabilitation plan:

1. Overall, yet specific, rehabilitation goals for the patient are delineated. For example, a satisfactory goal might be, "Two years from now the patient will be living independently in his own apartment."

2. Long-term (that is, monthly or yearly) and short-term (such as daily or weekly) goals are set. For example, to attain the overall goal of living on his own in his apartment, the patient may need to learn grooming skills; consumer skills, such as shopping for himself on a limited budget; apartment maintenance skills; and medication management skills. These might be considered long-term goals, with the short-term goals being, for example, "to make progress in two of these areas during the next three weeks."

3. Skills to be acquired and resources to be mobilized are prioritized. For example, poor grooming and lack of bathing might preclude participation in groups and social settings designed to help the patient attain the short-term goals identified above. Therefore, acquiring grooming skills might be a high-priority goal. Learning apartment maintenance might be delayed until three to four months before placement is likely.

4. Time lines are set to help the rehabilitation team and the patient realize that progress is expected, does occur, and has definite value and satisfaction. However, it is important to remember that the progress of chronic patients is characterized by stops and starts; rarely is there a smooth learning curve in the acquisition of new skills and competencies.

5. The rehabilitation planning process includes the coordination of agencies and natural support groups. Typically, the case manager or social worker is assigned this coordination function. The case manager keeps track of goals, needs, resources, and progress, and reports back to the rehabilitation team. An example of coordination would be notifying the State Department of Vocational Rehabilitation that a patient will be ready to participate in their program in three weeks, so that an appointment for evaluation can be made. Typically, coordination may also include case advocacy, for example, convincing or lobbying some other agency to accept or provide for the needs of the patient.

6. Treatment and rehabilitation personnel who are to be responsible for the above-listed interventions are identified. Specific personnel are charged with liaison responsibilities to communicate and disseminate information on rehabilitation plans and their modifications over time.

MONITORING PROGRESS OF REHABILITATION

There is no more important component to functional assessment than the ongoing monitoring of a patient's progress through a rehabilitation program. The instruments and modalities of behavioral measurement, described in the sections above, form the wherewithal to carry out continuing assessment of the patient's clinical progress. Repeated assessment—conducted on a daily, weekly, or monthly basis—can be done with behavioral interviewing, direct observation of behavior, self-monitoring of behavior, or checklists and questionnaires.

One of the most convenient ways to monitor progress is through measuring attainment of regularly set goals. In giving patients "homework assignments" to carry out certain behavioral tasks, the completion or noncompletion of the assignment becomes the measure of progress. Information on goal attainment can be used to determine the readiness of a patient for new goals, continued work on current goals, and a new treatment intervention (Austin et al. 1976). The diagram in Figure 7 that shows the empirical approach to treatment and rehabilitation highlights the importance of ongoing assessment of progress in clinical decision making.

CASE EXAMPLE

Al's progress was assessed in a continuing way through methods that were integral to his treatment program. His getting up, dressing, grooming, and bed making were evaluated by the nursing staff, who noted the number of prompts required for his completing these tasks. In social skills training sessions, the counts of errors made to questions assessing his social perception and cognitive processing skills reflected his progress. Ratings made by the therapist in these sessions also monitored Al's improvement in verbal and nonverbal expressiveness. At one point, when he encountered interpersonal scenes in the training of assertion with his parents, his error rate went up and his nonverbal performance deteriorated. This was an indication to his therapists that these situations needed to be broken down into smaller steps and that he required more modeling and positive feedback for his efforts.

Perhaps the most important method of monitoring his progress in the social skills training was his completion of homework assignments. Al had little difficulty completing assignments related to interactions with hospital staff and agency officials in the community. When given assignments to converse with peers, however, he reported several failures to complete the assignment. Again, this was useful information for the therapists, who increased their level of intervention, accompanying Al into the "field" to provide closer prompts and feedback for his peer contacts.

In weekly family therapy sessions, Al and his parents were observed for signs of spontaneously using the communication skills that were taught in the therapy. The leaders looked for manifestations of giving positive feedback to each other for desired actions, making positive requests of each other, and expressing negative feelings directly and non-accusatively. When no signs of spontaneous expression of negative feelings were noted, the therapists prompted the family to practice making statements of their feelings in relation to common problems in the home.

In Figure 10, a Behavioral Progress Record is depicted that can be used in most clinical settings to chart ongoing clinical changes of patients. The attainment of goals in each of up to four dimensions of a rehabilitation plan is checked off in the small box provided at the bottom right corner of each week's record. Long-term or monthly goals are approximated by weekly short-term goals. The method section of the Record provides a small space to jot down the rehabilitation interventions being used to achieve the goal for that week. The Behavioral Progress Record shown in Figure 10 is filled out with monitoring data from the case of Al.

SUMMARY

The assessment of the symptoms of severe and chronic mental disorders, described in Chapter 2, leads to a reliable diagnosis, which is the necessary first step in the treatment and rehabilitation of the chronic mental patient. An appropriate diagnosis leads to the selection of the appropriate drug treatment for the patient's disorder. The selection and appropriate use of psychopharmacological treatments to address the patient's impairment are described in Chapter 4. Supplementing the assessment of symptoms is the functional assessment, which is also a prerequisite in the provision of appropriate services to the severely psychiatrically disabled. Functional assessment assists in the identification of behavioral assets, excesses, and deficits that help or hinder performance in social and occupational roles. As was noted in this chapter, treatment and rehabilitation of the chronic mental patient should begin with an accurate inventory of a patient's capacities, that is, what he or she has been able to do in every-day life and what he or she is currently doing.

In this chapter we examined a variety of case examples and learning exercises regarding the use of functional assessment to identify treatment needs, determine rehabilitation goals, and monitor the progress and outcome of rehabilitation efforts (such as the skill-building approaches in social skills training, family management, and vocational rehabilitation described in Chapters 5, 6, and 7).

A general framework for functional assessment operationalizes problems in behavioral terms, using as dimensions the frequency, in-

Behavioral Progress Record

Name __A/__   Admission Date __10/17/86__

Long-Term Goals

Goal:	Arise, dress & groom	Tension reduced	Develop one new	Successful weekend
Expected Date:	independently	to "a little"	peer acquaintence	home visit
	11/10/86	11/16/86	11/16/86	11/16/86

Sub-Goals

Week of 10/26	Goal:	Up & groom with manual guidance from nurses	Tension below "very much"	Increase voice volume	Attend family education group
	Method:	Prompt, guide & praise compliance ✓	Neuroleptic drug titration, milieu therapy	Coaching during recreational therapy ✓	Praise for attending session ✓
Week of 11/2	Goal:	Up & groom with verbal prompts from nurses	Tension below "very much"	Converse with nurses once daily	Actively participate in family education
	Method:	Verbal prompts, Praise compliance, ignore Al's negativeness ✓	Same ✓	Social Skills Training ✓	Prompt and reinforce speaking up ✓
Week of 11/9	Goal:	Up & groom with no more than 1 verbal prompt	Tension below "pretty much"	Exchange info about selves with another patient	Participate in family communication skills
	Method:	Verbal prompt & Time to get dressed & groom, Use grooming checklist to rate ✓	Same ✓	Social Skills Training ✓	Behavioral rehearsal modeling and coaching ✓
Week of 11/16	Goal:	Up & groom without verbal prompt Self-monitoring of grooming	Tension at or below "a little"	Invite a patient to canteen for coffee	Make a "positive request" of parents
	Method:	Al will use grooming checklist & present himself for inspection prior to 0800 ✓	Same ✓	Prompt & reinforce on ward ✓	Coaching & feedback ✓

Notes: _____
_____
_____

FIGURE 10: The Behavioral Progress Record is used to monitor the progress of patients through the goal-setting steps of psychiatric rehabilitation. For Al, monthly goals were set in the domains of self-care skills, social interactions, tension and anxiety, and family relations. Each week, a subgoal was established with Al's collaboration that would serve as approximations to the longer term monthly goal in each of the four domains of functioning. The responsible therapist or clinician indicated the intervention method that was to be used to achieve the subgoal during the coming week. When a subgoal was attained, the clinician placed a checkmark in the relevant box. The Behavioral Progress Record enables the rehabilitation practitioner or therapist to track progress and make informed decisions on pacing treatment and on choice of interventions.

tensity, duration, latency, and form or quality of the patient's actions and verbalizations. This framework uses a multimodal approach in which all levels of human behavioral expression and subjective experience are examined in a comprehensive manner, with attention provided to the reliability, validity, and utility of the assessment process. Multimodal dimensions include thought and affect, social-interpersonal skills, and independent living skills. Intervention targets are defined in terms of behavioral deficits, excesses, and assets in order to define and prioritize goals for intervention.

Once the presenting problems are clearly defined, the assessment process focuses on the identification of biological and environmental determinants of the problems. The process of gathering information on the environmental conditions that typically occur before the problematic behavior and the consequences that tend to follow it is called functional analysis. A functional analysis specifies the antecedents and consequences of problem behaviors in the patient's present and past environments that contribute to the initiation and maintenance of the multimodal pattern of behavioral problems.

A variety of methods and instruments exist for use by the clinician to gather functional assessment information. Behavioral interviewing provides one method of assessment. A second method for functional assessment is the direct observation of behavior. Self-observation approaches provide a third method of obtaining a reliable picture of the frequency and context of the patient's problems. A fourth method of functional assessment involves the use of paper-and-pencil checklists, questionnaires, and rating forms that are related to specific skills and competencies. Methods must be in place to monitor and evaluate the ongoing progress of a patient through a rehabilitation program. Information gained from regular and periodic reassessments can be used to make clinical decisions about goals, interventions, and pacing of rehabilitation.

REFERENCES

American Psychiatric Association: Diagnostic and Statistical Manual of Mental Disorders (Third Edition). Washington, DC, American Psychiatric Association, 1980

Austin NK, Liberman RP, King LW, et al: A comparative evaluation of two day hospitals: goal attainment scaling in behavior therapy vs. milieu therapy. J Nerv Ment Dis 163:253–261 1976

Baker R, Hall JN: Rehabilitation Evaluation of Hall And Baker (REHAB). Aberdeen, Scotland, Vine Publishing, 1983

Brown M, Gordon WA, Diller L: Functional assessment and outcome measurement: an integrative review, in Annual Review of Rehabilitation. Edited by Pan EL, Backer TE, Vash CL. New York, Springer-Verlag, 1983

Burnes AJ, Roen SR: Social roles and adaptation to the community. Community Ment Health J 3:153–158 1967

Cautela JR: Behavior Analysis Forms for Clinical Intervention. Champaign, IL, Research Press, 1977

Ciarlo J, Riehman J: The Denver Community Mental Health Questionnaire: development of a multidimensional program evaluation, in Program Evaluation for Mental Health: Methods, Strategies, and Participants. Edited by Coursey RD, Spector GA, Murrel SA, et al. New York, Grune and Stratton, 1977

Clement PW, Richard RC, Hess AP: Reinforcement Survey for Adults. Pasadena, CA, Fuller Graduate School of Psychology, 1971

Ellsworth RB, Foster L, Childers B, et al: Hospital and community adjustment as perceived by psychiatric patients, their families, and staff. J Consult Clin Psychol 32:1–41 1968

Endicott J, Spitzer RL: What! Another rating scale? The psychiatric evaluation form. J Nerve and Ment Dis 154:88–104 1972a

Endicott J, Spitzer RL: Current and Past Psychopathology Scales (CAPPS): Rationale, reliability, and validity. Arch Gen Psychiatry 27:678–687 1972b

Goldstein MJ: Premorbid adjustment, paranoid status, and pattern of response to phenothiazines in acute schizophrenia. Schizophr Bull 1:24–37 1970

Guy W: ECDEU: Assessment Manual for Psychopharmacology, Rockwell, MD, U. S. Dept. of Health, Education, and Welfare, revised 1976

Harding CM, Strauss JS: The Course of Schizophrenia: An Evolving Concept, in Controversies in Schizophrenia. Edited by Alpert M. New York, Guilford 1985, pp 339–350

Harding CM, Brooks GW, Ashikaga T, et al: The Vermont Longitudinal Study of persons with severe mental illness: II. Long-term outcome of subjects who retrospectively met DSM–III criteria for schizophrenia. Am J Psychiatry 144: 727–735 1987

Harris JG: An abbreviated form of the Phillips rating scale of premorbid adjustment in schizophrenia. J Abnormal Psychology 84:129–137 1975

Harrow M, Grinker RR, Silverstein ML, Holtzman P: Is modern-day schizophrenia outcome still negative? Am J Psychiatry 135:1156–1162 1978

Hersen M, Belleck AS (Eds): Behavioral Assessment: A Practical Handbook, New York, Pergamon Press 1981

Katz MM, Lyerly SB: Methods for measuring adjustment and social behavior in the community: I. Rationale, description, discriminative validity and scale development. Psychological Reports 13:502–535

Keller MB, Shapiro RW: "Double depression" superimposition of acute depressive episodes on chronic depressive disorders. Am J Psychiatry 139:438–442 1982

Liberman RP, King LW, DeRisi WJ, McCann M: Personal Effectiveness: Guiding People to Assert Themselves and Improve Their Social Skills. Champaign, IL, Research Press 1975

MacPhillamy DJ, Lewinsohn PM: The pleasant events schedule. Studies of reliability, validity, and scale intercorrelation. J of Consulting & Clinical Psychology 50:363–380 1982

Overall J, Gorham D: The Brief Psychiatric Rating Scale. Psychol Rep 10:799–812, 1962

Paul GL, Lentz RJ: Psychosocial Treatment of Mental Patients. Cambridge, MA, Harvard University Press 1977

Platt S, Weyman A, Hirsch S, Hewett S: The Social Behavior Assessment Schedule (SBAS): Rationale, contents, scoring, and reliability of a new interview schedule. Social Psychiatry 15:43–55 1980

Power CJ: The time-sample behavioral checklist: observational assessment of patient functioning. J of Beh Assessment 1:199–210 1979

Serrban G: Social Stress and Functioning Inventory for Psychotic Disorders (SSFIPD): Measurement and prediction of schizophrenics' community adjustment. Comprehensive Psychiatry 19:337–347 1978

Spitzer RL, Endicott J, Fleiss JL, Cohen J: The Psychiatric Status Schedule: A technique for evaluating psychopathology and impairment in role functioning. Arch Gen Psychiatry 23: 41–55 1970

VanPutten T, May PRA, Marder SR, Wittman LA: Subjective response to antipsychotic drugs. Arch Gen Psychiatry 38:187–190 1981

Wallace CJ: Functional assessment in rehabilitation. Schizophrenia Bulletin (In press 1986)

Weissman MM, Paykel ES, Siegal R, Klerman GL: The social role performance of depressed women: comparisons with a normal group. Am J of Orthopsychiatry 41:390–405 1971

Wolpe J, Lang PJ: A fear survey schedule for use in behavior therapy. Behavior Research and Therapy 2:27–30 1964

CHAPTER 4

PRACTICAL PSYCHO-PHARMACOLOGY

BYRON J. WITTLIN, M.D.

*Use new drugs while
they still continue to act.*
Ancient Egyptian physician

While there are no known ways to directly alter the neurobiological vulnerability to schizophrenia, there is empirical evidence that antipsychotic drugs buffer patients' vulnerability to relapse. Antipsychotic drugs certainly reduce symptoms, caused or exacerbated by the superimposition of life stressors or poor coping ability on underlying psychobiological vulnerability. From the viewpoint of the stress-vulnerability-coping-competence model, then, antipsychotic drugs may be seen as conferring protection against the combined noxious effects of stress and vulnerability.

This chapter is a practical guide to the use of medications with the chronic mental patient. Although not meant to be a comprehensive text, it will cover significant points in the appropriate use and specific application of psychiatric drugs, specifically, antipsychotics. An overview will be given on the effects of antipsychotics—both desirable and undesirable—and practical tips on maximizing compliance while utilizing minimal effective dosages. Guidelines will be offered for use of specific medications to achieve therapeutic effects, use of drugs to treat side effects, and the importance of individualizing drug treatment to the patient. Approaches to patient and family education about medication will also be outlined.

RATIONALE—WHY MEDICATIONS?

Since the introduction of the antipsychotic chlorpromazine (Thorazine) in 1954, psychotropic medications have become the mainstay of treatment for schizophrenia and other psychiatric illnesses. They have helped enable the vast reduction of our inpatient state hospital population from approximately 550,000 in 1955 to under 200,000 today. Many people who might otherwise be in long-term psychiatric facilities are now functioning members of their communities, families, and workplaces, in part because of the beneficial effects of medication.

Many studies have documented the efficacy of antipsychotics in the treatment of schizophrenia and lithium and antidepressants in the treatment of affective disorders (Schatzberg and Cole 1986). Neuroleptics, as antipsychotics are also called, have proved effective as both acute treatment of psychotic symptoms and prophylaxis for relapse. For example, maintenance antipsychotic drugs reduce relapse rates during the first year after an acute episode from 70 percent to about 30 percent. Similarly, lithium has been effective in reducing the severity of, and in the prevention of, manic episodes in 70 to 80 percent of patients with bipolar disorders.

Some new areas of research question old assumptions about our approaches to initial treatment and maintenance therapy of schizophrenia. For example, "rapid neuroleptization"—rapidly repeating administrations of high-potency antipsychotic agents over a few hours until symptoms are controlled—has been shown to be safe and effective. However, there is now question whether these commonly used high doses produce better symptom reduction and control than do more modest and conservative medication doses. Recent studies suggest that many schizophrenic patients can benefit from much lower doses of maintenance medication—one fifth to one tenth of a "usual dose"—than was thought possible (Kane 1983; Marder et al. 1984). This has implications for reducing the risk of tardive dyskinesia, which afflicts 15 to 25 percent of patients who have taken antipsychotic medications (Baldessarini 1980). Since the incidence of tardive dyskinesia is thought to be proportional to a person's total lifetime exposure to neuroleptics, lower dose drug strategies have major advantages. Another approach that reduces a patient's overall exposure to neuroleptics is intermittent targeted use, in which drugs are used only during times of increased stress, decreased social support, or signs of impending exacerbation (Herz and Szymanski 1982).

I will discuss these new approaches as well as the standard methods developed over the last 30 years of medication use. They are important in overall treatment and community maintenance of the chronic mental patient. When prescribed and supervised by a psychiatrist for clearly documented disorders and taken reliably by a patient, psychotropics can help improve problems and symptoms in

thinking
feeling
socializing
working and playing
caring for self.

The usefulness, specific actions, and unwanted side effects of these medications must be thoroughly understood by the individuals who are taking them and by their families.

Several types of drugs are used in psychiatry, and each type is aimed at specific illnesses or problems (see Table 17). Because the majority of chronic mental patients suffer from schizophrenia, I will focus on the antipsychotic (or neuroleptic) drugs used to help treat the problems and symptoms of this disorder. The beneficial and therapeutic effects of neuroleptics will be described as well as the unpleasant side effects. Information will be given on choosing the best drug and dose for a person suffering from schizophrenia and on minimizing side effects. Regarding psychotropics in general, a drug that is helpful to a person suffering from one kind of illness or disturbance is usually not helpful to a person suffering from a different kind of illness. It is important to understand that a neuroleptic drug, such as haloperidol, might reduce

TABLE 17: Types of Psychiatric Drugs

Type of Drug	Generic Name (Trade Name)	Specific Use
Neuroleptics or antipsychotics	Chlorpromazine (Thorazine) Haloperidol (Haldol) Thioridazine (Mellaril) Trifluoperazine (Stelazine) Fluphenazine (Prolixin)	Schizophrenia Mania or "highs" in bipolar disorders, major depressive episodes with psychosis, and organic psychotic states
Mood stabilizers	Lithium Carbamazepine (Tegretol)	Bipolar disorders, depression
Antidepressants	Imipramine (Tofranil) Amitriptyline (Elavil) Doxepin (Sinequan) Desipramine (Norpramin, Desyrel) Chlordiazepoxide (Librium)	Moderate to severe depression Anxiety
Minor tranquilizers	Diazepam (Valium) Oxazepam (Serax) Lorazepam (Ativan) Phenobarbital	
Sedative-hypnotics	Seconal, Nembutal, Dalmane, Hydrate, Restoril, Chloral, Halcion	Insomnia
Stimulants	Amphetamines (Dexedrine) Methylphenidate (Ritalin)	Attention deficit disorder (childhood hyperactivity); narcolepsy

anxiety in a person suffering from schizophrenia but may have little effect and serious adverse effects in a person with a phobia.

THE ANTIPSYCHOTICS

Antipsychotics are useful specifically for the characteristic symptoms of schizophrenia. They come from five separate families of chemicals, but all share the same beneficial or therapeutic effects. There is no difference in the efficacy or therapeutic effects of one type of antipsychotic versus another. However, each drug has special side effects, and the choice of a neuroleptic drug is often made on the basis of producing the least bothersome side effects for the individual. Table 18 lists most of the currently available neuroleptics.

THERAPEUTIC EFFECTS OF ANTIPSYCHOTIC DRUGS

Antipsychotics relieve, reduce, and in many cases eliminate the symptoms of schizophrenia. These drugs are also effective in preventing relapse.

TABLE 18: Currently Available Antipsychotics

Class	Generic Name	Trade Name	Equivalent Dose (mg)	Recommended Daily Dose Range (mg)
Phenothiazine/ aliphates	Chlorpromazine	Thorazine	100	50–2000
Pipridines	Thioridazine	Mellaril	100	50–800
	Mesoridazine	Ferentil	50	25–400
	Piperacetazine	Quide	10	10–160
Piperazines	Prochlorperazine	Compazine	10	5–150
	Perphenazine	Trilafen	8	4–80
	Trifluoperazine	Stelazine	5	2–60
	Fluphenazine	Prolixin, Permitil	2	2–80
Thioxanthenes	Chlorprothixene	Taractan	25	10–600
	Thiothixene	Navane	4	2–80
Butyrophenones	Haloperidol	Haldol	2	1–100
	Droperidol*	Inapsine	2	**
	Loxapine	Loxitane	10	10–250
Lihydroindo-lones	Molindone	Moban	10	10–225

*IM only.
**Not recommended for regular or maintenance use.

As noted previously, symptoms return in 65 to 70 percent of schizophrenic patients within one year of stopping medication. There is a relapse rate of 5 to 10 percent per month for those patients not taking maintenance antipsychotic medication (Donaldson et al. 1983). This can be reduced to a 30 percent relapse rate for an entire year through continuing maintenance use of medication. It may be necessary to continue using the medication, though possibly at a reduced dose or frequency, for many years or a lifetime. For some patients the medication is necessary indefinitely, like insulin for a diabetic or thyroid replacement for a person with Graves's disease, to control symptoms, prevent relapse, and facilitate social and occupational functioning.

Antipsychotic medications are most effective in reducing the "positive" symptoms of schizophrenia, or those which can be detected by their obvious presence. They are less effective in helping the "negative" symptoms, or an absence or deficiency of adaptive and functional behaviors (see Table 19). It is also important to remember that medication is not a complete treatment program by itself. Medication reduces or eliminates symptoms. It facilitates cognitive functions and improves the patient's ability to learn from his treatment environment. It enables the patient to acquire new skills and utilize other forms of therapy (Liberman et al. 1984). Medication cannot teach a patient how to make and keep friends, get a job, or live in the community. Other forms of rehabilitation, such as behavior therapy, psychotherapy, and family and social therapy (see Chapters 5 through 8 for descriptions of these therapies in the context of our model for psychiatric rehabilitation), are necessary in combination with medication to produce the best results.

TABLE 19: Symptoms of Schizophrenia

Positive Symptoms	Negative Symptoms
Hyperactivity	Apathy, disinterest
Agitation, pacing	Depressed mood
Aggressiveness, hostility	Social withdrawal and isolation
Delusions	Poverty of speech
Anxiety	Motor retardation
Somatic complaints	Anhedonia
Hallucinations	Intellectual impairments
Cognitive disorganization (poor concentration, loose associations, nonsensical talk)	Poor grooming and self-care
Suspiciousness	

CASE EXAMPLE ———————————————————————————————

Joe was admitted to the hospital dirty, disheveled, and worried that the police had "bugged" his house and planned to harm him. He had spent the last month isolated in his room, refusing to go outside. Six days after initiation of antipsychotic medication, he no longer feared the police and decided that he had been having "crazy ideas." After two more weeks of medication and hospital therapy, Joe's delusions had not reappeared, but he continued to need constant encouragement and reinforcement from staff to bathe, wash his clothes, and participate in activities. When left alone, he preferred to lie down in bed, avoiding other patients and staff. These negative symptoms continued for the remainder of his hospital stay.

SIDE EFFECTS OF NEUROLEPTIC MEDICATIONS

Side effects are the most significant cause of poor compliance with antipsychotic medications. As shown in Table 20, side effect profiles of low- and high-potency medications tend to be complementary: High-potency drugs are associated mainly with extrapyramidal neuromuscular side effects, while low-potency drugs are plagued by sedative side effects. The most common side effects of antipsychotic drugs are

Tardive dyskinesia
Hypotension
Extrapyramidal symptoms

Sedation
Endocrine effects
Anticholinergic symptoms

or THE SEA.

TABLE 20: Incidence of Extrapyramidal Symptoms and Anticholinergic Effects of Commonly Used Antipsychotics

Generic Name	Trade Name	Extrapyramidal (Motor Activity)	Anticholinergic (Sedation)
Thioridazine	Mellaril	+	+ + + +
Chlorpromazine	Thorazine	+	+ + + +
Loxapine	Loxitane	+ + +	+ +
Trifluoperazine	Stelazine	+ + +	+ +
Perphenazine	Trilafen	+ + +	+ +
Fluphenazine	Prolixin	+ + + +	+
Thiothixene	Oavane	+ + + +	+
Haloperidol	Haldol	+ + + +	+

Tardive Dyskinesia

This group of abnormal involuntary movements is thought to be proportional to total lifetime exposure to the dopamine-blocking actions of neuroleptics. Patients who have had prior exposure to electroconvulsive therapy, who have been treated with lithium, who are older, and who have had a higher maximum dose have been shown in some studies to be at slightly higher risk (Baldessarini 1985). The abnormal muscle movements are usually buccal-lingual but also include waving of fingers or toes, and even truncal and diaphragmatic movements. The symptoms can often be masked by increasing the dose of neuroleptic medication, but may break through.

Although the actual prevalence rate of tardive dyskinesia is the subject of some disagreement, few would argue with a figure of 15 to 20 percent of those now receiving antipsychotic medication. In the only prospective study of tardive dyskinesia, the incidence of the syndrome was reported to be 12 percent after four years of cumulative neuroleptic exposure (Kane et al. 1982). These movements may be very apparent to the doctor, relatives, and friends, yet not be perceived by the patient. Most patients with tardive dyskinesia have mild or minimal movements and are unaware of their presence.

Treatment of tardive dyskinesia is a difficult and evolving issue (Jeste and Wyatt 1982). There is increasing evidence that it abates or subsides over time even with continued exposure to neuroleptics. Some schizophrenic disorders may manifest abnormal movements as part of the natural history of the illness. Such unusual movements or gesturing was described in 19th century psychiatric texts long before the advent of neuroleptic treatment. Thus mild, nonintrusive dyskinesias that do not interfere with a patient's psychosocial functioning may be best documented and then monitored by the treating physician.

There are no currently effective antidotes or preventives for tardive dyskinesia. The literature has many reports of failed treatment with various medications. Two approaches have helped reduce the movements. Biofeedback can reduce the severity of the involuntary movements by promoting the patient's awareness of the movements through visual or other cues.

Medication reduction or cessation may reduce the severity of the movements, often after an initial exacerbation or unmasking of the movements. Reduction of medication to the lowest effective dose is always desirable. Absolute discontinuation of medication exposes the patient and his or her relatives and social support system to the risk of an exacerbation of the illness. Such a decision requires careful weighing of risks and benefits of the tardive dyskinesia vis-à-vis neuroleptic medication. The physician, patient, and relatives should conjointly consider these factors before a decision to discontinue medications is made. In general, only dyskinesias that are severe enough to interfere with social and self-care functioning require absolute discontinuation of antipsychotic medications. If an individual is the sole wage earner in the family and his employability would be more threatened by a relapse of symptoms of schizophrenia than by tardive dyskinesia, then maintaining the neuroleptic therapy may be indicated, even in the face of mild to moderate dyskinesias.

Hypotension

More commonly associated with high-dose, low-potency agents (for example, chlorpromazine, thioridazine), this side effect is seen less often now because of increased use of low-dose, high-potency drugs. Hypotension can lead to fatigue, loss of balance, and potential injury from falls, especially in older patients. Concurrent use of alcohol, sedative-hypnotics, or sedating street drugs can potentiate the risk of hypotension.

Extrapyramidal Symptoms

A direct result of blocking dopamine receptors in the nigro-striatum subcortical part of the brain, the area affected in Parkinson's disease, extrapyramidal neuromuscular symptoms are produced to varying degrees by neuroleptics. These symptoms are tremor of hands or arms, rigidity of extremities, akinesia (lack of motivation, listlessness, lack of spontaneous movements), akathisia (internal restlessness—"I have a motor running inside me"—or restless movements of legs), and dystonic reactions.

Reported prevalence rates of extrapyramidal symptoms are from 23 to 88 percent, clustering around 40 percent (Johnson 1984). Dystonic reactions, commonly occurring in young patients during the first week of drug therapy, consist of spasms in muscles controlled by the cranial nerves. They occur in the neck, throat, or tongue. Spasm of the extra-ocular muscles is known as an occlo-gyric crisis. Dystonic reactions are frightening to both patient and relatives and can be both painful and life threatening. Fortunately, they can be readily aborted by injections of antidotes such as antihistamines or anti-Parkinson drugs.

Sedation

Often this side effect can be a useful therapeutic effect in the hyperactive, agitated, or manic patient, or the patient with insomnia. It becomes a problem when it interferes with cognitive and social functioning, as is the case with patients who drive or work in proximity to machinery. Fortunately, sedation often decreases as the patient adapts to the medication. The newer high-potency, low-dose medications tend to be less sedating, but they can still cause significant psychomotor slowing if not used judiciously. In many cases, administration of most or all antipsychotic medication at bedtime can relieve or lessen daytime sedation.

Endocrine Disturbances

These include decreased erections, delayed or absent ejaculation, anorgasmia, menstrual irregularities, galactorrhea, weight gain, and appetite increase.

Patients may be reluctant to tell you about these effects, especially sexual dysfunctions. Yet this can be particularly distressing, especially for younger (teenage) patients, for whom appearance and bodily function have special importance and mystery. It is important to ask about these effects and reassure your patients that these symptoms are often transient and are certainly reversible by changing the type or dose of antipsychotic drug. These side effects are among the most common reasons for noncompliance. Although they occur with all antipsychotics, they are most often associated with the aliphatic, piperidine and piperazine phenothiazine.

CASE EXAMPLE _____

Donna, age 17, seemed suddenly more agitated and worried during her session with her physician. Ten days earlier she had been hospitalized with anxiety, disorganization, and hallucinations after smoking phencyclidine (PCP) at a party. With antipsychotic medication and supportive therapy she had greatly improved, until today. Now she again appeared disorganized, insisting that she had a newborn child, clearly a delusion. After careful questions, Donna told her physician that she was having breast soreness and galactorrhea. Donna responded to reassurance, factual information about side effects, and a reduction in dosage of her medication.

Anticholinergic Symptoms

Anticholinergic symptoms include dry mouth, blurred vision, constipation, nausea, urinary retention or reduced force of urine stream, and memory disturbance. They are most often associated with high-dose, low-potency medications. They can be exacerbated by use of anti-Parkinson agents, such as benztropine mesylate (Cogentin) and triexyphenidyl hydrochloride (Artane).

Other less common side effects include skin rash, skin photosensitivity (chlorpromazine), retrograde ejaculation (which can be very disturbing to the male patient who may think he is "dried up"—associated with thioridazine), blood dyscrasias, and jaundice.

Coping With Side Effects

The sedative, anticholinergic, hypotensive, and even some endocrine side effects tend to appear after days or weeks on neuroleptic medication as the body adjusts and compensates. Advising the patient to "stick with it," with reassurance about the temporary nature of these side effects, may be all that is necessary.

For extrapyramidal symptoms, the so-called anti-Parkinson agents can be used either orally or by intramuscular injection, as in the case of dystonic reactions or severe akathisia. These antidote drugs are listed in Table 21.

There has been debate over prophylactic use of anti-Parkinson agents with antipsychotics. Always prescribing an anti-Parkinson agent with an antipsychotic will help prevent onset of these distressing symptoms, and therefore increase compliance. However, not all patients have these side effects, and waiting for onset of symptoms may save some patients from taking an unnecessary medication that also has its own hazards. Although this decision is best left for the practitioner, the high frequency of these uncomfortable (and even frightening) side effects, as well as the relative safety of the anti-Parkinson agents, favors prophylactic use. Although anti-Parkinson drugs are frequently prescribed for extrapyramidal side effects, in over half of patients who experience extrapyramidal symptoms, reduction of the neuroleptic dose results in disappearance of these side effects without loss of therapeutic control (Johnson 1984).

Two other methods to reduce or eliminate side effects are a) reduction of medication dose and b) switching to another drug that doesn't have the same side effect. For instance, switching from a low-dose, high-potency agent to a high-dose, low-potency agent can reduce or eliminate extrapyramidal symptoms in many patients (but possibly at the price of other side effects).

Patients can learn to cope with or prevent most minor side effects. For example, mild photosensitivity will respond to use of sunscreens,

TABLE 21: Anti-Parkinson Drugs Used in Treating Extrapyramidal Symptoms

Type	Generic Name	Trade Name	Usual Daily Dose (mg)
Anticholinergic agents	Benztropine	Cogentin	2–8
	Biperiden	Akineton	2–6
	Procyclidine	Kemadrin	7.5–20.00
	Trihexyphenidyl	Artane	2–16
Dopamine agonist	Amantadine	Symmetrel	200–300

visors, and avoidance of sun exposure. Patients with dry mouth or mild constipation, from cholinergic inhibition, can be instructed to increase fluid intake, use sugarless gum or hard candies, increase physical exercise, and add bulk to their diet. Educational programs and medication management groups are appropriate avenues to provide this information. In the learning exercise below, you can apply an educational approach to improving your patient's understanding of and coping with side effects.

More troublesome and potentially disabling side effects, such as tremors, dystonias, excessive sedation, or severe constipation, require intervention by the prescribing physician. Patients should be encouraged to seek medical attention for these problems.

LEARNING EXERCISE

Interview a patient you are seeing who is receiving medication. Ask him or her to select three side effects that he or she has experienced. Suggest common side effects associated with the medications the patient is taking if he or she is unable to identify three. Ask the patient to identify the steps to take to alleviate each one and to explain how these steps would be implemented.

GETTING THE BEST DOSE OF THE NEUROLEPTIC

Whenever possible, a period of drug-free evaluation and careful rediagnosis and assessment should precede treatment with antipsychotic drugs. This helps the doctor to confirm the diagnosis of schizophrenia and to fully observe the patient without drugs.

When starting an antipsychotic drug, it should be realized that its actions and effects take time. The drug must be absorbed from the stomach, transported through the bloodstream, cross the blood-brain barrier, and reach the neurons in the brain. This obviously takes time, sometimes as much as two to four weeks to achieve therapeutic effects. Individual differences in drug absorption, transportation, elimination, body weight, and metabolism lead to great individual variation in dose, onset of action, and ultimate efficacy. In fact, recent evidence indicates that when injectable long-acting neuroleptics are administered, steady-state levels of the drug in the blood stream are not reached for as long as 6 to 9 months after initiation of treatment.

Individuals vary in how they absorb and metabolize neuroleptic medication because of differences in cellular physiology and body storage. Some people use up the drug more quickly and therefore need higher doses than other people. The same dose of a drug may produce a thousandfold difference in blood levels of that drug in two different people. This means that *the best dose must be carefully tailored to each individual's needs.* An occasional patient may need huge doses of a medication—for example, up to 300 mg fluphenazine or 10,000 mg chlorpromazine daily—to get the same beneficial effects as another patient who does well with very small doses of the same drug.

During the first two weeks of treatment, it may help to give oral neuroleptic medication several times a day, particularly if the patient is severely psychotic and behaviorally out of control. However, within two to three weeks on oral neuroleptic therapy, stabilization begins and the entire daily dose can be given in a single bedtime dose. There are three advantages to giving the entire daily dose once at bedtime:

First, some of the drug is kept in storage in the body and is slowly released during a 24-hour period to keep a relatively constant blood level whether the drug is given once a day or several times a day. Though the blood level may drop somewhat during the hours after a single dose, the antipsychotic therapeutic effect remains intact for many days and weeks because of the slow metabolism of these drugs.

Second, side effects, like drowsiness, can be maximal while the patient is sleeping and thus not be so bothersome.

Third, the patient is less likely to forget to take the drug if it only has to be taken once a day and is kept in a single place in the home.

A usually reliable sign that a person is getting too much medication is excessive sedation. If the person is becoming drowsy or falling asleep during the day, despite an adequate number of hours of sleep at night, then the dose might be lowered.

The only way to arrive at the best or optimal dose is by gradually increasing the dose until no further improvement occurs. When the patient reaches a plateau and stops showing any further signs of improvement in psychopathology in spite of increasing the dose, the optimal level has been achieved. Methods for determining psychopathology in titrating neuroleptic dose are given in Chapter 2. The use of repeated administrations of the Brief Psychiatric Rating Scale can sensitively reveal optimal drug effects on the psychotic and other symptoms of schizophrenia.

The best way of determining the optimal dose level is to increase the dose of the drug only when the patient has stopped showing signs of improvement at the previous dosage level. This may mean leaving the dose at a relatively low level for many weeks. In fact, a surprisingly large number of patients never need an increase (and can even do well with a decrease) from the initial low dose level. They continue to improve until psychotic symptoms are gone or greatly decreased. This is a change from the previous practice of aggressively increasing the dose of medication to quickly eradicate symptoms. Rapid dose increases do not alleviate symptoms more quickly and may predispose patients to more side effects.

Insomnia and agitation are often the first symptoms to show improvement with antipsychotic drug treatment. Insomnia is also often the earliest warning signal that a relapse is about to occur. The patient, relatives, and the doctor together should collaborate on finding the right dose. The patient knows best how he or she feels and thinks; relatives are in an excellent position to observe changes in behavior; and the doctor knows best how the patient looks, sounds, and acts.

It usually takes four to six weeks at the maximal dose range with a particular drug before a doctor and patient can conclude that the drug has received a fair trial. Doctor and patient should not switch to a different drug unless they have tried a four- to six-week period at the highest dose possible without having intolerable side effects.

About 20 percent of patients with schizophrenia are refractory to treatment with antipsychotics in spite of trials with various medications at various dosages. They respond only in limited ways and persist in experiencing major symptoms of the disorder. It may be harmful to expose these patients to potential short- and long-term side effects in the hope of illusory improvement (Gardos and Cole 1976). Avoiding irrational high doses, providing a trial of low-dose neuroleptic therapy, limiting side effect hazards, and considering alternate pharmacologic approaches are important principles to adhere to. Some new drugs, when used in combination with neuroleptics, have been found to help individuals who are limited responders to neuroleptics alone. These drugs include lithium, carbamazepine, reserpine, clonidine propranolol, naltrexone, and benzodiazepine tranquilizers.

Drugs in the antipsychotic class have different potencies, as is evident in Table 18. This means that 2 mg of haloperidol or fluphenazine have approximately the same effectiveness as 100 mg of chlorpromazine or thioridazine. However, in the best or optimal dose range for each, they all have the same therapeutic effectiveness. There is no reason to prefer high-potency to low-potency drugs unless very high dosage treatment is required or the side effect profile is more favorable. In that case, the doctor would usually choose the high-potency drug for the sake of convenience.

The dose of antipsychotic medication needed by a person for optimal response varies with the stress and stimulation in his or her life. If a person is moving to a new home, leaving the hospital to live in the community, starting a new job, getting married, or living and working in a more crowded or active environment, then the need for a larger amount of medication may develop. It is important to be flexible in increasing and decreasing the dose as changes occur in the patient's life.

Guidelines for instituting neuroleptic therapy for antipsychotic effects are given in Table 22.

The best guideline in finding the optimal dose of an antipsychotic drug is to use the lowest dose that still produces the maximum amount of improvement in thinking, feeling, socializing, work and play, and self-care. Using a dose that is high enough to produce maximum benefit but low enough to minimize side effects requires close contact, trust, and mutual working together by the patient, the doctor, and the family.

TABLE 22:   Guidelines for Instituting Antipsychotic Drug Therapy

1. Whenever possible, a period of drug-free evaluation and careful diagnosis should precede treatment.
2. Most acute schizophreniform illnesses should be treated with antipsychotics.
3. Adequate sedation and control of even acutely agitated patients can be achieved with any antipsychotic medication. All antipsychotic medications are equally effective in equivalent doses.
4. In general, high-potency drugs are to be preferred. At adequate antipsychotic doses, their side effects are less problematic than those of low-potency drugs.
5. In an acutely psychotic patient, underdosing is a more serious error than excessive dosing. However, the lowest effective medication dose is always the goal.
6. Individuals have been shown to vary widely in their drug absorption, distribution, and metabolism patterns. Adequate doses for some patients will therefore be too little or too much for a significant number of other patients.
7. An adequate antipsychotic drug trial can be considered to be four to six weeks of a single drug at or near maximal dose range.
8. Polypharmacy has not been shown to be more effective than single drug treatment and carries increased risks. The same antipsychotic that the patient receives on a daily basis can be used orally or intramuscularly as needed for agitation.
9. Rapidity of dosage increments depends upon the persisting psychotic symptomatology (insomnia, agitation, hallucinations, delusions) and the need for extra doses.
10. Single daily bedtime doses are preferred.
11. If patients are excessively lethargic or an acute organic brain syndrome develops, decrease or temporarily discontinue medication.

TABLE 22:   (continued)

12. Reduced doses are required for children and older patients.
13. If an adequate trial produces no response to treatment, consider the following:
    a) parenteral therapy (rapid metabolizer or covert noncompliance)
    b) diagnostic error
    c) a different antipsychotic class
    d) high-dose therapy (2 to 4 times maximal dose) with consultation and guidance
14. Use anti-Parkinson drugs as necessary. Prophylactic use is preferable to potentially unrecognized side effects and lack of drug maintenance.
15. Acute extrapyramidal side effects are not necessarily an indication to decrease, discontinue, or change medication. Treatment should be focused on adequate doses to control psychotic symptoms, not side effects.
16. Treatment should be continued for six months after a first schizophrenic episode. Two or more episodes probably require maintenance antipsychotic therapy.

MAINTENANCE DRUG THERAPY

One of the most important causes of relapse in schizophrenia is the failure to continue taking medication after the symptoms subside. On the average, 40 percent of patients stop taking their prescribed medication within the first year after leaving the hospital (Van Putten 1974). This produces the "revolving door" phenomenon, with patients being admitted to and discharged from the hospital repeatedly.

There are many reasons for prematurely stopping antipsychotic drug therapy:

- Many patients experience uncomfortable and often disabling side effects, the most disturbing of which are not easily seen by the doctor or by relatives—uneasiness and feelings of internal jumpiness (akathisia), feeling slowed down and lifeless, and lacking spontaneity (akinesia). Other side effects of drugs include general feelings of discomfort. These side effects are often overlooked by the physician, but not by the patient, who then abandons medications only to suffer a relapse.
- Many patients never fully or even partially comprehend the nature and seriousness of their illness, nor do they appreciate the need to take antipsychotic medication indefinitely.

LEARNING EXERCISE

Interview a patient you are treating with antipsychotic medication. Ask the patient what he or she considers positive effects of the medication, negative effects, and why he or she considers it important to take the medication. After your interview, consider what the chances are that this patient will continue to take the medication in the future. Why?

Talk with a patient who does not want to take medications. How many of his or her reasons are based on

a) side effects
b) unrealistic fears (damaging, addicting, and so on)
c) lack of information
d) trust and control issues
e) environmental factors

Consider these factors in your own patients. What can you do to enhance compliance for them?

- Taking medication reminds a person that he or she is sick, which produces low self-esteem. Some patients stop taking medication so they can deny that they have a problem. Because of the social stigma of mental illness, some patients refuse to take their medication in the presence of others.
- Some patients leave the hospital or are discharged before their symptoms have been controlled, so they may be too ill to take their medication properly. The very nature of schizophrenia may affect a patient's judgment, insight, and stability. The concentration and cognitive grasp required for reliable drug taking may be deficient.
- Some patients never understand the delayed connection between stopping drug therapy and relapse because it often takes weeks or even months for the body to use up and metabolize all the medication that has been stored. A patient will temporarily feel very well without taking the prescribed drug because the medication continues to exert its effectiveness and the side effects are somewhat less. It may take three, four, or even more relapses before a patient realizes that the relapse occurs weeks or even months after stopping the medication.
- Patients who return to using street drugs such as marijuana, LSD, PCP or angel dust, amphetamines, cocaine, or diet drugs can suffer a relapse since they mistakenly believe that these drugs can help their symptoms.
- It is difficult to remember to take medication every day. Unless a person gets into a routine, with a special place for the medication and

a special time to take it, it is very easy to forget. It is a bother to have to be reminded of the medication, and some patients rebel against family members who try to help by reminding.

Well-grounded and tried and tested principles for maintenance neuroleptic drug therapy are provided in Table 23. This table also includes suggestions on when and how a patient might be withdrawn from his or her neuroleptic drug therapy or have the drug dose significantly reduced. Adherence to these principles will enable the clinician to avoid pitfalls leading to either unnecessary relapses or excessive side effects.

CASE EXAMPLES ——————————————————————————
Carol's new job, her first since her hospital discharge three months earlier, brought on new feelings of confidence. She preferred to forget that her antipsychotic medication had eliminated the hallucinations and fears she recently experienced during her third psychotic episode in the past four years. Taking medication three times daily, she hated to look at the bottles. Each dose reminded her of unpleasant memories. She felt good, she was working, she was making new friends. "Maybe," she thought, "I don't need these medications any more. After all, look how well I am doing. These medicines can stay in the medicine cabinet 'just in case.'"

Pete lost his job when he insisted that other employees were trying to persecute him and sabotage his work. An increase of his neuroleptic medication resolved these symptoms without hospitalization, but now he felt bored and seemed to have less energy and motivation. He began drinking with the guys at the corner bar to relieve his boredom and help him relax. One day he was introduced to cocaine, which increased his energy and made him feel confident. Two weeks after he began using cocaine, he felt that his neighbors were spying on him and reporting his activities to the police. He was sure he could hear them laughing at him. After Pete barricaded himself in a friend's home, his physician arranged to have Pete hospitalized.

TABLE 23: Principles for Maintenance Antipsychotic Drug Therapy for Schizophrenics

1. Only treatment-resistant patients benefit from high or megadose therapy—these patients are mostly under the age of 40 with less than 10 years' cumulative hospitalization.
2. High doses produce more side effects, especially in older patients.
3. Placebo or no medication is effective in maintaining a sizable minority of patients.

TABLE 23: *(continued)*

4. Low-dose antipsychotic therapy deserves consideration since it may be activating for the apathetic, withdrawn, and depressed patient who does not have florid psychotic symptoms, and it is often sufficient to maintain remission for many patients.
5. There are marked interindividual variations in drug absorption and metabolism, so dose level is a poor indicator of active levels in the central nervous system, or plasma. Use each patient as his or her own control rather then referring to arbitrary standards or dosages.
6. Every chronic schizophrenic person maintained on antipsychotic medication should have the benefit of an adequate trial without drugs.

Suggested guidelines for reducing or discontinuing antipsychotic medications:

1. When a patient's drug history reveals that discontinuance or reduction of antipsychotic drugs was followed by relapse, it is safe to conclude that any new attempt to withdraw drugs is likely to fail.
2. Withdrawal of antipsychotic medication can be implemented in the following ways:
   a) Gradual withdrawal (versus abrupt)
   b) If the patient is on more than one antipsychotic, they should be stopped one at a time
   c) If a patient is on an anti-Parkinson drug, it should be continued for 1 to 2 weeks after antipsychotic drug withdrawal to protect against withdrawal-emergent dyskinesias
   d) If the patient (and family or staff) is anxious and reluctant about withdrawal, reduction to a low, token dose may be preferable to total withdrawal.
3. Closely follow patients successfully withdrawn from medication for a year, since clinical relapse may be expected to occur at any time during the first 12 months.
4. If clinical deterioration occurs upon withdrawal, resume antipsychotic medication at the lowest effective dose.
5. If dyskinesias appear or worsen upon withdrawal, judicious drug management must take into account both the dyskinesia and any subsequent clinical deterioration. Withdrawal-emergent dyskinesias often appear spontaneously in 6 to 22 weeks.
6. It is important to distinguish among
   a) withdrawal-emergent dyskinesias (these eventually disappear),

TABLE 23: (continued)

    b) covert dyskinesias (irreversible and unmasked by neuroleptic withdrawal), and

    c) tardive dyskinesia (irreversible; present during therapy).

LEARNING EXERCISE

All of us have had to take medication at one time or another in our lives. Think of the last two times you were prescribed medicine by your doctor. For each medicine, write down on a piece of paper answers to the following questions:

    1) What was the name of the medicine?

    2) Why was it prescribed?

    3) Did you finish the prescription?

    4) If not, why not? List your reasons.

Share your answers with three other colleagues. Do you see any patterns that explain medication noncompliance?

DIVERGENT DRUGS FOR SCHIZOPHRENIC DISORDERS

Antipsychotic drugs remain the mainstay of pharmacologic treatment for schizophrenia. Recent studies suggest that other medications may also be useful. Lithium, an effective treatment for mania, bipolar disorders, and perhaps other affective disorders, seems to benefit treatment of psychosis with acute onset and remitting cause, especially if accompanied by affective symptoms, but it is not effective as the sole maintenance medication.

Propranolol, a beta-adrenergic receptor blocker commonly used for hypertension and cardiac disease, was claimed in the early 1970s to yield dramatic improvements in psychosis. Some chronically ill schizophrenic patients showed remission on high doses of propranolol. A series of controlled studies over the last 10 years have failed to find consistent evidence of effectiveness for propranolol in chronic schizophrenia.

Carbamazepine, an anticonvulsant commonly used for partial-complex seizure disorder, has demonstrated effectiveness in rapid-cycling bipolar disorders but not in chronic schizophrenia. Clonazepam, a benzodiazepine, also shows promise for treating affective psychosis and is now receiving trials for schizophrenia. Reserpine was used in the treatment of schizophrenia prior to the introduction of chlorpromazine in the mid-1950s. There is renewed interest in reserpine. Although these alternate medications have shown promise for augmenting the therapeutic activity of neuroleptics in treatment-refractory psychoses, the neuroleptic antipsychotic drugs remain the primary pharmacological agents for treatment and maintenance of chronic schizophrenia.

DEPOT INJECTABLE NEUROLEPTICS

Where do the long-acting depot neuroleptics fit into the treatment of schizophrenia? How can they help accomplish the goal of developing a long-term strategy for maintenance treatment?

For the past 20 years, experience has been accumulating with depot neuroleptics, and their advantages in maintenance therapy have become clear. Among these advantages are the promise of a guaranteed drug delivery, possible reduction in the dose administered, predictable and constant plasma drug level, and treatment of patients who are refractory to oral medication because of absorption difficulties.

Once maintenance therapy with depot injections has begun, subsequent drug defaulting—which amounts to refusing injections—is estimated to be 10 percent to 15 percent over a two-year period, a fraction of the high rate seen with oral medication. Moreover, it appears that relapse rates with depot neuroleptics are less than with oral medications, especially after the first year of drug use (Hogarty et al. 1979).

Improved Adherence Rate

One of the primary reasons for this improved rate is that a long-acting drug can be given at two- to four-week intervals. The patient is freed from the daily concern of drug taking. The opportunity for forgetting to take medication is substantially reduced with depot neuroleptics.

Thus, the patient's adherence to prescribed medication is improved. The probability that schizophrenic symptoms will reappear and affect the patient's insight or motivation to continue taking medication is reduced.

Should a relapse occur while the patient is receiving depot neuroleptic medication, the treating physician knows that the relapse is due to factors other than failure to take medication as prescribed. As a rule, with the oral route of administration, the physician has no way of accurately knowing whether the patient was taking his or her medication. And although routine blood level measurements will confirm the presence or absence of a drug in the body, they cannot accurately measure whether the patient is taking the medication as prescribed. Although pill counts are a technique often used for assessing adherence to medication in patients with schizophrenia, they can be misrepresented by the patient.

With depot neuroleptics, knowing that the medication was received could greatly aid the psychiatrist in understanding the circumstances surrounding a patient's relapse and in developing an appropriate treatment strategy.

Reduction in Dose and Relapses

It is theorized that the total amount of drug needed with the depot injection technique to achieve comparable antipsychotic efficacy may be less than that required with oral administration. This is possible, in part, because parenterally administered drugs bypass the initial biotransformation process of the gut and liver (Johnson 1981). More important, there are indications that equivalent clinical efficacy can be achieved at lower plasma drug levels with depot neuroleptics than with oral therapy. This finding may be related to the ability of depot drugs to overcome problems associated with oral drug absorption and thus provide more constant and predictable plasma drug levels. Furthermore, the different pharmacokinetics of depot drugs compared with oral medication may contribute to these findings, in particular, the plasma level versus time profiles.

Recent data from clinical trials suggest that the doses of oral neuroleptics commonly used in the United States may be much higher than needed, perhaps double the required dose (Baldessarini and Davis 1980; Baldessarini et al. 1984). Furthermore, this overdosing appears to be greater with the high-potency than with the low-potency neuroleptics (Baldessarini et al. 1984). Evidence has accumulated that indicates that high-dose therapy is associated with an increase in unpleasant side effects, such as sedation and extrapyramidal symptoms. Thus, the current trend is toward finding the minimal effective dose—the balance point between therapeutic control and minimization of side effects in each patient.

However, the use of a minimal effective dose strategy heightens the need for patient adherence to medication because there will be no excess drug to compensate for missed or forgotten medication. Depot neuroleptics, which come closest to ensuring medication adherence as well as minimizing variations in drug absorption and bioavailability, become the logical treatment of choice in establishing minimum effective dosage regimens.

There is some indication that depot neuroleptics alter the nature of a relapse. In a study comparing the effects of oral and depot neuroleptics (Hogarty et al. 1979), patients who were taking oral medications and subsequently relapsed were significantly more impaired in terms of the characteristic symptoms of schizophrenia—hallucinations, thought disorder, conceptual disorganization, suspiciousness, hostility, uncooperativeness, and blunted affect.

On the other hand, patients who relapsed after having been treated with the long-acting injectable form of the same neuroleptic became significantly more impaired in the affective component of their illness—on measures of anxiety and depression. Furthermore, there is some evidence that among patients who relapse, the interval between relapses is lengthened with depot medications (Johnson 1982). Such findings suggest differences in patients' responses to the two methods of administration.

MAXIMIZING COMPLIANCE

Compliance with a neuroleptic drug regimen can be seen as a complex set of behavioral responses that must be learned by each patient. Often, little education or explanation takes place in the hospital, where the focus is on symptom control and return to the community. Factors such as cost, inconvenience, side effects, and delayed return of symptoms after stopping medications all conspire against compliance in the community. Despite these factors, patients may learn regular drug-taking behavior with some straightforward strategies:

1. Facilitating attendance at aftercare clinics. Not attending clinic appointments is the most frequent cause of drug noncompliance after hospital discharge. Simple techniques such as written appointments, telephone or mail reminders, nonthreatening clinic staff, presence of food, or other reinforcers can improve attendance.
2. Educating families and caregivers. Patients who share positive attitudes about the value of medication with household members are more likely to adhere to long-term drug therapy. Education allows the patient and his or her support network to become informed consumers and co-participants in the active monitoring of the use and effects of medication.
3. Using a systematic incentive program. Rewards such as food, praise, or "credits" have been shown to effectively increase compliance.
4. Cognitive restructuring. Rehearsing rationales for drug therapy with the patient may gradually reduce continuing doubt about the merits of continued medication. Many patients with schizophrenia have residual cognitive and memory deficits. Regular reminders, discussion, and repetition are useful techniques to deal with these problems.
5. Use of medication self-management training. Directive and active training strategies have been developed to educate patients and caregivers in the above-mentioned strategies.

A program using these strategies has been developed at the Rehabilitation Service of the Brentwood Psychiatric Division of the West Los Angeles Veterans Administration (VA) Medical Center, and the University of California at Los Angeles Department of Psychiatry. The Medication Management Module consists of four skill areas: a) identifying the benefits of antipsychotic medication, b) learning reliable self-administration, c) identifying and coping with side effects, and d) negotiating changes in medication with health care providers.

The Medication Management Module utilizes learning principles and behavioral techniques to teach and reinforce the acquisition of knowledge of and reliable use of neuroleptic drugs. The training methods include goal setting, repeated practice and overlearning, use of multimedia, positive reinforcement and shaping techniques, role-playing, modeling, checking for assimilation of presented material, and assignments to promote transfer of learned skills to the patient's real-life setting. Since 1982, over 500 patients have participated in the training of medication self-management. Completion of skills training has correlated with total time spent in psychiatric hospital over the last five years and level of motivation at the start of training. It appears that patients with longer cumulative periods of hospitalization have gained more insight into their illnesses and a more favorable attachment to treatment staff, thereby enhancing their motivation to participate in the medication self-management training. Severity of disability or symptoms has not correlated with completion of the program.

A large-scale field test in a variety of mental health facilities has evaluated this innovative program for teaching patients to be more responsible consumers of their antipsychotic drugs. Twenty-eight facilities in the United States and Canada have documented the efficacy of the training methods, effects on compliance, as well as "user friendliness" of the training materials.

The following principles help maximize compliance and prevent relapse:

1. Use the drug that is most acceptable to the patient. Choose a drug that is best tolerated by the patient and has the least side effects. Remember: All the available antipsychotic drugs are equally effective when properly prescribed.
2. Prescribe the lowest effective dose.
3. For patients who are not reliable in taking oral medication, try long-acting depot medication (such as fluphenazine decanoate or haloperidol decanoate), which can be given once every two to four weeks. Small doses of these injectable medications can be effective in preventing relapse without producing serious side effects. As little as 6.25 mg (¼ cc) or less of injectable fluphenazine or 12.5 mg of injectable haloperidol per month can be effective.
4. Incorporate drug holidays into the regimen in which a patient does not take the drug for one weekend each month. This may reduce side effects and can raise the patient's hopes.
5. The patient must understand that treatment should be continued for six months after the first episode of schizophrenia. Two or more episodes/relapses probably require maintenance anti-psychotic drug therapy for an indefinite period of time.

6. Make it easy for a person to remember to take the medication by keeping the bottle in a visible location that can be reached easily. Also, prescribe the entire daily dose once a day at bedtime.
7. Discuss medication, its effects, and its side effects frequently with the patient and the patient's family. It is important for everybody to be informed of the importance of drug therapy and for the doctor to know how the patient is responding.
8. Use medication self-assessment forms, side-effect check sheets, information pamphlets, and medication management groups. If the patient is included in the treatment process, he or she is more likely to take an active interest and report compliance.
9. Polypharmacy (the use of more than one antipsychotic drug at a time) is not advised because it a) unnecessarily exposes the patient to the potential side effects of each drug group, b) exposes the patient to the hazards of adverse drug interactions, c) complicates the treatment program and makes it more difficult to take medication reliably, and d) is not any more effective than taking proper doses of a single drug.

THE INTERACTION BETWEEN THE ENVIRONMENT AND MEDICATION

While there is no question that antipsychotic drugs have both therapeutic and preventive effects in schizophrenia and manic-depressive disorders, these effects depend to a considerable extent on the nature of the treatment environment. Medications are never prescribed or ingested in a psychosocial vacuum. The impact of the environment at home as well as in hospitals and clinics is understandable, since the symptoms and signs of schizophrenia are themselves strongly influenced by the patient's surroundings. The qualities of certain environments have been found to have an impact on the beneficial effects of antipsychotic medications.

For example, overly stimulating environments, in which excessive social demands, social censure, noise, and unrealistically high expectations for performance impinge upon a schizophrenic person, can provoke exacerbations of delusions, hallucinations, agitation, and thought disorder. On the other hand, understimulating and socially impoverished environments, such as custodial settings in the back wards of large state hospitals, can increase the negative symptoms of schizophrenia, such as withdrawal, muteness, poor self-care, and apathy. From research done with schizophrenic patients who have received antipsychotic drugs, it appears that medication is most helpful in protecting against the symptoms associated with over-stimulating environments. In treatment or rehabilitation settings in which the level of stimulation is optimal—that is, where there are structured, clear, and reasonable expectations for performance with lavish positive feedback and encouragement for small improvements—medication may be somewhat less important. When older, very chronic schizophrenic patients who have been on medication for many years move from custodial, understimulating settings to more active treatment, antipsychotic drugs may even hinder social and instrumental learning, due to excessive sedation or akinetic, apathetic effects (Liberman et al. 1984).

For patients who return to live with families that are excessively critical or emotionally overinvolved, maintenance antipsychotic medication confers protection against relapse. On the other hand, those patients who return from the hospital to live with relatives who are more tolerant, accepting, and supportive are not as likely to need medication for prophylactic purposes, at least during the first nine months after discharge. Thus the patient, the drug, and the social environment must be considered together in planning and predicting drug effects.

LEARNING EXERCISE

Think of a patient with chronic schizophrenia whom you recently treated for a relapse. List factors that may have led to his or her relapse. Did the relapse result from noncompliance? What could you have done to minimize the chance of relapse? Don't forget environmental factors! What would you tell your patient's family or caretaker? Develop your own approach to working with families and caretakers. You will use it many times during your professional career.

Thus there are a number of factors related to individual differences among patients and their environments that must be considered in selecting the patient's drug dose and form of administration. As with nonpsychiatric drugs, effectiveness may depend on absorption, metabolism, storage, and excretion of the drug. Also, the sensitivity of the illness to the drug will affect the dose required. Environmental factors, family involvement, exposure to stressors, and the availability of coping mechanisms in the patient also conspire to affect the efficacy of drug treatment and dosages required. Often, then, your experience, flexibility, and attention to drug-person-environment interactions are important in the successful treatment of your patient.

There are two overriding principles for prescribing and adjusting antipsychotic medications. The first is to *individualize treatment*. Match the medication type and dosage to the particular patient and his or her problems, stresses, supports, and environment. The second is *listen to the patient*. He or she will tell you what works best. The meaning of a drug effect or side-effect to an individual can affect the outcome of treatment.

LEARNING EXERCISE

As a physician, your patients and your treatment team consider you the expert on the use and effects of medication. How would you educate your patients and staff about optimal medication use? Can you design a medication teaching group or seminar? What material would you cover? What techniques would you use? Would you provide articles? handouts? Be specific. Then, get together with a colleague and try to design and implement an educational process for patients. Through instructions and group discussion, hospitalized psychiatric patients learn the indications, effects, and side-effects of psychotropic medications (Redman 1978).

The staff of the Rehabilitation Service of the West Los Angeles VA Medical Center, Brentwood Psychiatric Division, have developed, validated, and field-tested a medication education program called the Medication Management Module. The Module consists of a trainer's manual, a patient's workbook, and a videocassette that demonstrates the key areas of managing maintenance antipsychotic medication. A mental health or rehabilitation practitioner guides a group of patients through the curriculum using directive teaching techniques such as problem solving, in vivo exercises, and homework (Wallace et al. 1985; Liberman and Evans 1985).

The objectives of this module are as follows:

1. Increase patients' knowledge about therapeutic and prophylactic effects of their medications.
2. Give patients general information about the effects and side effects of antipsychotic drugs.
3. Emphasize the importance of continuing prescribed medications after hospital discharge.
4. Decrease the chance of medication error while patients are self-administering drugs.
5. Give patients a better understanding of why they are taking their drugs, what the drugs are doing for them, and how long they will have to take the drugs.
6. Offer suggestions to help patients deal with minor side effects.
7. Help patients recognize symptoms that should be reported to a nurse, pharmacist, or physician.
8. Teach patients how to effectively and constructively discuss their medication concerns with their health care providers with the aim of a collaborative relationship in pharmacotherapy.

The Medication Management Module is available from the Psychiatric Rehabilitation Consultants, Camarillo-UCLA Research Center, Box A, Camarillo, CA 93011.

SUMMARY

Psychiatric drugs help improve problems and symptoms that a person experiences in thinking, feeling, socializing, working and playing, and caring for self. There are six major types of drugs used in psychiatry, and each is aimed at specific illnesses or problems: They include neuroleptics or antipsychotics, mood stabilizers, antidepressants, minor tranquilizers, sedative-hypnotics, and stimulants. Antipsychotic medications are useful in treating some of the symptoms of schizophrenia. There is no difference in the efficacy or therapeutic effects of one type of antipsychotic versus another.

Side-effects are the most significant cause of noncompliance with medication regimens. The most common side-effects of neuroleptic drugs are tardive dyskinesia, hypotension, extrapyramidal symptoms, sedation, endocrine effects, and anticholinergic symptoms. Educational programs and medication management groups help to provide information about medications and side-effects to patients.

When possible, a period of drug-free evaluation and assessment should precede treatment with antipsychotic drugs. When starting an antipsychotic drug, it is important to remember that its actions and effects take time. Individual differences in drug absorption, transportation, elimination, body weight, and metabolism result in great individual variation in dose, onset of action, and ultimate efficacy. The optimal dose is determined by increasing the dose of the drug only when the patient has stopped showing signs of improvement at the previous dosage level. Use the lowest dose that still produces the maximum amount of improvement in thinking, feeling, socializing, work and play, and self-care.

REFERENCES

Baldessarini RJ: Clinical and epidemiological aspects of tardive dyskinesia. J Clin Psychiatry 46:8–13, 1985

Baldessarini RJ: Tardive Dyskinesia (APA Task Force Report No. 18). Washington, DC, American Psychiatric Association, 1980

Beaver F, Doran E: Patient Health Education Program. Los Angeles, CA, Brentwood Veterans Administration Medical Center, 1980

Donaldson SR, Gelenberg AJ, Baldessarini RJ, et al: The pharmacologic treatment of schizophrenia: A progress report. Schizophr Bull 9:504–527, 1983

Falloon IRH, Boyd JL, McGill CW, et al: Family management in the prevention of exacerbation of schizophrenia. N Engl J Med 306:1437–1440, 1982

Gardos G, Cole JO: Maintenance antipsychotic therapy: is the cure worse than the disease? Am J Psychiatry 133:32–36, 1976

Gardos G, Cole JO, Tarsy D: Withdrawal syndromes associated with antipsychotic drugs. Am J Psychiatry 135:1321–1324, 1978

Herz MI, Szymanski HV, Simon JC: Intermittent medication for stable schizophrenic outpatients: an alternative to maintenance medication. Am J Psychiatry 139:918–922, 1982

Jeste DV, Wyatt RJ: Understanding and Treating Tardive Dyskinesia. Washington, DC, American Psychiatric Press, 1982

Johnson DAW: Observations on the use of long-acting depot neuroleptic injections in the maintenance therapy of schizophrenia. J Clin Psychiatry 45:13–21, 1984

Kane JM: Low dose medication strategies in the maintenance treatment for schizophrenia. Schizophr Bull 9:29–33, 1983

Kane JM, Woerner M, Weinhold P, et al: A prospective study of tardive dyskinesia development. J Clin Psychopharmacol 2:345–349, 1982

Liberman RP, et al: Drug-psychosocial interactions in the treatment of schizophrenia, in The Chronically Mentally Ill: Research and Services. Edited by Mirabi M. New York, Spectrum Publications, 1984

Liberman RP, et al: Protective intervention in schizophrenia: combined neuroleptic drug therapy and medication self-management training, in Treatment Strategies in Schizophrenia. Edited by Goldstein MJ, Hand I, Hahlweg K. New York, Springer Verlag, 1986

Marder SR, Van Putten T, Mintz J, et al: Costs and benefits of two doses of fluphenazine. Arch Gen Psychiatry 41:1025–1029, 1984

Redman BK: Curriculum in patient education. Am J Nurs 78:1363–1366, 1978

Schatzberg AF, Cole JO: Manual of Clinical Psychopharmacology. Washington, DC, American Psychiatric Press, 1986

Van Putten T: Why do schizophrenic patients refuse to take their drugs? Arch Gen Psychiatry 31:67–72, 1974

CHAPTER 5

SOCIAL SKILLS TRAINING

ROBERT PAUL LIBERMAN, M.D.

Psychiatry is the study of processes that involve or go on between people. The field of psychiatry is the field of interpersonal relations. . . . A personality can never be isolated from the complex of interpersonal relations in which the person lives and has his being.

Harry Stack Sullivan
Conceptions of Modern Psychiatry, 1947

I n our society, there are schools and educational opportunities for almost every conceivable human skill, from cooking and foreign languages to sporting events, dancing, and computer programming. Systematic training and apprenticeships are available for people who want to learn how to become a carpenter, a truck driver, or a dental technician.

However, for those people who lack social and emotional skills, there is a void of learning opportunities. Unless one has been blessed with parents, siblings, friends, or significant others who have modeled social effectiveness and emotional expressiveness, these skills may never be acquired. Individuals who have the insidious onset of process schizophrenia from the time of adolescence are examples of those whose social skills are poorly developed and stunted. Even when some semblance of skills has been initially acquired, however, intercurrent symptoms of severe mental disorder—such as major depressive episodes or psychotic illnesses—can displace the skills and render an individual unable to use those skills potentially available in his or her repertoire. Still others, after long years of institutionalization in hospitals or community back streets, have their social and emotional skills wither from disuse.

Fortunately, for the mentally ill individuals with social disabilities, over a decade of research and development has yielded effective methods for social skills training. Social skills training is available and effective for a wide range of chronic and acute psychiatric patients, including those from minority population groups and those with little education or verbal skills, who need to learn emotionally expressive and social skills (Liberman et al. 1985).

Almost by definition of the *Diagnostic and Statistical Manual of Mental Disorders (Third Edition-Revised)* (American Psychiatric Association 1987) patients suffering from chronic schizophrenic, affective, and anxiety disorders who cross the thresholds of hospitals, clinics, or consulting offices suffer from deficits in social skills. For example, deterioration in social relations is a key diagnostic criterion in the schizophrenic disorders, and persistent fear of interaction with others is a major feature of social phobias. Without the ability to communicate and engage in relationships, patients have difficulty in meeting their material and affiliative needs. They are often exploited, victimized, pushed aside, or simply ignored in the bustle of everyday life. Sometimes, frustrated in their failure to obtain their needs, they lash out with aggression or hostility. Rather than taking an active part in their environments, they are acted upon by others.

SOCIAL SKILLS PRODUCE PERSONAL EFFECTIVENESS THROUGH COMMUNICATION

The problems in living experienced by chronic mental patients stem in large part from their inability to express their feelings or to communicate their interests and desires to others who are important to them. Person-to-person communication is one of the most essential of our human capacities. Each day, patients must satisfy their emotional, social, and biological needs by interacting effectively with physicians, nurses, social workers, relatives, operators of residential care facilities, police, store-keepers, and employers. When needs go unmet because of social and communication deficits, these patients' quality of life is diminished. Patients lacking social skills are thereby shut off from satisfying relationships with others and feel stifled, lonely, frustrated, depressed, and isolated. In a study of several hundred chronic mental patients living in board and care homes in Los Angeles, it was found that compared with a control sample of normals, their greatest-felt deficiencies in "quality of life" related to their lack of friends, jobs, and family ties (Lehman 1983).

CASE EXAMPLE ──────────────────────────────────────

Improvements in social skills allow patients to more effectively pursue their interests, capitalize on opportunities, and live more rewarding lives. Consider the following examples of individuals who were referred for social skills training:

> Jerry, a 25-year-old clerk with two hospitalizations for schizophrenia, has no friends. He is shy and withdrawn from peers and talks in an inaudible tone of voice.

> Mary has lived in a succession of board and care homes, and has just been ejected from another. She is belligerent with authority figures and does not distinguish between assertion and aggression.

> Tim can't get a job, and feels depressed and demoralized. He rarely smiles and freezes when asked about his poor job history.

DEFINING SOCIAL SKILLS

While the general concept of social skills is often limited to interpersonal behaviors, the definition used in current training approaches is broader in nature. Social skills include affective, cognitive, and motoric domains of functioning. They comprise the transactions between people that result in attainment of one's tangible and social-emotional goals. Skills must be demonstrated in a large variety of interpersonal contexts and require the coordinated delivery of appropriate verbal and nonverbal responses. As pointed out by Hersen and Bellack (1977), "the socially skilled individual is attuned to the realities of the situation and is aware when he is likely to be rewarded for efforts. The overriding factor is effectiveness of behavior in social interactions" (p. 175).

Social skills may be viewed as the coping process by which social competence is achieved. The skills—verbal and nonverbal communication, internal feelings, attitudes, and perceptions of the interpersonal context—mediate successful outcomes of social interactions that are reflected in the achievement of the individual's goals and the favorable impression made on others (Liberman 1982; Wallace et al. 1980). Social competence can be equated with a high frequency of successful social outcomes and a satisfying quality of life. The skills required for competence include 1) accurate social perception or receiving of the relevant characteristics of an interpersonal situation, that is, being aware of the feelings and aims of the person with whom one is speaking as well as one's rights and responsibilities in the situation; 2) cognitive processing or translating of social perceptions into alternate courses of action and deciding upon the best alternative; and 3) implementing or sending the chosen alternative response back to the other person using appropriate verbal and nonverbal behaviors. Consider how the patient in the vignette below experiences deficits in receiving, processing, and sending skills.

CASE EXAMPLE ———————————————————————————————
"I am convinced that when I make the effort I can be quite an effective person, and I am good at disguising the difficulty I often have in picking up what people say, especially if I am distracted by something. I have typically been overzealous about expressing my point of view or feelings about things, and suffered later, regretting much that I have said. But often what I do say is appreciated by other people, and is quite appropriate to what is being discussed.

"Problems with my normal facade arise mainly when other people expect me to become emotionally involved with them. I find emotions tremendously complex, and I am quite acutely aware of the many over- and undertones of things people say and the way they say them. Generally, I like direct, honest, kind people, and I have difficulty handling social situations that require me to be artificial or too careful.

"Intimacy is an interesting problem in my life. In a way, I am capable of the deepest spiritual intimacy with people, yet I am less capable than most people of handling the demands of relationships. I cannot share negative feelings other people have, because I am too sensitive to them" (Anonymous 1981).

IMPORTANCE OF SOCIAL SKILLS TRAINING FOR CHRONIC MENTAL PATIENTS

There are four sources of empirical data that recommend social skills training as a method for improving chronic patients' competence. Research evidence has shown that 1) premorbid social adjustment powerfully predicts subsequent course and outcome of psychiatric disorders, 2) social function appears to be deficient in children who are at risk for schizophrenia, 3) the deficits in social skills pervasively present in persons with major mental disorders are prognostic for relapse and rehospitalization, and (4) skills training within the family context can reduce stressful emotional climates and relapse rates in schizophrenia.

Many studies have found that premorbid social competence is a predictor of outcome in major mental disorders (Liberman 1982a). These extremely well-replicated findings suggest that long-term prognosis might be improved if the postmorbid level of social functioning of chronic mental patients could be raised, such as through social skills training.

Investigations of children who later became schizophrenic, or who were at high risk for schizophrenia because of having a schizophrenic parent, have revealed that poor social competence typically precedes the onset of the core symptoms of the disorder, often by many years. Preschizophrenic children tend to be characterized by their teachers as disagreeable, aggressive, socially insecure, angry, and socially anxious (Goldstein 1982). These findings suggest that social skills deficits may comprise part of the person's psychobiological predisposition to schizophrenia. An intriguing implication is that social skills training may be a potentially effective means of preventing schizophrenia in children and adolescents at risk for the disorder.

The magnitude of deficits in social and living skills has been well documented in chronic psychiatric patients. Such patients have poor eye contact, inappropriate facial expression, poor gestures and posture, poor response timing or synchrony, and very low rates of spontaneous social interaction (Liberman et al. 1974; Paul and Lentz 1977; Liberman 1982a). Schizophrenic patients also have greater difficulty and perform more poorly in interpersonal judgment and in recognizing emotions in others (Wallace et al. 1980; Liberman et al. 1980). In one study, major functional deficits in social and personal areas were found in over 50 percent of a sample of chronic psychiatric patients (Sylph et al. 1978). A multihospital study of schizophrenic patients placed in foster homes after relatively brief hospitalizations found that relapse rates at one year after discharge were significantly higher among those patients who had prerelease deficiencies in social skills (Linn et al. 1982). This finding was extended by a study in the United Kingdom that found release rates from a large psychiatric hospital best predicted by the levels of social adjustment of the patients (Presly et al. 1982).

These research data suggest that social skills training might help to remediate deficits in areas of functioning that are important for successful tenure in the community. Moreover, since tension and stress within the family system has been found to powerfully predict relapse in schizophrenic and depressed patients (Hooley 1985), it would appear reasonable to try to improve the communication and problem-solving skills of patients and their relatives. In fact, as is described in the next chapter on family management, skills development in families containing a mentally ill member does have a profoundly beneficial impact on relapse, family burden, and social adjustment.

In summary, then, social skills training appears to be a fruitful avenue for strengthening the psychobiologically vulnerable individual against the stressful effects of life events, challenges of community adjustment, and family conflict and tension. Skills training can be oriented around the instrumental role needs of the individual: medication self-management, home finding and maintenance, recreation and leisure skills, money management and consumerism, and use of public agencies. Training of affiliative skills can also be the focus of training, with intervention efforts focusing on upgrading the individual's conversational, peer and friendship, and family relationship skills.

In pursuing social skills training, it is important to realize that skills will be most efficiently and durably acquired if the training is embedded in a broad and comprehensive program of rehabilitation. Chronic mental disorder does not yield easily to unidimensional treatments or interventions; thus, skills training is but one component in a multidimensional program that should include judicious use of antipsychotic medication, psychosocial supports (for example, self-help clubs), a continuing and stable therapeutic relationship with caregivers and agencies, case management, crisis intervention, family management, residential services, and vocational rehabilitation. Indeed, the other chapters of this book describe the boundaries of comprehensive psychiatric rehabilitation, especially Chapter 8, "Community Support."

The following case vignettes illustrate the utility of social skills training when it is provided in the context of a comprehensive rehabilitation program. Do you have any patients under your care that have problems similar to those of these patients?

CASE EXAMPLES—SOCIAL SKILLS TRAINING IN ACTION _____

Steve was a 20-year-old junior college student who had suffered a psychotic episode while in summer maneuvers with the National Guard. He heard voices deriding him and felt that his thoughts and actions were being controlled by his father. He was a religiously scrupulous young man who held very high expectations for himself. After neuroleptic medication brought his psychotic symptoms into remission, Steve and his therapist worked on several social skills that would have the effect of strengthening his recovery. He felt awkward at work when his supervisor praised his efforts, because he felt he should be doing even better. One goal, then, was to practice in sessions how to verbally accept a compliment and then to apply this at work. A corollary to this was learning how to say to his supervisor, "I'm not quite getting this new procedure. Can you go over it again with me please?" In this manner, he was able to reduce the stress he experienced at work. In a similar fashion, he role-played asking a girl out for a date and then, upon getting the date, how to ask open-ended questions and reflect back interest and empathy to sustain heterosocial conversations. After six months of social skills training and neuroleptic maintenance therapy, Steve was able to attend a college away from home. He wrote to his therapist a month after starting his junior year at college, "My ability to meet people and socialize is good. I've made lots of friends. I have a really swell roommate and we get along well."

Tom, after being discharged from his third psychiatric hospitalization in four years of schizophrenic relapses, soon found himself in a bind with his father, who managed his Social Security disability pension. Tom wanted to control the money himself and use it to purchase a car and place a down payment on an apartment. His father felt he wasn't ready to assume those responsibilities and balked at turning the funds over to his son. They battled verbally over this issue repeatedly, failing to make progress and increasing the tension in the household.

Finally, Tom's case manager decided to teach Tom how to carry out problem solving and negotiation with his father. Over five sessions, Tom learned to empathize with his father's point of view through reflecting back to his father the latter's statements and assertions. This was followed by his making a request of his father to listen carefully to his viewpoints. Tom then was taught to suggest brainstorming alternatives for managing the funds, in addition to sole management by Tom or by his father. When Tom actually used this problem-solving technique in a subsequent discussion with his father, much to his amazement he found a new flexibility and responsiveness in his father. After some discussion, they decided on a compromise, which was that Tom would control half of his monthly funds for two months on a trial basis. If after that period it was mutually agreed that Tom had managed the funds well, he would be given full rein of his money. This worked out well, with some continued coaching by the case manager for constructive communication between Tom and his father. Within six months, Tom had found a job and was able to finance a car and an apartment.

Marjorie had recurrent depressions that were so frequent they almost were continuous. They inhibited her long-felt desire to return to college after raising four children and study for a career in accounting. She obtained some symptomatic relief with antidepressant medication but was unable to mobilize herself to apply to college, go through the entrance examinations and interviews, and work out accommodations with her husband and children for home maintenance, cooking, and chores. With her therapist, she role-played college admission interviews, including sham interviews in which she was stressed and asked embarrassing questions (for example, "Why would a mother of four children want to become an accountant?"). She practiced asserting her desires and goals and also reviewed her rights and responsibilities as a mother, wife, and individual. She also learned how to engage her family in a problem-solving process that led to plans for managing the household tasks without her full-time involvement. Five years later, she had completed college and was a junior executive in an auditing firm.

LEARNING EXERCISE

Reflect for a moment and think of a patient of yours, past or present, who suffers from a chronic mental disorder and who might benefit from social skills training. On a piece of paper, or in conversation with a colleague, answer the following questions as you formulate a skills-training plan for that patient.

1. As specifically as possible, what is the current level of social skills that the patient possesses in both instrumental and affiliative domains of life? For example, can the patient initiate conversations with strangers? Make a positive request of an agency worker? Go through a job interview? Give appropriate levels of self-disclosure?
2. What behavioral goals or targets for training could be established in preparation for social skills training for this patient? Again, be as specific and operational as possible in pinpointing what the patient might be able to do, with whom, where, and when.
3. Would you be willing to engage this patient in social skills training?

SKILLS TRAINING BUTTRESSES COPING AND COMPETENCE AGAINST THE ONSLAUGHT OF STRESS AND VULNERABILITY

Psychotic symptoms and their accompanying behavioral disabilities emerge or are exacerbated when stressors impinge upon an individual with an underlying and enduring biobehavioral vulnerability. The symptomatic and social status of a person with the biological vulnerability for schizophrenia at any point in time is determined by the way in which the individual and his or her social support network are able to modulate the impact of interpersonal, financial, and biological stressors. Either too much environmental change, stressors, and ambient tension, or, on the other hand, deficient coping skills and social support can lead to breakdown and exacerbation.

In addition to the relapse or exacerbation of psychotic symptoms such as hallucinations or delusions, the negative or deficit symptoms of schizophrenia and other chronic mental disorders pose a major challenge to practitioners. Social withdrawal, apathy, anergy, slovenliness, and anhedonia do not respond well to neuroleptic drugs. Neither do drugs teach life and coping skills, except indirectly through removal or reduction of positive symptoms, such as delusions, thought disorder, or hallucinations. Most schizophrenic persons need to learn or relearn social and personal skills for surviving in the community.

The learning of living skills is usually facilitated by the concurrent administration of psychotropic drugs and psychosocial treatment. As described in Chapter 4, "Practical Psychopharmacology," recent studies have suggested that much lower doses of neuroleptics than are ordinarily prescribed can avert relapse and sustain community tenure, while producing fewer side effects. Drugs and psychosocial interventions can be viewed as complementary elements in treatment, with drugs ameliorating and preventing symptoms and psychosocial interventions building skills and coping capacities. Another way of examining this relationship between drugs and psychosocial treatments is to view the impact of drugs on the central nervous system as facilitating the patient's ability to focus and process information from the environment, thereby promoting the acquisition and generalization of skills being trained. One type of psychosocial treatment that has proved to be effective with chronic mental patients is social skills training.

For example, a person who learns good social and assertiveness skills can galvanize assistance and support from friends and relatives that, in turn, will aid in coping efforts, community survival, and instrumental problem-solving. Repeated many times over the course of months and years, these mastery experiences may also favorably affect neurotransmitters or other aspects of central nervous system function. Evidence from various laboratory experiments has clearly documented that environmental enrichment, learning experiences, conditioning, and behavioral training can influence both the function and structure of the central nervous system (Kandel 1983; Rosenzweig et al. 1968; Lesse 1959).

COPING AND COMPETENCE CAN DISPLACE PSYCHOTIC SYMPTOMS

It is a maxim in the science of human behavior that the development of prosocial skills can displace or replace symptomatic or deviant behavior. This has been shown clearly in classrooms where hyperactive and disruptive behavior of children markedly diminishes when the teacher prompts and reinforces more appropriate academic and attentive behavior. It has been shown in many studies of chronic mental patients as well. In the landmark research carried out by Gordon Paul and his colleagues at a state hospital in Illinois, severely disruptive and crazy behaviors were supplanted by appropriate social and self-care skills when a social learning program was introduced that structured the daily activities of the ward and provided immediate and consistent token reinforcement for improvements in the patients' behavior (Paul and Lentz 1977). The following vignette describes how nursing staff can use two basic principles of learning—prompting and reinforcement—to bring about significant improvements in conversational skills, which in turn displace social isolation, destructiveness, and tantrums in a young adult chronic patient.

CASE EXAMPLE

Jack, a 20-year-old with schizophrenic symptoms beginning at age 15, had retreated into a seclusive life marked by negativism and tantrums whenever his family or professionals would attempt to solicit his engagement in life's activities. He wore out his welcome on several community psychiatric units because he would destroy property whenever encouraged to participate in the milieu. One of his favorite targets for destruction was the unit's TV set, which earned him the enmity of staff and patients alike. As a last resort, he was hospitalized on the Clinical Research Unit of the Camarillo-University of California at Los Angeles Research Center at Camarillo State Hospital in California.

Because Jack found social contact so aversive, it was chosen as a negative reinforcer to motivate his learning some basic conversational skills. That is, a behavior therapy program was established in which Jack could successfully escape from social contact with nursing staff by first uttering some simple verbalizations. Since he was practically mute and incoherent, it was felt that this was a suitable starting point for his basic level, and it was predicted that he would gradually find social contact more reinforcing. The goals of this program were to get Jack to make eye contact, to speak loudly enough to be heard at a distance of 10 feet, to sit straight up and place his hands at his side (this goal was set to reduce Jack's tendency to seize the arms of the chair and rock it back and forth in self-stimulatory rituals), and to respond to selected questions with answers that lasted at least 15 seconds. Questions included, "Jack, what did you eat for breakfast?" and "Jack, tell me what you plan to do today." Nursing staff took turns approaching Jack three times daily to engage him in these simple conversations. If he responded with appropriate verbal and nonverbal behaviors, then the nurse would immediately leave him and allow him to have his privacy. The program was carried out over a six-month period with over 1,800 learning trials required before Jack was ready to reenter the community and participate in a day hospital. His seclusiveness gradually diminished, and there were no tantrums or destructive acts during the last three months of his hospitalization. On the day he left the Research Unit, he came on his own to the nurses' station, looked the staff in the eyes, and said firmly, "I'm really glad to get out of this place. I'm never coming back!" The staff broke out into spontaneous applause!

Jack made further progress in a social skills training group in the local community mental health center and was able to live semi-independently in a board and care home. He began to accompany the patients and staff of the mental health center to weekly bowling activities and attended a social club twice weekly. He was able to make an appointment himself to see an optometrist to obtain a new pair of glasses to replace the ones he had demolished months before. After a year or so of alienation from his family, he was able to resume visits to their home. They were delighted with his new-found willingness to socialize and interact. A complete research report has been published describing the procedures and results with Jack (Fichter et al. 1976).

The next case example also illustrates how prosocial behavior can replace bizarre symptoms of psychosis. In this case, recreational skills were taught as a means to reduce deviance. It should be noted that appropriate use of leisure time with recreational activities is extraordinarily important in the treatment and rehabilitation of chronic mental patients since many of them are unable to work and have long periods of free time on their hands. "Idle hands are the devil's workshop" is an old folk expression that has profound implications for individuals who lapse into delusional and hallucinatory experiences unless they have alternate social and recreational activities to engage their attention.

CASE EXAMPLE

Jerry was a 37-year old male diagnosed as suffering from refractory schizophrenia who engaged in mumbling and solitary laughter ranging in volume from soft and barely audible to loud and highly disruptive. When asked why he mumbled, Jerry would vacillate between attributing the sounds to voices outside of himself and denying that the behavior occurred. Jerry was in his fourth hospitalization within a 12-year period. As part of his psychiatric treatment regimen, Jerry was given thiothixene (Navane) 30 mg/day during the inpatient period.

A study was carried out to determine whether immersion in recreational tasks would displace Jerry's bizarre mumbling and self-vocalizations. He wore a wireless FM microphone in his shirt, and staff monitored his vocalizations through portable FM receivers. A time-sampling procedure was used in which every 15 seconds during one-hour sessions an observer would listen to Jerry and record the occurrence or nonoccurrence of stereotypic vocalizations. The patient was given an explanation of the procedure and fully consented to its implementation.

During open-ended sessions, Jerry was free to wander throughout the ward and had access to the recreational material freely available. But no instructions or reinforcement were given to him regarding engagement in recreation activities. During the structured recreational therapy sessions, also an hour in length, Jerry was instructed to involve himself in self-selected recreational tasks and was given reinforcement (tokens exchangeable for cookies, soda, cigarettes, candy) for participating. A varied set of recreational activities was made available, including art projects, model construction, and card games. The activities were supervised by nursing staff and a recreational therapist who provided the instructions, encouragement, and social and token reinforcement.

Results were striking. The average mumbling rate occurred much less frequently during structured recreational therapy sessions than during unstructured "free" time. The mean percent of intervals in which bizarre vocalizations occurred was 71.65 during unstructured periods and 28 percent during recreational therapy sessions. Observations made immediately after the end of the recreational therapy sessions indicated a near doubling of the rate of inappropriate vocalizations. Thus, it appears that the engagement in recreational activities actively displaced symptomatic behavior in the psychotic patient, providing a rationale for scheduling such activities throughout much of the patient's waking hours in psychiatric facilities.

EXPLICIT VERSUS IMPLICIT SOCIAL SKILLS TRAINING

While many psychosocial programs pronounce that social skills training is carried out as a component of the program, it is important to distinguish between nonspecific group activities that engage patients in "socialization" and methods that deliberately and systematically use behavioral learning techniques in a structured approach to building skills. Socialization activities are valuable of course, both for their own sake and for the incidental learning that can take place when people spontaneously socialize and interact. However, with chronic mental patients who have cognitive and motivational deficits because of their psychobiological vulnerability it is often necessary to design special learning environments for the training of social skills. In this chapter, we shall limit our definition of social skills training to those methods that harness the specific principles of human learning to promote the acquisition, generalization, and durability of skills needed in interpersonal situations.

WHAT ARE PRINCIPLES OF LEARNING?

In order to be truly effective with the wide spectrum of cognitively impaired chronic mental patients, social skills training is designed around a framework that contains the following basic principles of human learning:

Problem Definition. The therapist or trainer must translate the patient's obvious presenting symptoms and problems into deficits of socially appropriate behavior.

LEARNING EXERCISE

Try to put yourself in the place of a chronic mental patient who has too much time to dawdle and become self-absorbed. An approximation to this situation is when you are forced to wait for some activity or service and have not anticipated the wait. For example, getting caught in an unexpected traffic jam when you are already late for an appointment. Or having to stand in line at some public agency to file an application. Can you remember the feelings generated by these frustrating instances when you had time on your hands? Did you feel angry? Anxious? Did you begin to talk to yourself? Other approximations are during times of severe illness when physical debility enforced lengthy time periods when you were unable to participate in your usual activities. Remember your last flu episode or when you had to spend time idle after surgery? What types of unpleasant symptoms did you experience? How did you cope with the limitations on your activities? You can carry out this exercise through self-reflection or through discussing mutual experiences with a colleague, relative, or friend.

Example: Jenny was often involved in self-destructive and humiliating sexual relationships with men because she lacked the ability to develop relationships based on companionability and was unable to refuse sexual advances with self-assertiveness.

Inventory of Assets. During the evaluation of a patient for social skills training, it is important to take note of the person's strengths and capabilities in social relations. Does the person know how to meet people? Has the person maintained a friendship for a period of months or years? Can the person sustain a conversation by using appropriate levels of self-disclosure and asking open-ended questions?

Example: Desmond, although suffering from frequent hallucinations that caused anguish, was able to engage in conversations that were rational and coherent for 15 to 20 minutes at a time. During conversations, he showed good active listening skills and appeared to absorb the information he was receiving.

Establish a Reinforcing Therapeutic Alliance. The initial task of the therapist or treatment team is to engage the patient and the patient's family or significant others in a warm, accepting, and mutually respectful relationship. This requires establishing rapport, showing concern, expressing empathy, and demonstrating competence. A therapeutic alliance with its associated reinforcing qualities is earned, not automatic.

Example: Prior to the first meeting with the patient, the therapist makes certain that directions for finding the clinic are clear, by sending a map if necessary and informing the patient about public transportation or parking. During the first visit, the therapist checks to find out how the patient prefers to be addressed—by first or last name—and takes special care to describe details of the treatment contract and plan. The therapist points out why the prescribed treatment or training is distinctive and gives a rationale for its value and utility. When the patient leaves the clinic, the therapist always says, "Goodbye . . . Have a nice week. . . . I'll see you next time."

Goal Setting. It is important to move quickly from the patient's problems to formulating positive goals to be sought in the social skills training sessions. Undue focusing on and discussing of problems can inadvertently reinforce them. Setting specific and concrete interpersonal goals is perhaps the most challenging step in the behavioral procedures comprising social skills training. Therapists must ask, with the patient's active involvement, "What feeling or interpersonal need is not being expressed or obtained?"; "With whom do you need to improve your relationship?"; "What are your short- and long-term goals in this relationship?"; "Where and when does this interaction occur?"

Example: Lily decided she needed to be able to tell her adult daughter that she understood her needs for money, but that she would not be able to give her a loan or a gift because she needed it for herself. Jeff wanted to be able to tell visitors at the condominium he managed not to park their cars in spaces reserved for residents. Cindy chose to practice telling her boyfriend that she appreciated his concern for her emotional distress, but that she wanted to work on her problems with the help of a psychiatrist and felt pressured by his advice. Joe wanted to be able to sign up for the Social and Independent Living Skills Program and had to learn how to introduce himself to the intake worker and describe his needs for the program.

Behavioral Rehearsal. Much of the training of social skills takes place in simulated situations that approximate, through role-playing, the patient's real life circumstances. Other members in the group, or a therapist, take the part of figures in the patient's ordinary life, and scenes related to the patient's goals are practiced or rehearsed.

Example: Jean said that Sam looked a little like the shopkeeper that she wanted to be able to strike up a conversation with, and Sam, another member in the group, agreed to take the shopkeeper's part. The short-term goal here was for Jean to be successful in engaging the shopkeeper in a brief, casual conversation about the neighborhood; her long-term goal was to reduce her feelings of isolation and loneliness.

Positive Reinforcement. All steps along the way, from showing interest in participating in social skills training to completing homework assignments, are met with positive feedback or reinforcement by the therapist or trainer. An advantage of conducting social skills training in groups is that the reinforcement, or praise, can be multiplied manyfold and delivered by credible peers as well as professionals. Positive reinforcement has several behavioral components—looking at the person; coming close; making a pleasant facial expression; having a warm tone of voice; praising the behavior, not the person.

Example: After Jean completed rehearsing the scene with Sam, the trainer solicited positive reinforcement for her efforts from the other group members by asking, "What did you folks like about the way Jean started that conversation?"

Sam replied, "When she began speaking, I could tell that she was interested in me because she made good eye contact and smiled. That was a good job, Jean."

Shaping. Shaping is the building of complex sequences and chains of social behavior through successively reinforcing small steps along the way. It requires the therapist to break down long-term goals into small steps and to reinforce the patient's progress in accomplishing these small subgoals.

Example: Before undertaking the demands of asking a girl out for a date, Paul practiced going into shops and libraries and simply striking up conversations with young women working in those places. He practiced asking open-ended questions such as, "Do you like working here?" and "I often wonder what it's like to have a job like yours. How is it for you?" As he rehearsed these encounters in the social skills training group and then completed them in homework assignments, he was given liberal praise by the group leader and group members.

Prompting. Often, it's not possible to wait for some desirable behavior to occur and then to reinforce it. Prompting or cueing a patient to use elements of speech or phrases and to employ effective nonverbal behaviors can be a shortcut to teaching social skills. This requires the therapist or trainer to be very active—more like an athletic coach than a nondirective professional.

Example: Gayla, the group leader, rose from her chair and moved next to Paul as he practiced making a phone call for a date with a girl. As he paused, Gayla said, "Now, speak in a firm tone of voice and tell her how much you would enjoy spending the evening with her." Almost immediately, Paul's voice firmed up and he paraphrased the affirmative content in Gayla's prompt.

LEARNING EXERCISE

Can you outline the use of learning principles in the treatment of one of your patients? Think of a patient with a particular set of problems or symptoms. Ask yourself, "What adaptive behaviors does this patient lack that, if they were taught and reinforced, might supplant some of the social deviance and behavioral defects of the patient?" Once you target one or more specific adaptive behaviors that are not too great a leap beyond the patient's current capacity, think of some reinforcer that you could use to strengthen those behaviors. Reinforcers can be tangible items (food, drink, cigarettes, money) or social rewards such as praise and a pat on the back. For some patients, privacy may be a reinforcer, as it was in the case of Jack, described above.

A good rule of thumb to help you to choose a suitable reinforcer for a patient is the "high frequency" rule. Any behavior that occurs at high frequency (and hence is likely to be preferred by the individual) can be used to reinforce other more adaptive behaviors that are not occurring frequently enough. For example, with patients who have a high rate of talking about their delusions, a reinforcement program can be designed that increases the amount of coherent and rational conversation through contingent opportunities to have an open-ended chat that permits "crazy talk." This approach has been effectively used with patients having neuroleptic-resistant delusions (Liberman et al. 1973). Try to design a simple reinforcement program for one of your patients using these learning principles.

Modeling. By demonstrating a particular skill or component of a skill, the therapist (or other group members who have the skill to demonstrate) can teach the patient to improve. It's important to highlight the specific behavioral components being demonstrated and to make sure that the patient understands what is being pinpointed for learning. Modeling is particularly useful for chronic patients with cognitive deficits. Such patients have great difficulty learning social skills through instructions, prompts, and reinforcement alone.

Example: Gayla asked Joe to demonstrate to Desmond how to make good eye contact and to gesticulate with his hands while speaking forcibly about his loss of Social Security payments to the social worker. While Joe was modeling this behavior, Gayla stood closely by Desmond and said, "Watch how Joe is looking straight at the person and using his hands to get his point across."

Homework and In Vivo Practice. The proof of the pudding is whether a patient actually uses the skills practiced in the training session in his or her real life settings. For this reason, homework assignments are regularly given at the completion of each patient's rehearsal in the group. And homework assignments are consistently followed up on by the therapist, who inquires at the very start of each session about assignment completion. Sometimes it is necessary to bridge the gap between session and real life practice by having the therapist or trainer accompany the patient part of the way toward carrying out a homework assignment.

Example: After doing well in the behavioral rehearsal, Desmond was given a homework card by Gayla to visit his local Social Security office and request an appointment with a social worker. It was the first step toward actually filing an appeal for what he felt was an invalid suspension of his Social Security income.

VARIATIONS IN SOCIAL SKILLS TRAINING TECHNIQUES

It is important to tailor social skills training procedures to the needs of the individual patient, since all patients present different constellations of social abilities, deficiencies, and learning rates. Several training models, as well as variations on each model, are available to the clinician. Most widely known and used is the "basic training" approach, which includes instructions to the patient, modeling of appropriate use of skills, behavioral rehearsal, prompting, and positive feedback with homework. Incorporated into the basic training model are methods for improving the patient's perception of the social situation; understanding of the needs, desires, rights, and responsibilities of himself and the other person in the situation; processing of these perceptions for consideration of options for responding in the situation; and finally, the sending of a response back to the other person.

A somewhat more recent innovation in social skills training has been the design of "modules" for highly prescribed development of skills for achieving affiliation and independent living (Goldstein et al. 1976; Wallace et al. 1985). An advantage of a modular approach to skills training is its "exportability" to other practitioners. A module is self-contained, with a trainer's manual, a patient's handbook, and videocassettes or audiocassettes that serve to demonstrate, or model, appropriate skills. In the modules for training social and independent living skills being offered at the Brentwood (Psychiatric) Division of the West Los Angeles VA Medical Center, groups of 4 to 12 patients are led by one or two trainers. Trainers are occupational therapists, mental health associates, social workers, nurses, psychiatrists, and psychologists. Modules have been designed for teaching medication self-management skills, leisure and recreational skills, conversation skills, social problem-solving skills, money management, home maintenance, and grooming.

Some chronic patients, particularly those with thought disorders and distractibility, cannot sustain attention to the variants of social skills training described above. Such patients would have great difficulty, for instance, sitting quietly for 45 to 90 minutes in a group in which the training takes place. For the more regressed, incoherent, and floridly psychotic patients, an "attention-focusing procedure" for training basic conversational skills has been devised (Liberman et al. 1985).

THE BASIC TRAINING MODEL

Social skills training is generally conducted in a group room, but a hospital or community mental health center day room or recreation room can double for training purposes. Training can also take place in natural settings, such as in the patient's home, on the job, or in community facilities. The therapeutic process is designed to gradually shape the patient's behavior by reinforcing approximations or components of the ultimately desired skill. For example, the following are specific behavioral components to three general social skills that can be trained in sequence (Goldstein et al. 1976):

Starting a Conversation

1. Choose the right time and place.
2. Greet the other person.
3. Make small talk about the immediate situation or some common interest.
4. Judge if the other person is listening and wants to continue the chat.
5. Open the main topic you want to talk about.

Responding to a Complaint

1. Listen openly to the complaint.
2. Ask the person to explain anything you don't understand.
3. Show that you understand the other person's thoughts and feelings.
4. Tell the other person your thoughts and feelings, accepting responsibility if appropriate.
5. Summarize the steps to be taken to resolve the complaint by each party.

Asking for Help

1. Define the problem that troubles you.
2. Decide if you want to seek help for the problem.
3. Identify the people who might be available to help you.
4. Make a choice of a potential helper to approach.
5. Tell the helper about your problem.

6. Make a positive request for assistance, indicating how you would value the help.

SETTING GOALS FOR SOCIAL SKILLS TRAINING

At the beginning of the training session, the patient formulates, with the help of the counselor or trainer, the goals and scenes to be used in the training process. Patients, and their relatives or caretakers, are encouraged to participate actively in choosing their behavioral goals for the session. Some patients, however, need much guidance and direction in the selection of appropriate goals, particularly in the early stages of training. The counselor, therapist, or trainer should not shrink from sharing the responsibility for goal setting and choosing scenes. Ethical precepts and knowledge of developmental milestones, age, and culture-appropriate goals and values can guide the therapist in this responsibility.

When helping the patient decide on training goals, the therapist should make use of all information that he or she has on that person—including mental status, psychiatric and social history, behavioral assessments, family reports, and current assessment of assets and deficits. Practice scenes usually overlap with real life assignments that are to be subsequently given to the patient. Some scenes and goals are better than others. The following criteria for selecting goals and scenes may be useful to the practitioner:

1. Positive and constructive behaviors should be chosen rather than the tack of decreasing the frequency of some unwanted behavior or interaction. For example, requesting a desired change in the actions of a relative is preferable to complaining about past frustrations.
2. Functional behaviors should be chosen whenever possible, rather than "convenience" behaviors. Functional refers to those skills that if acquired, would provide maximum payoff to the patient in his or her real life situations. For example, practicing how to compromise and negotiate with a social service worker in a community agency that the patient must deal with subsequent to discharge from the hospital is preferable to practicing negotiation skills with a nursing staff member with whom the patient has had a conflict.
3. High-frequency interactions should be chosen over those that occur only occasionally, since this provides more practice opportunities to consolidate the skills into one's repertoire. For example, initiating conversations would be preferable to learning how to return defective merchandise for a socially withdrawn individual; similarly, asking the boss to repeat instructions on a task would be better to practice than would asking the boss for a raise. Greeting a relative at the end of a work day would be a better scene to practice than giving birthday greetings.

LEARNING EXERCISE

Consider a patient that you have worked with clinically. Pretend that this patient has come to you for social skills training. What goals and scenes might you propose or expect the patient to present as grist for the social skills training mill? From among the many possible goals and interpersonal scenes, choose one that has positive, functional, and high-frequency features.

THE BASIC TRAINING PROCESS

In a typical session, the patient is requested to role-play a problematic interpersonal situation with another patient or the trainer. Formulation of a scene that simulates the problem may be aided by determining a) the goal of the interaction, b) the most effective way to achieve the goal, and c) with whom and in what situations the problem occurs. Ideally, scenes should be selected that mirror, as much as possible, the real and significant life events, although standard role-play scenes are used in many programs. The stepwise procedures for employing basic social skills training are depicted in the flow chart in Figure 11.

The following is an example of training that uses the basic social skills model. Bob, a 32-year-old patient with chronic schizophrenia who has had multiple admissions to psychiatric hospitals over the past 10 years, has difficulty in conversing with other people. Training focuses on conversation. At an early stage of training, the therapist (T) is working with Bob to ask questions of others and on making appropriate self-disclosures, so friendship might develop. Nonverbal behaviors like eye contact and expressing appropriate affect will be targeted for later stages of training.

Therapist: Alright Bob, I want you to practice having a conversation with Jim [another patient in the group]. Talk to Jim for a few minutes about whatever you want, but remember to ask him questions and tell him about yourself. Do you understand, Bob?

Bob: Yes, I understand, but I don't think I can do it.

Therapist: I'd like you to try. Just do the best you can.

Bob: Good. Jim, you start the conversation off.

Jim: Okay. Hi Bob, how are you today?

Bob: I'm fine, Jim. How are you?

Jim: Very well, Bob. Thanks for asking.

Bob: What have you been doing today?

Jim: I've been working hard. Later today I'm going to the beach with a friend.

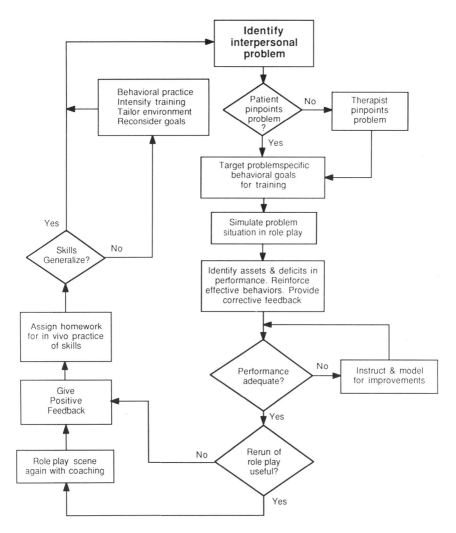

FIGURE 11: Flow chart describing steps in the structured and systematic method of basic social skills training. The response of the patient to each step in the sequence determines the extensiveness of training required. Basic social skills training can be done in individual, family, or group therapy modes.

Bob: That sounds like fun. Do you go to the beach often?
Jim: Yes, I do. I really enjoy the ocean.
Bob: What else do you like to do?
Jim: I like to go to the movies.
Bob: Have you seen any good movies lately?

Jim: No, I haven't been able to afford the movies lately.
Therapist: Okay. That's fine. Let's review your performance, Bob.

At the conclusion of the scene, the therapist gives feedback to the patient. Positive aspects of the performance are emphasized, along with areas that need improvement. Feedback is often accompanied by playback of a videotape of positive segments of the patient's performance.

Therapist: Let's look at the videotape, Bob, to see how well you did. In general, you asked a lot of good questions. When Jim said he likes to go to the beach, you asked, "Do you go to the beach often." Then when he said he likes to go to movies, you asked if he has seen any lately. Those are excellent questions, Bob. You are making great progress in asking questions to get to know others better.

Two points need to be made about this positive feedback. First, it is very specific. The trainer noted exact instances when the skill was appropriately applied. Second, the patient was praised or reinforced for using the skill correctly. Next, the therapist points out ways in which the patient may improve his performance.

Therapist: Bob, you asked some good questions, but you did not make any self-disclosures. For example, when Jim said he enjoys the beach, you could have said, "I like the beach, too" instead of asking him what else he likes to do. Telling people about yourself is very important because people will get to know you better and maybe make friends with you.

Again, the corrective feedback is very specific and constructive, to help the patient know exactly how he could have improved. A brief rationale for using the skill is also usually given. The next step in training might involve the trainer modeling the correct usage of the skills while the patient observes closely.

Therapist: Bob, you have been making great progress on making self-disclosures. Pay close attention now. I'm going to have a conversation with Jim. I will ask him questions and tell him some things about myself. Listen carefully so you can learn how to have better conversations.

Following the modeling scene, the patient would be asked to repeat the role-play scene. Feedback is provided after the scene, and then the session is terminated. Progress is usually measured by assessments taken each day of training. Role-play conversations are often used to assess changes in the targeted skills. Sometimes the role-plays during training are used for assessment purposes; other times, assessments are taken after training. Training usually continues until a criterion for adequate performance is met. One clinically sound criterion is the completion of a "homework assignment" in a natural setting that is linked to the practiced skill.

Social skills training is a very active and directive therapy. The therapist or trainer must prepare for the sessions in advance and be able to quickly determine relevant interpersonal goals and scenes to use in the training. Goal setting can be accomplished prior to the social skills training session, for example, in a planning meeting (Liberman et al. 1975) or through consultation with a patient's case manager or primary therapist. Alternatively, goals and scenes can be set through focused interviewing of the patient at the start of the skills training session.

The process of training requires movement and activity on the part of the therapist. The therapist, as shown in Figures 12 and 13, is out of his or her seat, in a coaching stance ready to provide prompts, verbal rewards, and encouragement to the patient as the interaction unfolds.

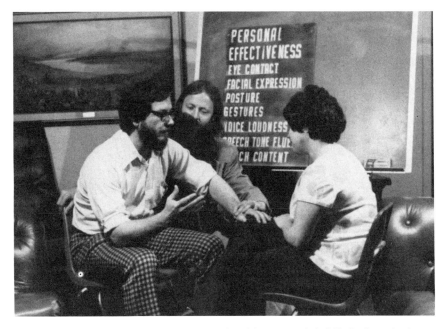

FIGURE 12: A patient is being coached by a social skills trainer to lean forward and use his hands more effectively in practicing communication skills. Note that the trainer, in this case a psychiatric nurse, is situated close to the patient in a kneeling position and is manually guiding the patient's hand during a practice trial, or behavioral rehearsal. Posters such as the one in the picture are typically used to visually prompt appropriate elements of nonverbal expression.

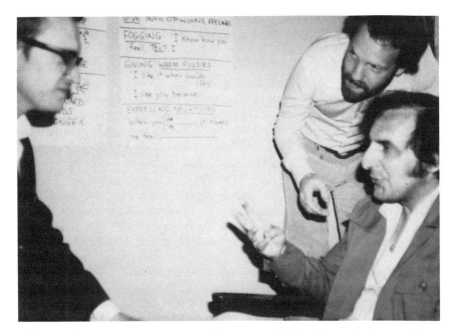

FIGURE 13:   Social skills training is being carried out by a trainer or therapist who is prompting and giving "on line" feedback and encouragement to a patient who is practicing conversation skills. The therapist takes an active and directive role in training and observes the interaction as it unfolds to determine interventions to use. Posters on the wall serve to remind patients and therapists of the components of social skills to be mastered.

A practitioner who is tied to the nondirective and reflective mode of therapy would have great difficulty adopting social skills training into his or her armamentarium.

CASE EXAMPLE ⸻⸻⸻⸻⸻⸻⸻⸻⸻⸻⸻⸻⸻⸻⸻⸻

Manny was a 54-year-old Mexican-American who had been previously hospitalized with a diagnosis of schizophrenia. He reported hearing voices that told him to write nonsensical phrases in a notebook he carried and on the walls of his home and his workplace. After a period of remission, he suffered a relapse of his symptoms despite maintenance use of neuroleptic drugs. Concomitantly, he began withdrawing from social contact and spent increasing periods of time alone or meandering the streets, muttering to himself and scribbling in his notebook. When he began to write on the walls of the factory where he worked, his supervisor laid him off. However, because Manny had a long and faithful employment record, the supervisor communicated to the mental health center that he would be willing to save his job if his symptoms were controlled. Manny also had a supportive and concerned family who were willing to cooperate in his treatment.

As part of his treatment plan, Manny participated in a thrice-weekly social skills training group in the mental health center's day hospital. The broad goals for Manny in social skills training were 1) to reestablish social contact with friends, 2) to take his wife and children out to visit relatives and to social gatherings, and 3) to return to work when ready. These goals were felt to be functional alternatives to his symptomatic behaviors. It was predicted that as he increased his social participation, his symptoms would abate.

The following scenes were role-played by Manny during the social skills training group sessions and were then subsequently carried out in homework assignments:

1. Telephoning a friend to ask how he is doing.
2. Telephoning a friend to ask him to go to wrestling matches.
3. Dropping by a friend's home to say hello.
4. Inviting friends over for dinner with Manny's family.
5. Having a 10-minute conversation with each of his daughters.
6. Having a family discussion to plan a weekend social outing.
7. Calling the city recreation department to get information about free recreational activities for families in the community.
8. Visiting his work supervisor to tell him of his improvement and activities at the day treatment center.
9. Visiting his work supervisor to ask for his job back.
10. Starting a conversation with co-workers on coffee break.

Manny had to practice some of the scenes three or four times before he was able to successfully complete the assignment in the community. Especially with patients like Manny who are not very verbal, social skills training is a deliberate and sometimes arduous process. The principle of shaping must be used along with the corollary of "starting where the patient is." For individuals like Manny who have seldom been reinforced for initiating or maintaining interpersonal interaction, progress during training may come slowly. The skilled therapist is prepared for this and is on the lookout for small improvements in the patient to reinforce. Manny showed steady progress and eventually returned to his job. His symptoms cleared and he was able to resume normal social and family routines.

Positive changes in the social skills levels of patients must eventually be maintained in the natural environment, otherwise the patient's newly acquired skills will deteriorate. One means for enhancing transfer of skills to other environments is by training the patients in general strategies for dealing with a variety of social situations. This form of social skills training focuses on developing problem-solving capacities in the patient.

TRAINING IN PROBLEM-SOLVING SKILLS

Inadequate performance in social situations may, in part, result from deficits in cognitive problem-solving abilities. Since chronic psychiatric patients have been found to be deficient in basic problem-solving skills, teaching components of problem solving can be added to the basic training model. Interpersonal communications is viewed as a three-stage process, requiring

1. "Receiving" skills—attending to and accurately perceiving cues and contextual elements of interpersonal situations.
2. "Processing" skills—generating response alternatives, weighing the consequences of each alternative, and selecting optimal options.
3. "Sending" skills—using the chosen option for an effective social response, integrating both verbal and nonverbal skills.

As in the basic training model, an interpersonal scene is role-played and videotaped. After the role-play, the therapist asks specific questions to assess the patient's receiving skills. The following is an example of an interchange between therapist and patient at the conclusion of the role-play.

Jim, 38 years old and diagnosed as a chronic schizophrenic, has been hospitalized on several occasions. Currently an outpatient, Jim has just become part of a social skills training group that emphasizes heterosocial or dating skills. A role-play conversation between Jim and Trudy, another patient, has just been completed, and the therapist is about to assess Jim's receiving skills.

Therapist: That was good, Jim. You participated well in the conversation with Trudy. I think this will be a good start for training. I want to ask you a few questions first, though. Jim, what was Trudy talking about?

Jim: She was talking about walking on the beach and enjoying sunsets and cool drives.

Therapist: How did she feel?

Jim: I think she felt relaxed. She seemed comfortable with me.

Therapist: Very good. What was your goal in this interaction, Jim?

Jim: I think it was to get to know Trudy better.

Therapist: That is right. To get to know Trudy better and to feel comfortable enough to ask her for a date. You are doing very well so far, Jim. You are paying attention, and you have a good idea of what you need to work on.

The therapist asked specific questions of Jim to be able to assess if he was accurately perceiving the situation. After completion of the receiving skills stage, processing skills are assessed and trained, if necessary. This stage involves generating response options and identifying positive and negative consequences of the potential options. The patient again role-plays a conversation with the trainer or another patient and is asked another series of questions following the scene.

Jim has just completed a role-play conversation with Trudy, in which he asked her for a date. In the following sequence, Jim's processing skills are assessed.

Therapist: That was a very good conversation, Jim. You seemed relaxed, for the most part. What could you have done when Trudy said she already had plans for Saturday night?

Jim: I'm not sure. I guess she didn't want to go out with me.

Therapist: That may not be right, Jim. What could you have done to check that out?

Jim: Maybe I could have asked her out for another night.

Therapist: Exactly. How do you think Trudy would have felt if you had asked her out for another night?

Jim: I guess that I am too interested in her.

Therapist: Possibly, but more than likely she would have been flattered that you were really interested in her. What could she have done if she was interested in going out with you?

Jim: She could have said that she was busy for that night but she would like to go out with me another time.

Therapist: Very good. How could you have achieved your goal of making a date with her?

Jim: I guess by being more persistent and not feeling rejected when she said she was busy.

Therapist: Exactly right, Jim.

The therapist asked specific questions to gauge Jim's processing abilities and prompted alternative responses within Jim's repertoire of skills. The next step is to assess the patient's sending skills. If video equipment is available, the therapist and patient view the videotape of the role-play and the patient is asked to assess his or her performance in response to the therapist's questions.

Therapist: I want to ask you some more questions now, regarding the conversation you had with Trudy. How was your voice volume, Jim?

Jim: It was all right. Maybe it was too soft.

Therapist: Good. I think you could have spoken a little louder also. That's something we can work on later. How was your facial expression?

Jim: I think it was good. I looked interested in Trudy and I was smiling quite a bit.

Therapist: Right. Maybe you felt a little nervous, but your face showed relaxation. What about your posture?

Jim: It looked all right to me.

Therapist: Well, maybe you could have leaned closer to her more. That would show interest. Do you think you made enough eye contact?

Jim: I guess I was looking down a bit too much, but I did make some eye contact.

Therapist: You did make some good eye contact. We can work on increasing the eye contact that you make. Jim, basically you are able to look at yourself on the screen and have a good idea of your strengths and weaknesses. That is a very good start.

The therapist again asked specific questions to determine how the subject perceived his sending skills. As in all stages of social skills training, reinforcement is given for appropriate responding. In all three stages of this model, the therapist may prompt or model correct responses or ask that the scene be role-played again. When the patient performs the sending skills at an acceptable level, assessment and training continue with a new scene.

LEARNING EXERCISE

Now you should be ready to take the plunge and try to employ some of the social skills training techniques with one of your patients. Plan your strategy in advance of a therapy session, which might more easily be an individual session for your initiation into the fraternity of social skills trainers. Consider all the steps required for training an interpersonal skill and be modest in the goal or scene you select in conjunction with the patient. The guidelines listed below may be helpful cues to you as you prepare for the session and then go through the steps.

STEPWISE GUIDELINES FOR TRAINING OF SOCIAL SKILLS

Behaviorally oriented social skills training is highly structured, and the training process follows a prescribed set of steps, each based on social learning principles. The following guidelines set out the training steps that can be used by neophyte therapists and trainers. It is important to recognize that the structure involved in the training procedure actually frees the therapist or trainer to instill his or her own personal style into the interactions with the patients. In this manner, the systematic nature of the training procedure promotes spontaneity and liveliness in the therapist-patient relationship and ensures cohesion and active participation in the group.

1. Specify the interpersonal problem by asking
   - What emotion or communication skill is lacking or not being appropriately expressed?
   - What social and living situations are causing problems or challenges?
   - What daily life situations must the individual be able to manage and master?
   - With whom does the patient want and need to improve social contact or obtain life needs?
   - Where and when does the problem situation occur?

2. Formulate a scene that simulates or recapitulates the features of the real life problem situation.

3. Elicit the patient's short-term and long-term goals in the situation. Goals may be related to instrumental needs (obtaining or satisfying a tangible need) or affectional needs (acquiring or maintaining friendship or social support). Ask:
   - What is your short-term or immediate goal?
   - What is your long-term goal with this person and situation?

4. Identify the assets, deficits, and excesses in the patient's performance during the "dry run" by focusing on receiving, processing, and sending skills. Ask the patient the following questions:
   - Who spoke with you in that situation?
   - What did the other person say?
   - How was the other person feeling?
   - Did you get your short-term and long-term goals met?
   - Name alternative ways you might have handled the situation.
   - For each alternative, consider whether or not your short-term and long-term goals would have been met.
   - Which alternative would be the most reasonable and most likely to lead to your meeting your goals? Why?

5. Give positive feedback for specific elements that were well done or correctly expressed. Give constructive feedback with correct responses for deficits and errors.

6. Arrange for a model to demonstrate more adaptive alternatives and prompt the patient to again give a rationale for the chosen alternative.

7. Direct the patient's attention to the behavioral elements being modeled through on-line annotation.

8. Engage the patient in replay of scene or rerun, offering instructions and prompts as needed to initiate action and remind the patient of behaviors for remediation.

9. Provide on-line support, prompts, and positive feedback in coaching the patient to improve performance during rerun of scene.

10. Give generous praise to reinforce progress or even effort after the patient rehearses the rerun.

11. Focus on all dimensions of social competence in social skills training, including
    • Topical content and semantic choice of words and phrases
    • Nonverbal components of expression
    • Timing and reciprocity
    • Appropriateness of context, cues, and expectations
    • Receiving (social perception) and processing skills
    • Social problem solving

12. Shape behavioral changes in small increments, starting with where the patient has assets and without expecting much improvement at any one time.

13. Instigate implementation and follow-through of social problem solving by giving a homework assignment that the patient can carry out in the natural environment.

14. Ensure that the patient comprehends the problem, the short- and long-term goals, and the plan of action by reviewing these systematically at the end of training.

15. Generalize improvements in social skill into real life settings and strengthen durability over time through
    • Repeated practice and overlearning
    • Specific, attainable, and functional homework assignments
    • Positive feedback for successful transfer of skills to real life
    • Training in use of self-instructions, self-evaluation, and self-reinforcement
    • Involving significant others in the training and implementation
    • Fading the structure and frequency of the training

THE TEACHING INTERACTION

A variation of the social skills training model, useful for spontaneous teaching of patients in natural settings like inpatient wards or board-and-care homes, is called the Teaching Interaction. The Teaching Interaction is a sequence of training steps that helps to manage and contain minor disruptive and preaggressive behaviors. Originally developed to supplement the token economy motivational systems in group homes for delinquent youths, the Teaching Interaction both inculcates new interpersonal skills and strengthens relationships between staff members and patients.

The Teaching Interaction consists of 10 components that are implemented at the first indication of conflict, strife, or aggression between two individuals. If the responsibility for the initial agitation can be ascertained, the person having that responsibility goes through the Teaching Interaction procedure first. Many times it is impossible to attribute responsibility and so both patients need to go through the training steps. The 10 components or steps for a residential care operator, therapist, or nursing staff member are as follows:

1. Express positive affect to the offending patient (using a smile, a special greeting, or warm physical contact).

LEARNING EXERCISE

To gain greater empathy for patients who participate in social skills training, choose one of the following real life assignments and carry it out. Your experiences, objective and subjective, in completing these homework assignments can be discussed with relatives, friends, or colleagues.

1. Go to a coffee shop or bar, sit down, and request a glass of water without ordering any food or beverage.
2. Drive into a service station and ask the attendant to check your oil and water without purchasing any gasoline.
3. Go into an expensive clothing store or boutique and tell the salesperson that you don't wish to purchase anything, but you would like to try on one of the expensive garments.
4. Walk into an auto dealer's showroom and tell the salesperson that although you aren't interested in buying a car now, you would like to have a test drive.

These exercises may create for you an approximation of the tension and anxiety experienced by patients as they try out assignments that may appear easy to you but that are major challenges to their level of skill. The assignment card, depicted in Figure 14, is an example of an aid for encouraging patients' compliance with homework. Having a card, personally filled out and signed by their therapist or trainer, can boost patients' morale and serve as a bridge between training sessions. Patients can be instructed to carry the card with them in their pocket, wallet, or purse.

```
┌─────────────────────────────────────────────────────────────┐
│                 PERSONAL EFFECTIVENESS                        │
│                 ASSIGNMENT–REPORT CARD                        │
│                                                               │
│   Name_____        │
│   Date assignment given _____        │
│   PE Assignment _____        │
│   _____         │
│   _____         │
│                                                               │
│   Date assignment due _____(____)       │
│   (check when completed)                                      │
│                      Counselor's initials_____        │
└─────────────────────────────────────────────────────────────┘
```

Front of card

```
┌─────────────────────────────────────────────────────────────┐
│                                                               │
│          CUES FOR PERSONAL EFFECTIVENESS                      │
│                                                               │
│          1. Maintain EYE CONTACT                              │
│                                                               │
│          2. Use your HANDS                                    │
│                                                               │
│          3. Lean TOWARD the other person                      │
│                                                               │
│          4. Pleasant FACIAL EXPRESSION                        │
│                                                               │
│          5. Speak with FIRM TONE and FLUENT pace              │
│                                                               │
└─────────────────────────────────────────────────────────────┘
```

Back of card

FIGURE 14:   Homework assignments are an integral step in the social skills training process. By carrying out in real life what has been practiced in the training session, patients can generalize and internalize the new skills they have learned. Homework assignments are more likely completed if reminder cards or slips are handed out at the time of the session. The 2 × 4 card shown can be carried in a wallet or purse and serves to bridge the gap between training session and real life.

2. Praise what the patient has been able to accomplish in the recent past, or some positive progress or recent adaptive behavior.
3. Describe the inappropriate and disruptive behavior.
4. Describe the appropriate alternative behaviors that could be used in a similar situation.

5. Give a rationale to the patient for using the appropriate behavior.
6. Describe the consequences that must be imposed for the inappropriate behavior.
7. Request the patient to acknowledge what has happened.
8. Practice the situation that was conflict laden, using more appropriate alternatives to threats and violence.
9. Give feedback to the patient during the time he or she is practicing alternative behaviors, offering both praise and corrective feedback.
10. Reward the new and more appropriate behavior with praise and tangible reinforcers.

MODULES FOR TRAINING SOCIAL AND INDEPENDENT LIVING SKILLS

Because many chronic mental patients share a common spectrum of skills deficits for community living, it is feasible and efficient to "package" a generic set of training materials to cover these areas. One approach to generic packaging of skills training is modules that can be used by a wide diversity of mental health and rehabilitation professionals and paraprofessionals. Modules provide step-by-step instructions and can be used with little orientation and training for the practitioner. The trainer or therapist teaches the skills using a combination of videotaped demonstrations, focused instructions, specialized role-plays, social and videotaped feedback, and practice in the "real world."

For the practitioner, modules offer a structured protocol for teaching skills to patients that allows rapid and faithful delivery of the essential training while still permitting leeway for the personality and individual style of the trainer. For the patient, the module format mandates active and increasing degrees of participation in the therapeutic process, with the goal of enhanced ability to function autonomously.

Each module consists of a set of sequential exercises that

1. Introduces the patients to the purpose and rationale for the module and heightens their motivation to participate,
2. Trains the skills required to fulfill their needs in the subject area of the module,
3. Teaches the patients how to gather the resources they will require to put their skills to use,
4. Teaches them how to anticipate and solve problems that might be encountered as they try to employ their skills, and
5. Arranges for practice of the skills in the "real world."

As shown in Table 24, each module comprises a number of skill areas that when integrated and cumulatively learned, provide the abilities and knowledge to cope with the challenges presented by living in the community by that segment of life in the community. Thus, the skill

TABLE 24: Examples of Modules and Skill Areas Within Modules for Training Social and Independent Living Skills

---

Module: **Home Finding and Maintenance**
Skill Areas: Resources for discovering housing leads
Factors in selecting appropriate residences
Phone and in-person contacts
Moving in—cleaning, utilities, rent
Decorating the house

Module: **Money Management**
Skill Areas: Budgeting and record-keeping income and expenditures
Savings and checking accounts
Best buys for the consumer
Reducing consumer debts

Module: **Conversational Skills**
Skill Areas: Active listening skills
Levels of self-disclosure
Identifying others' emotions
Open- and close-ended questions
Changing the topic of conversation

---

areas composing the Money Management Module should enable a patient who learns the skills to function with a limited amount of funds in a community residence.

In the Medication Management Module, the following cluster of skills is deemed important for accomplishing goals in reliable use of neuroleptic drugs:

- obtaining and using basic information about the benefits of neuroleptic antipsychotic medication,
- learning safe methods of self-administration of medication,
- identifying and coping with side effects, and
- negotiating medication issues and problems with physicians.

Within each skill area, as depicted in Figure 15, a set of component behavioral competencies are taught that are required for coping with others in the community. In the case of the Medication Management Module's skill area "Negotiating medication issues with a physician," requisite competencies for a patient to learn include greeting the physician pleasantly, specifying the problem and its duration that relates to the medication, and making a positive and courteous request for assistance in managing the side effect.

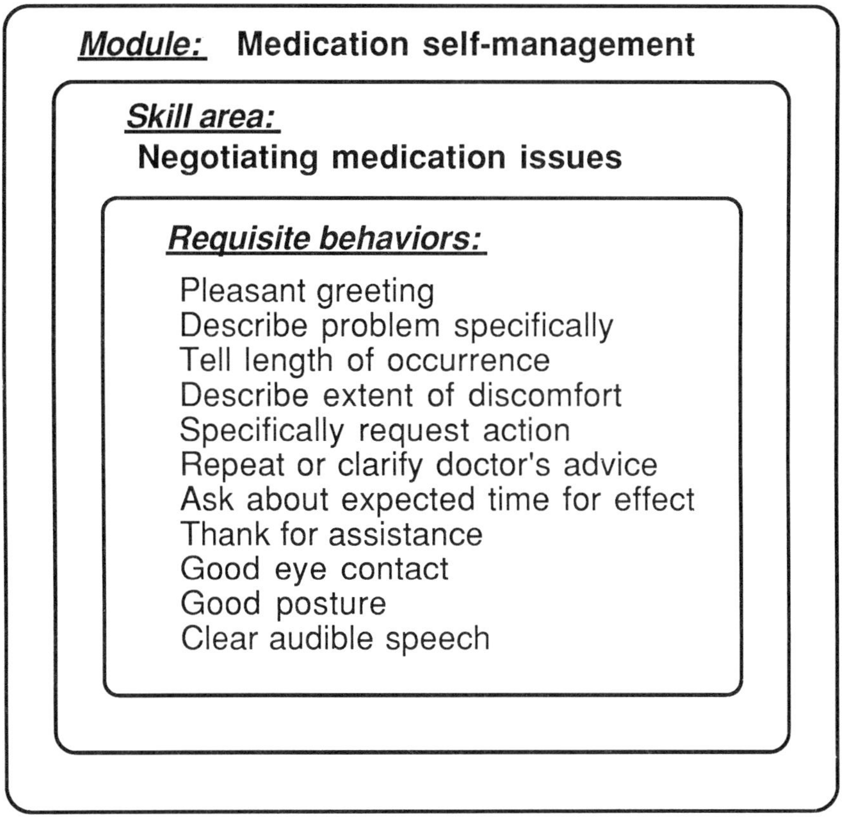

> ### *Module:*   Medication self-management
>
> > ### *Skill area:*
> > **Negotiating medication issues**
> >
> > > ### *Requisite behaviors:*
> > > Pleasant greeting
> > > Describe problem specifically
> > > Tell length of occurrence
> > > Describe extent of discomfort
> > > Specifically request action
> > > Repeat or clarify doctor's advice
> > > Ask about expected time for effect
> > > Thank for assistance
> > > Good eye contact
> > > Good posture
> > > Clear audible speech

FIGURE 15:   A diagrammatic representation of the interlocking elements of a skills-training module depicts the specific behavioral criteria required for patients in negotiating medication issues and problems with health care providers. Each module is divided into separate skill areas, with each area having specific, target behaviors for training.

The modules are designed to teach patients two types of competencies—the ability to perform skills necessary for successful community adjustment and the ability to solve problems that arise as obstacles to the use of these skills. The skills taught in each module have been identified as important for functioning by health and rehabilitation professionals. The skills in each module are taught through seven highly prescribed learning activities, which are repeated in each skill area. The learning activities are infused with principles of learning, delineated earlier in this chapter, that facilitate patients' acquiring the know-how of the module. One might view the learning activities of a module as tantamount to special education for the mentally disabled. The learning activities are

- Introduction to the skill area
- Videotape and questions/answers
- Role-play
- Resource management
- Outcome problems
- In vivo exercises
- Homework assignments

In order to help guide trainers through the complexities of the seven learning activities, each activity is preceded by explicit directions to the therapist/trainer, a list of materials needed, and a summary of the steps to follow.

Introduction to the Skill Area
In the introduction, patients are encouraged to identify the goals of the module and of each skill area, the steps necessary to achieve the goals, and the benefits that will accrue if the goals are achieved. The aim here is to motivate the patients to participate actively. In addition, the exchange of questions and answers in this exercise introduces patients to the terminology used in various aspects of the training.

Videotape and Questions/Answers
In the second learning activity, patients view videotaped demonstrations of correct performance of the skills. The tape is stopped periodically to allow the trainer to ask questions that assess the patient's attentiveness and comprehension. (Here, as in most of the exercises in the modules, both the questions and the gist of the answers are provided in the trainer's manual.) If there are incorrect answers, feedback is provided and the videotape is replayed. Presenting the information until it is understood allows patients to proceed at their own pace, thereby individualizing the training even though it is offered in a group.

Role-Play
In the third learning activity, patients are asked to role-play or practice the skills they have just viewed. Videotaping this performance for subsequent review is recommended. When reviewing the role-play, the trainer and other patients evaluate the performance for the presence of such behavior as good eye contact, alert posture, and audible voice volume—in other words, good communication skills. Feedback is presented in a positive light, minimizing the destructive consequences of criticism. Role-plays are repeated as many times as needed for patients to demonstrate the knowledge and skills depicted in the videotape.

Resource Management

After each skill has been correctly role-played, patients are taught how to obtain and manage the resources required to use that particular skill. Resources must be gathered for patients to implement a particular community living skill. For example, even if an individual has the skills to perform competently during a job interview, he or she needs money, clothes, a typed resume, and transportation to effect the interview. The training methods consist of role-played exercises and interactions designed to assess the patient's ability to process the various alternatives open for effective resource management. The trainer describes the skill and then asks a series of questions designed to have patients actively consider the resources (for example, time, money, people, places, materials, transportation, telephone) they might need to perform the skill. For each resource mentioned, patients discuss how they could go about obtaining it (for example, how they could find a phone for calling the doctor or pharmacist, how they could arrange transportation to the hospital or clinic). Patients then evaluate each resource by deciding what the advantages and disadvantages might be.

Outcome Problems

After patients have been trained to marshall the necessary resources, they are taught to solve the problems presented when the environment fails to respond as expected and unanticipated barriers to effective use of knowledge and skills must be overcome. Inevitably, patients will encounter unexpected obstacles to obtaining their goals, despite their best presentation of skills. For example, if an individual arrives for a job interview or for a medication appointment, but the employer or physician is not there as planned, the patient needs to have strategies for responding. Many patients will respond to such baffling and frustrating experiences with hostility, passivity, or stereotyped symptoms. By teaching the patient a variety of alternative response modes (such as asking to see a surrogate, requesting another appointment as early as possible, asking to wait), the patient becomes more resilient and better able to meet short- and long-term needs. Here, as for resource management, problem-solving skills are systematically applied.

The trainer begins by reading a description of an attempt to use the skill and the response made by the environment. Then the trainer asks the patients questions designed to have them consider a variety of alternatives that might remove the obstacle. The entire problem-solving process is aided by the use of a form listing seven steps for problem solving.

Again, there are no predetermined answers; however, the trainer does try to steer the patient toward using alternatives that minimize expenditure of resources (including time and money). The use of the systematic problem-solving process for each skill area helps the patient to internalize and generalize the process.

In Vivo Exercises

It is imperative that patients have the opportunity to practice in the natural environment the skills they have learned. The in vivo exercises take the patients out of the training group—but not too far out. Patients perform the skills in their world, with the trainer along to observe and collect data regarding performance as well as to provide prompting, encouragement, and positive feedback. An example of an in vivo exercise is to have the patient ask questions about his or her medication to the program nurse, with the module trainer along as backup.

Homework Assignments

Finally, patients are given the opportunity to perform independently the skills they have learned. Since it is the goal of the program to teach them to function independently, this represents the ultimate step in training. Wherever possible, their performances are evaluated by examining tangible evidence or permanent products of the patients' efforts. For example, if the assignment is to obtain information about medication from a community pharmacist, the patient can report the information to the therapist and bring back the pharmacist's business card.

CASE EXAMPLE

Ben is a 26-year-old black veteran who joined the army after dropping out of high school in the 11th grade. He served as a communications specialist, enjoyed the work, and received his high school equivalency certificate while in the army. Since his discharge from the army, on a medical disability, Ben has lived in a variety of places. At times he has existed in a homeless state, living on handouts and soup kitchens while sleeping on the streets of the city. He has also lived in board and care homes. He has worked at several part-time jobs, for example, as a dishwasher and cook in a fast-food shop, as a clerk and stockman in a drug store, and, most recently, as a taxi driver.

Ben's social support network was limited. His family lives in a distant state and he has only limited contact with them. Of a handful of friends, only one is seen more often than once a month. Ben has had two psychiatric hospitalizations during the past five years. His most recent hospitalization occurred just prior to his entry into the social and independent living skills program. At that admission, he had delusions and hallucinations characteristic of schizophrenia that responded readily to neuroleptic drugs. Ben had a long history of failure to adhere to his medication regimens. After two months in the hospital, he was referred to the skills training program to help him prepare for community reentry. The initial evaluation by the skills program found several areas of skill deficits—home finding, leisure and recreational skills, medication management, job-seeking skills, and conversation skills. Ben and the skills trainers agreed to prioritize medication management as the first order of business.

A typical introductory session of the Medication Management Module, with the therapist, Ben, and a fellow patient named George, is as follows:

Therapist: Today we are beginning the Medication Management Module. The goal of this module is to provide you with the information and skills necessary for you to manage your medication properly and safely. This is important for you to know since you are taking these medications. In the module, you will see videotapes that present the important information to you. Pay close attention, because I will ask you questions whose answers will highlight the skills that are being taught.

Therapist: Ben, what is the goal of this module?

Ben: To learn about my medication.

Therapist: Right! George, why would you need to learn this information?

George: Because I'm taking the meds and I need to know how to take them . . . to tell me what they are supposed to do.

Therapist: That's very good George. If you take your meds right, what positive consequences will happen?

George: I won't hear any voices or see things.

Therapist: Yes. How about you Ben?

Ben: They make me think clearer.

Therapist: Excellent.

Following the general introduction to the module, training progresses through the various skills in the module that patients have just identified. Training includes a combination of behavioral techniques including role-played practices, social and videotaped demonstrations, and social and videotaped feedback. Following an introduction to the skill that emphasizes the relationship of the skill to the overall goal of the module, training involves two basic sets of procedures.

First, patients view a videotaped demonstration of the correct performance of the skill. The tape is periodically stopped and patients are asked questions to assess their attentiveness to and comprehension of the information conveyed in the demonstration. Incorrect answers result in replaying the videotape and highlighting the information needed to correctly answer the question when it is repeated. Evaluation data are collected about the number of correct and incorrect answers as a means of monitoring each patient's progress through the modules.

In the second set of procedures, patients are asked to practice the skills they have just viewed in a role-play. This performance is videotaped for subsequent review by the patient and therapist. Positive feedback is provided for the performance of criteria behavior and suggestions for improvement to highlight absent criteria behaviors are made. The role-play is then reenacted and the process is repeated until the client exhibits 100 percent of the criteria behavior included in the scene's skills.

To illustrate the training process, excerpts are given here from the skill area on negotiating medication problems with physicians. Training begins with an introduction to the goals of the scene.

Therapist: In this scene, you will learn how to present information about a side effect of your medication to your doctor in a way that will maximize your chances of obtaining positive action toward relief of the problem. What is the goal of this scene?

Ben: To learn how to talk to a doctor about my side effects.

Therapist: Right, and what is the goal of this module?

Ben: To learn how to manage my medication.

Therapist: You've got it! Let's watch the tape.

The modeling tape is shown to the group at this point. The tape depicts a patient discussing a side effect of his medication with a doctor. Edited pauses appear on the tape, and the therapist asks questions about what had just been demonstrated. Two kinds of questions are asked, some that are primarily attentional and others that highlight the relevant criteria behavior.

Therapist: Ben, who is in this scene?

Ben: A doctor and a patient.

Therapist: Right. George do you remember their names?

George: Dr. Smith and . . . Frank.

Therapist: Exactly right. You two are really paying close attention. George, what did Frank do when he first met the doctor?

George: Said hello to him.

Therapist: Yes, did you notice anything else?

George: He introduced himself.

Therapist: Right! It's important to greet the doctor pleasantly and to be sure and introduce yourself, especially if the doctor hasn't seen you in a while or if he is a new doctor for you. Ben, what was Frank's problem in the scene?

Ben: He was drowsy at work.

Therapist: Yes. What information did he tell the doctor about this drowsiness?

Ben: That it's bothering him.

Therapist: OK, was there anything else?

Ben: No.

Therapist: How about you, George?

George: He just said he was drowsy and it was interfering with his work.

Therapist: Good. It's important to describe very carefully what the problem is and how much it's bothering you. But that's not all you should tell him. Let's view that tape again. Watch closely for all the information he tells the doctor.

Patients are then asked to practice, in a role-play, the skills they have observed in the video. In this example, instructions are to describe the side effect and request action to help alleviate a side effect if possible. In many instances, other patients provide extremely good suggestions for improvements in performance.

The following excerpt illustrates a typical patient's performance and the way in which the therapist provides feedback to the patient.

Ben: Hello, doctor. I wanted to talk to you about a problem I've been having that I think is a side effect of my medication.

Doctor: OK.

Ben: For a few days, my right hand has been shaking. I can't seem to make it stop and it's really bothering me. Could you do something about it?

Doctor: Let's increase your side effect medication to three tablets per day instead of one.

Ben: OK, how long should it be before the shaking stops?

Doctor: Very soon . . . a day or two at the most.

Ben: I hope it works, doctor. Thank you for your help.

Therapist: You did a really nice job there. Let's start with your nonverbal behavior. Your eye contact, voice volume, and speech fluency were excellent. In fact, I couldn't have done a better job myself. What do you think?

Ben: Well, I tried hard to remember the things we discussed. I wish I'd sat up straighter.

ATTRIBUTES OF CLINICIANS USING SOCIAL SKILLS TRAINING

Trainers of social and independent living skills should have the basic assets required of any good therapist who works successfully with patients with chronic mental illness: excellent interpersonal skills, familiarity with behavior therapy principles, enthusiasm for working with severely disabled people, capacity both to follow detailed procedures and to adapt them to situational constraints, and the ability to collect behavioral data. Trainers must learn the basic elements used in teaching social skills: modeling, behavior rehearsal, prompting, feedback, reinforcement, and homework assignments. An agency adopting skills-training modules must also provide administrative and organizational support to meet the demands of this unique service delivery system.

ATTENTION-FOCUSING SOCIAL SKILLS TRAINING

A patient's ability to attend to relevant features of the training situation for periods of 30 to 90 minutes is assumed in both the basic and problem-solving training models. However, a significant number of chronic psychiatric patients are characterized by such severe cognitive, memory, and attentional impairments that they cannot participate collaboratively in a group-based training procedure. A method for training social skills based on procedures that help to focus the patient's attention on relevant training materials while minimizing demands on cognitive abilities has recently been developed at the Camarillo/University of California at Los Angeles Clinical Research Center.

The attention-focusing procedure is characterized by multiple, relatively short training trials, in which each discrete trial has a discriminable beginning and end. A highly structured training situation minimizes distractibility by carefully manipulating the teaching components in each trial. This procedure has been used to train conversational skills in highly distractible, institutionalized chronic schizophrenics. While role-playing, corrective feedback, modeling, prompting, and reinforcement are important elements, the attention-focusing model is distinguished by the controlled and sequential presentation of the training components. A trainer initiates a conversation with the patient by making a statement. If the patient makes a correct response, he or she is praised and the response is sometimes reinforced with something to eat or drink. If a correct response is not forthcoming, the trainer implements a prompt sequence. The patient is praised if he or she responds appropriately following the prompts. The same statement is presented by the trainer until the patient responds correctly four times in succession. Then, responses to new conversational statements are trained.

CASE EXAMPLE ————————————————————————————————

The following is an example of attention focusing with a patient named Sue, a chronic schizophrenic hospitalized continuously for 15 years, who has been described as socially isolated and highly distractible. Social skills training is directed toward training Sue on how to compliment other people, among other skills. Sue is being trained individually by a therapist and an aide named Tom.

Tom: I just bought this shirt yesterday.
Sue: (no response)

Therapist: Sue, give Tom a compliment.
Sue: (no response)
Therapist: One compliment you can give is "That's a nice shirt."
Sue: (no response)
Tom: I just bought this shirt yesterday.
Sue: (no response)
Therapist: Sue, give Tom a compliment.
Sue: (no response)
Therapist: One compliment you can give is "That's a nice shirt."
Sue: That's a nice shirt.
Tom: Thank you very much.
Therapist: Very good, Sue. That is a nice compliment.
Tom: I just bought this shirt yesterday.
Sue: (no response)
Therapist: Sue, give Tom a compliment.
Sue: I like your shirt.
Tom: I'm glad you like it.
Therapist: That is a very good compliment, Sue.
Tom: I just bought this shirt yesterday.
Sue: That is a nice shirt.
Tom: Thank you, Sue.
Therapist: Very, very good Sue. Now you are making nice compliments.

Typically, patients are taught to make 8 to 12 alternative responses, or exemplars, in each domain of conversational skills. Steps are then taken to promote transfer of training to other appropriate situations, if generalization does not occur spontaneously. The attention-focusing model of skills training has been validated by training a group of patients on three conversational skills: asking questions, giving compliments, and making requests for engagement in activities with others. Results indicated that this highly structured procedure is effective for training social skills in withdrawn, thought-disordered, low-functioning chronic schizophrenic patients.

LEARNING EXERCISE

Now that you have been exposed to the various models for conducting systematic and structured social skills training, it is time to evaluate your own skills in using this modality with your patients. Review the following checklist of therapist competencies before and after applying the methods of social skills training to one or more of your patients. Then check off those skills that you feel you've gotten under your belt.

CHECKLIST OF THERAPIST SKILLS

☐ Actively help the client in setting and eliciting specific goals.

☐ Assist the patient in building possible scenes in terms of "What emotion or communication?"; "Who is the interpersonal target?"; and "Where and when?"

☐ Instruct the patient about rationale and procedure, to promote favorable expectations and orientation before role-playing begins.

☐ Structure patient role-playing by setting the scene and assigning roles to the patient and surrogates.

☐ Engage the patient in behavioral rehearsal—getting the patient to role-play with others.

☐ Model more appropriate alternatives for the patient.

☐ Prompt and cue the patient during the role-playing.

☐ Coach or "shadow" the patient—being out of your seat and closely supporting the patient.

☐ Give patient corrective feedback for specific behaviors.

☐ Ignore or suppress mildly disruptive behavior.

☐ Get physically within one foot of the patient during role-play.

☐ Touch the patient, if appropriate, for support and positive feedback.

☐ Suggest an alternative behavior for a problem situation that can be used and practiced during the behavioral rehearsal or role-play.

☐ Give specific homework assignment.

EFFECTIVENESS OF SOCIAL SKILLS TRAINING

Well-designed and controlled research studies have convincingly documented that psychiatric patients' deficient interpersonal behaviors can be improved by engaging them in highly directive instructional sessions, infused with learning principles, that aim at teaching, generalizing, and maintaining specific behavioral and cognitive skills. Over the past 15 years, more than 50 studies have been published on social skills training with psychiatric patients (for reviews, see Wallace et al. 1980; Liberman et al. 1985; Brady 1984). These studies provided the first evidence that social skills training was a feasible treatment strategy for major mental disorders and laid an empirical foundation for recent innovations in training techniques.

The results of these studies can be summarized by three conclusions:

1. Psychiatric patients can be trained in behaviors that will improve their social skills in specific interpersonal situations. The types of skills that have been learned through training include discrete behaviors, such as eye contact and conversationally relevant questions and responses, as well as a broader array of verbal and nonverbal interpersonal behaviors, such as problem solving, anger control, appropriate affect, and "overall assertiveness."
2. Patients show moderate to substantial generalization of trained behaviors to untrained scenes and relationships. Behavioral generalization to different and novel situations appears to be more difficult and labored for patients who are regressed, suffer from chronic long-standing thought disorder, and have attentional deficits. Generalization or transfer of training also is more difficult to achieve with complex behaviors, such as requesting a change in another person, than with simpler behaviors, such as eye contact or giving a compliment. This presents a special problem for social skills training with chronic mental patients living in the community, for whom complex social behaviors may be necessary to be able to use accessible resources and generate social support.
3. Comprehensive, intensive social skills training can reduce clinical symptoms and relapse in psychiatric patients. Among neuroleptic-stabilized schizophrenic inpatients, intensive social skills training significantly lowered symptoms (Liberman et al. 1984; Wallace and Liberman 1985). Similarly, schizophrenic patients who participated in a day hospital program and concurrently received social skills training showed symptoms reduction that was more durable over a six-month follow-up period than that of patients who attended the day program but did not receive social skills training (Bellack et al. 1984). Social skills training alleviates depression for unmedicated depressed outpatients (McKnight et al. 1984), has clinical effectiveness equivalent to antidepressant medication, and is associated with a lower rate of dropout from treatment than is antidepressants treatment (Bellack et al. 1983).

The most convincing evidence for the efficacy of social skills training in schizophrenia comes from a study in which 103 patients, most of whom received guaranteed neuroleptic drugs through long-acting depot injections, were randomly assigned to social skills training, an educationally oriented and practical form of family therapy, a combination of family therapy and social skills training, or a medication-only condition (Hogarty et al. 1986). The goals of the social skills training were to increase patients' social competence, enabling them to relate more constructively in family and community-based relationships, thereby lowering stress and arousal that could provoke relapse. Sessions were held during regular outpatient visits throughout the entire one-year period following discharge from the hospital for an acute psychotic episode. Both the social skills training and family therapy programs lowered relapse rates from the 41 percent found in the drug-only group to approximately 20 percent in one year. These statistically significant reductions in relapse rates were independent of patients' compliance with neuroleptic maintenance medication. Interestingly, the protective effects of social skills training and family therapy were additive, in that no patients receiving both psychosocial interventions relapsed during the course of the first posthospital year.

Several caveats should be stated regarding the value of social skills training for patients with chronic mental disorders such as schizophrenia. First, it is most effective if the training can be provided after a patient has reconstituted from the cognitive disorganization and severe psychotic symptoms of an illness episode. This is true of schizophrenia, mania, or major depression. This means that full efforts should be made to find the type and dose of psychotropic drugs capable of controlling the patient's psychopathology, as highlighted in Chapters 2 and 4 of this book. Once symptoms are stabilized, maintenance medication should be provided to sustain a patient's ability to focus attention and engage productively in the training.

A second point relates to the importance of tailoring the form, frequency, and curriculum of the social skills training to the functional level of the patient. Many psychiatric patients manifest learning disabilities that require highly directive behavioral techniques for teaching social skills. Chronic patients often have information-processing and attentional deficits, and show hyperarousal or hypoarousal during psychophysiological testing. These patients may experience overstimulation from emotional stressors or even from training sessions that are not adequately structured and modulated. Chronic patients often fail to be motivated by customary forms of social and tangible rewards available in traditional therapy. The acquisition of social skills is impaired in many patients by their lack of conversational skills, an important building block to the attainment of social competence. Patients with schizophrenia often have deficiencies in their social perception and their ability to generate response alternatives for coping with everyday problems such as making an appointment or getting help with annoying drug effects. Patients with verbal dysfluencies, minimal vocal intonation, and poor eye contact may be further impaired in their social learning.

The wide variation in cognitive impairment and social deficits among psychiatric patients illustrates the importance of tailoring social skills training procedures to the needs of individual patients. Three training models that have been developed for use with psychiatric patients with different needs and functional levels have been described in this chapter.

A final point relates to the ways in which practitioners must reorient themselves to succeed in generalizing the effects of skills training. Social skills training is generally conducted in a setting, such as a clinic or inpatient facility, that is removed from the patient's natural environment. However, for an intervention to be considered clinically significant, generalization to other situations and to more natural settings is important. While social skills training has made considerable progress in enhancing skill levels of psychiatric patients, more work is needed in assessing and promoting generalization and long-term change.

There are several possible factors worth exploring that presently may be limiting the generalization of newly acquired skills. First, the situations presented in clinic or hospital role-plays may not be similar to the situations actually encountered in the natural environment. Most patients are probably aware that a simulated situation is not "real," and all the important stimulus characteristics of the situation may not be present during role-play training. It may be necessary to shift the focus of training from the clinic or hospital to more naturalistic environments where more relevant stimuli can be present while training, stimulus control, and performance observation continue to be carefully monitored. For example, the use of work therapy sites associated with hospitals could be employed to train both work and on-the-job social interaction skills. Similarly, in-hospital recreational and leisure activities could be used as a training ground for interpersonal-skills training.

Another challenge for social skills research is the problem associated with the situationally specific nature of behavior. There is an endless stream of social situations in life, and it is impossible to train all the possible responses required for all possible situations. In social skills training, a number of different role-play scenes and responses are practiced that prompt and reinforce various forms of the target skill. For instance, an unassertive patient might practice sending burnt food back in a restaurant, confronting a person who cut in front of him in line, and saying no to unreasonable requests. In the attention-focusing model, a patient may be trained to ask questions of a conversational partner when presented with statements like "I went to a movie last night," "I like to fly in planes," and "Baseball is my favorite sport." This method of training, which emphasizes a variety of uses of a particular skill, has been recommended as a way to establish generalized responses. It also may be necessary to train general skills by which patients learn to analyze novel situations, generate innovative responses, and analyze their performance in order to become more proficient in responding to the ever-changing flow of social situations. This problem-solving strategy for promoting the generalization of skills may direct research and rehabilitation to the information-processing skills approach, training patients not only in behavioral performance, but in cognitive processing skills as well.

A third area of development will be in validating the content of skills training programs. Much of the content of current programs has developed from "armchair" research about what the relevant situations and the most effective responses are. It may be possible that the patients are mastering the training material but that the skills taught are not functionally related to the skills required for effective performance in the community. More research is needed to functionally validate and match the environmental situation-response requirements of the population of chronically mentally ill. This involves systematic and naturalistic observation of the environment in order to determine what constitutes effective social and independent functioning and how this relates to training content areas.

With schizophrenic and other severely impaired patient populations, generalization is usually limited if efforts are not made to promote use of the skills in settings outside therapy. For instance, a patient may be well trained in skills that are important to a good conversation, such as making appropriate self-disclosures and asking good questions. However, generalization may be impeded because factors present in the training situation, such as attentiveness, responsiveness, reinforcement, and feedback, may not be available in the natural environment.

It may be expecting too much of the patient to use his or her newly learned skills in other environments and with people who are not always attentive and responsive. In natural situations, praise or rewards are rarely provided for asking questions or making self-disclosures. Usually inappropriate responses are not correct; rather, people tend to cut a conversation short if inappropriate things are said. Ideally, the skills would be maintained in other settings by the reinforcement qualities of engaging in interesting conversations. However, this is usually not achieved without active programming.

One way to establish a solid link between the training setting and extra-therapy settings is by issuing homework assignments to use the new skills in other settings and with other individuals. A number of clinical researchers have used such assignments with positive results. This tactic has proved to be more effective when accompanied by prompts and reinforcement in the other setting. Friends, family members, nursing personnel, and peers can aid in this process by prompting and reinforcing new social behaviors until they are established.

Once the trained skills are well established and maintained by natural reinforcements in the environment, prompts and external reinforcement may be withdrawn. Gradually delaying reinforcement and making its delivery more variable will minimize the likelihood that newly learned patterns of behavior will be disrupted. As shown in Table 25, conducting social skills training in groups provides distinct advantages for learning to take place.

TABLE 25: Advantages of Social Skills Training in Groups

Provides naturalistic and spontaneous opportunities for trying out skills

Provides arena for ongoing assessment of informally exhibited social skills

Reinforcement of learned skills is amplified through peer feedback

Modeling options are multiplied and are more credible through peers

Buddy system can be used to assist completion of homework assignments

Motivation to persist in training comes from more advanced, "veteran" clients

Orientation and favorable expectations for the training can be provided by peers as well as therapists

Training should not be separated from the patient's everyday world but, rather, fully integrated with it. Whenever possible, therapy should be taken out of the clinician's office and practiced in homes, wards, schools, stores, restaurants, and other environments where it is desirable to perform the target behaviors. Potent reinforcers such as praise, money, edibles, and privileges should be initially tied to successful performance of the behavior; only after the behavior is thoroughly ingrained and under the control of natural contingencies should prosthetic reinforcement be removed.

SUMMARY

Since the symptoms and disabilities of chronic and severe psychiatric disorders are in equilibrium with the coping and competence of a vulnerable individual, social skills training can improve a person's mastery over stress, reduce the probability of relapse, and elevate social adjustment. In this chapter, the salient issues for the clinician intent on applying social skills training for chronic psychiatric patients have been highlighted.

While the technology for social skills training has matured and the empirical validation for its efficacy has grown over the past 10 years, its use is still limited to a relatively small number of behaviorally oriented practitioners. Many institutions and clinics offer socialization groups and experiences for chronically mentally ill patients, but very few offer structured and systematic social skills training. A major challenge in the field

---

LEARNING EXERCISE

Respond to these decision-making requests to help you actually use what you have learned from this chapter.

List four individuals for whom social skills training would be appropriate. These can be either patients that you have primary clinical responsibility for or patients that you have clinical contact with during the week. Of these four patients, which one do you think you would be most likely to be successful with in using the social skills treatment methods?

What general problem area (for example, obtaining employment, meeting new friends, talking with a family member) would you choose to work on with this patient? Describe the specific scene and task that you would create to give the patient a chance to practice this new behavior. At what specific place and at what specific time would you be doing this social skills training? What behavior(s) could you or someone else model for the patient that he or she could learn from? What realistic, "outside the therapy session" assignment could you give the patient based on his or her performance?

---

is how to promote wider dissemination and faithful replication of social skills training.

The importance of carefully selecting the type of training model to fit the needs of individual patients is increasingly clear. Many patients may benefit from basic social skills training conducted in a role-playing format. However, patients who are functioning at a higher social level may derive more benefit from a format that emphasizes cognitive problem-solving strategies. Alternatively, highly withdrawn and distractable chronic patients may need a more structured type of training based on attention-focusing procedures.

Generalization and maintenance are of critical importance to the success of any social skills training program. One promising strategy for maintaining social skills in natural living environments is to follow the intensive training in a clinic or hospital with booster sessions in the aftercare period.

Another successful strategy for promoting social skills generalization and durability is the use of homework assignments. Homework assignments, or directing the patient to use newly acquired skills in his or her daily life, can effectively facilitate skill generalization. Minimal training, in the form of intermittent verbal prompts and reinforcement for trained responses in the naturalistic setting, can also induce transfer of learning. Once trained responses are established in the natural environment, gradual fading of prompts and gradual thinning of reinforcement will maximize the likelihood that the new responses will continue.

The application of social skills training for schizophrenic patients is a relatively new area: Its development began only after the advent of antipsychotic medication. To date, social skills training procedures have been relatively successful in teaching patients situationally specific behaviors within clinical and academic settings. As research continues, other necessary areas of program development will be identified, especially in the area of generalization. Recent studies have shown that patients who have undergone social skills training are viewed as more socially adept by individuals in the community. However, we are only beginning to document the extent to which social skills training leads to improved and durable social functioning, quality of life, and clinical remissions. The ultimate utility of social skills training may depend on the resolution of these issues. However, on the basis of current ongoing research and reviews of social skills training and assessment, there is no reason to assume that such challenges will not be met.

REFERENCES

American Psychiatric Association: Diagnostic and Statistical Manuals of Mental Disorders (Third Edition-Revised). Washington, DC, American Psychiatric Association, 1987

Anonymous: Problems of living with schizophrenia: first person account. Schizophr Bull 7:196–197, 1981

Bellack AS, Hersen M, Himmelhoch JM: A comparison of social skills training, pharmacotherapy and psychotherapy for depression. Behav Res Ther 21:101–107, 1983

Bellack AS, Turner SM, Hersen M, et al: An examination of the efficacy of social skills training for chronic schizophrenic patients. Hosp Community Psychiatry 35:1023–1028, 1984

Brady JP: Social skills training for psychiatric patients. Am J Psychiatry 141:491–498, 1984

Fichter M, Wallace CJ, Liberman RP, et al: Improving social interaction in a chronic psychotic using discriminated avoidance. J Appl Behav Anal 9:377–386, 1976

Goldstein AP: Structured Learning Therapy. New York, Academic Press, 1973

Goldstein AP, Sprafkin RP, Gershaw MJ: Skill Training for Community Living: Applying Structural Learning Theory. New York, Pergamon Press, 1976

Goldstein MJ: Preventive Interventions in Schizophrenia [Publication No (ADM) 82–111]. Washington, DC, U.S. Dept of Health and Human Services, 1982

Hersen M, Bellack AS: Assessment of social skills, in Handbook of Behavioral Assessment. Edited by Ciminero AR, Calhoun KS, Adams HE. New York, Wiley, 1977

Hogarty GE, Anderson CM, Reiss DJ, et al: Family psychoeducation, social skills training, and maintenance chemotherapy in the after-care treatment of schizophrenia. Arch Gen Psychiatry 43:633–642, 1986

Hooley JM: Expressed emotion: a review of the critical literature. Clinical Psychological Review 5:119–139, 1985

Kandel ER: From metapsychology to molecular biology. AM J Psychiatry 140:1277–1293, 1983

Lehman AF: The well-being of chronic mental patients. Arch Gen Psychiatry 40:369–373, 1983

Lesse H: Amygdaloid electrical activity during a conditioned response, in Electroence-phalography, Clinical Neurophysiology and Epilepsy. Edited by Va Bogant L, Rad-ermecker J. London, Pergamon Press, 1959

Liberman RP: Assessment of social skills. Schizophr Bull 8:62–84, 1982a

Liberman RP: Social factors in schizophrenia, in Annual Review of the American Psychiatric Association [volume 1]. Edited by Grinspoon L. Washington, DC, American Psychiatric Press 1982b

Liberman RP, DeRisi WJ, King LW, et al: Behavioral measurement in a community mental health center, in Evaluating Behavioral Programs in Community, Residential and Educational Settings. Edited by Davidson P, Clark F, Hamerlynck L. Champaign, IL, Research Press, 1974

Liberman RP, King LW, DeRisi WJ, et al: Personal Effectiveness: Guiding People to Assert Themselves and Improve Their Social Skills. Champaign, IL, Research Press, 1975

Liberman RP, Lillie F, Falloon IRH, et al: Social skills training with relapsing schizophrenics. Behav Modif 8:155–179, 1984

Liberman RP, Massel HK, Mosk MD, et al: Social skills training for chronic mental patients. Hosp Community Psychiatry 36:396–403, 1985

Liberman RP, Teigen J, Patterson R, et al: Reducing delusional speech in chronic paranoid schizophrenics. J Appl Behav Anal 6:57–64, 1973

Liberman RP, Wallace CJ, Vaughn CE, et al: Social and family factors in the course of schizophrenia: toward an interpersonal problem-solving therapy for schizophrenics and their relatives, in Psychotherapy of Schizophrenia. Edited by Strauss JS, Fleck S, Bowers M, et al. New York, Plenum, 1980

Linn MW, Klett CJ, Coffey EM: Relapse of psychiatric patients in foster care. AM J Psychiatry 139:778–783, 1982

McKnight DL, Nelson RO, Hayes SC, et al: Importance of treating individually assessed response classes in the amelioration of depression. Behavior Therapy 15:315–335, 1984

Paul GL, Lentz R: Psychosocial Treatment of the Chronic Mental Patient. Cambridge, MA, Harvard University Press, 1977

Presly AS, Grubb AB, Semple D: Predictors of successful rehabilitation in long stay patients. Acta Psychiatr Scand 66:83–88, 1982

Rosenzweig MR, Leiman AL: Brain functions. Annual Review of Psychology 19:55–98, 1968

Sylph JA, Ross HE, Kedwood HB: Social disability in chronic psychiatric patients. Am J Psychiatry 134:1391–1394, 1978

Wallace CJ, Liberman RP: Social skills training for patients with schizophrenia. Psychiatry Res 15:239–247, 1985

Wallace CJ, Boone SE, Donahoe CP, et al: Psychosocial rehabilitation for the chronically mentally disabled, in Behavioral Treatment of Adult Disorders. Edited by Marlow D. New York, Guilford Press, 1985

Wallace CJ, Nelson CJ, Liberman RP, et al: A review and critique of social skills training with schizophrenic patients. Schizophr Bull 6:42–63, 1980

CHAPTER 6

BEHAVIORAL FAMILY MANAGEMENT

ROBERT PAUL LIBERMAN, M.D.

Relatives must learn not to be consumed by their family member's illness. But this is easier said than done because living with schizophrenia is like living on the edge of a volcano.

Donald Richardson
President, National Alliance for the Mentally Ill

Several converging movements during the past decade have produced family-based approaches to the care of individuals with schizophrenia that have brought a new optimism into the management of a disorder that had carried a poor prognosis. The optimism is not generated by faddish attachment to a new ideology or philosophy of treatment, but rather by well-replicated, empirical data documenting highly significant reductions in relapse rates in patients living in different cities the world over. Replicated findings are scarce in psychiatry, so when clinical researchers report reductions in relapse from over 50 percent to less than 10 percent in the 9 to 12 months following a hospitalization, mental health and rehabilitation professionals have taken notice.

The movements converging to crystallize family management strategies in the care of schizophrenia include:

1. Deinstitutionalization, which has produced a mass exodus from mental hospitals, reduced accessibility to hospitals for even floridly ill psychotic patients, and increased responsibilities for care and support of the mentally ill by their relatives.
2. Stress and burden experienced by families who are unequipped to manage their mentally ill relatives at home.
3. Growth of a vital advocacy and self-help movement by relatives of mentally ill persons, which has organized nationally and spawned hundreds of local chapters and tens of thousands of members.
4. Disenchantment with reliance solely on maintenance antipsychotic medications, with their noxious side effects, for the treatment of schizophrenia.
5. Development of behavioral and educational methods for clinical problems in psychiatry that offer practical help for all social classes and that supersede less widely applicable psychodynamic and insight therapies.
6. Reduction of stigma of mental illness and increased public awareness and acceptance of mental disorders as bona fide illnesses that deserve treatment.

HOW EFFECTIVE IS FAMILY MANAGEMENT?

One type of family management that has been carefully evaluated in a controlled clinical trial is behavioral family management (BFM; Falloon and Liberman 1983). Its methods are derived from social learning theory and encompass highly structured and directive behavioral techniques, such as goal setting, modeling, behavioral rehearsal, reinforcement, and homework assignments. Patients and their relatives, in joint sessions, learn about schizophrenia and its treatments and about communication and problem-solving skills.

In a clinical experiment, 36 young adult schizophrenic individuals who were living at home in stressful and tense relationships with parents were randomly assigned to in-home BFM or clinic-based supportive individual therapy (Falloon et al. 1982, 1984). Before entering therapy, all patients had their psychotic symptoms stabilized with at least one month of neuroleptic drug treatment.

Regardless of treatment condition, all patients followed the same treatment schedule: weekly visits during the first three months, biweekly visits for the next six months, and monthly visits thereafter for a total of two years. In addition to their BFM or individual therapy—which was conducted by mental health professionals—all patients were seen monthly at the clinic by a psychiatrist or clinical pharmacist who was blind to the type of psychosocial therapy and was responsible for prescribing optimal doses of neuroleptic drugs.

The comparative effectiveness of the BFM and individual therapy was assessed by a battery of outcome instruments, including ratings of psychotic symptoms, community tenure, social functioning, family burden, and cost-effectiveness. Statistically significant advantages of BFM were noted in each of the outcome dimensions. The results for clinical outcome are depicted in Figure 16. While only 6 percent of the patients receiving BFM suffered a relapse or exacerbation of their schizophrenic symptoms during the first nine months of treatment, 44 percent of those receiving individual therapy did so. The 44 percent relapse rate actually compares favorably with the approximately 55 percent relapse rate in nine months of patients' returning to live in households marked by stress (Vaughn et al. 1984). The 6 percent relapse rate—accounted for by a single patient among the group of 18 assigned to BFM—is placed in even more hopeful light by the 56 percent of BFM patients who were in full remission of their schizophrenic symptoms at the nine-month point, many of them functioning relatively normally in social and vocational roles.

Two years after treatment had begun, at the point where the BFM had entered a "maintenance" stage, the relapse rates for the two treatment conditions were 11 percent for BFM and 83 percent for those in individual therapy. For patients hospitalized during the two-year period, the average number of days spent in hospital for the BFM patients was 1.8 days per year versus 11.3 days per year for those receiving individual therapy. Since symptoms are only one dimension of outcome, what did the BFM do to patients' social adjustment? Whether one evaluated overall social adjustment, leisure activities, family life, self-neglect, work, or friendships outside the family, the patients in the BFM had significantly better outcomes. Family burden was vastly reduced for the relatives receiving BFM, but little changed for relatives of patients getting individual therapy. Even though the costs for time and transportation of

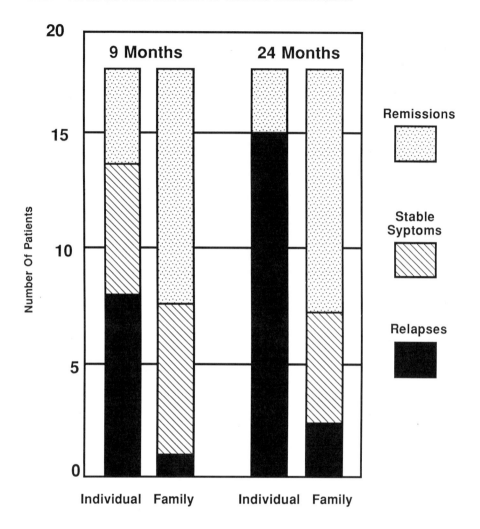

FIGURE 16: Comparison of outcomes of schizophrenic patients randomly assigned to behavioral family management or individual supportive therapy (N = 18 in each group) for 9 and 24 months after entry into the respective treatment programs. By the end of 24 months, 66 percent of family-treated patients were in full remission of their psychotic symptoms, compared with only 17 percent of the individually treated patients. Adapted from Falloon IRH, Boyd JL, McGill CW, et al: Family management in the prevention of morbidity of schizophrenia. Arch Gen Psychiatry 42:887–896, 1985.

therapists to the BFM home sessions were higher than the clinic-based program, the much lower rates of rehospitalization and other clinical services for the BFM patients yielded a much greater cost-effectiveness for BFM (Falloon et al. 1985; Falloon 1985).

At first glance, the results of this research study suggest a major breakthrough in the treatment of schizophrenia. Another interpretation might be, however, that BFM merely improved the medication compliance of patients, which in turn resulted in lower rates of relapse. Data from many other studies of treatment of schizophrenia, however, controvert this interpretation, since approximately 30 to 40 percent of patients relapse in a year even when reliable neuroleptic medication is assured. Moreover, in this controlled study, the actual amount of medication ingested by patients in the BFM was about 100 mg per day less, in chlorpromazine equivalents, than that ingested by their counterparts in individual therapy. Thus, even though the treatment outcomes for BFM were much superior, they were obtained with patients requiring much less antipsychotic medication.

Do not rush to the conclusion, however, that medication is not important for patients participating in BFM. That would be a false lead. Most patients in BFM did require continuation of their maintenance antipsychotic drug, albeit at a lower dose level. In fact, the only patient in the BFM group who relapsed during the first nine months was an individual who failed to take his medication regularly. The important lesson from this study that can be carried back into our clinics and mental health centers is that a combination of optimal drug therapy with family management can be a potent approach to the treatment and rehabilitation of chronic mental patients.

CAN FAMILY COPING AND COMPETENCE OVERRIDE STRESS AND VULNERABILITY?

Let's try to understand how the remarkable results from Dr. Falloon's study relate to the stress-vulnerability-coping-competence model of mental disorder. In that model, coping skills produce competence and mastery of life's challenges, thereby strengthening individuals against stressors and protecting them from their own psychobiological vulnerability. Behavioral family management aims to inculcate coping skills through teaching patients and their relatives better ways of communicating and solving daily problems. In fact, Dr. Falloon discovered that patients and their relatives did improve their coping and problem-solving skills as a result of being exposed to BFM. Those families that displayed the greatest improvements in coping also had the best clinical outcomes. We might postulate, therefore, that the enhanced problem-solving capacity of patients and their relatives in the BFM program blunted the pathogenic impact of stressors on the schizophrenic disorder. Moreover, improved coping and competence in these families enabled patients to remain out of the hospital with little in the way of schizophrenic symptoms and with less need for the protective antipsychotic effects of medication.

In the stress-vulnerability-coping-competence model, psychobiological vulnerability is an enduring trait that changes slowly, if at all, in response to environmental, personal, or biological events. If vulnerability did not change significantly and yet medication needs were reduced, how then did BFM-induced coping and competence promote such positive outcomes? By referring to Figure 17, we can see how the relapse threshold is more easily exceeded by patients living in households where tension and stress are at a high pitch. Given the unpredictable and unsettling experience of living with schizophrenia at home, most families understandably struggle with high levels of tension and stress. Behavioral family management, by providing patients and relatives alike with problem-solving skills, enabled the family group to directly address sources of stress, such as finding ways to allow each other needed privacy or having more effectiveness in dealing with social agencies. Whether the sources of stress emanated from within or outside the family boundaries, they could be deflected by active coping and use of constructive alternatives. In this manner, both ambient levels of tension and external threats to the integrity of the family unit were defused, and the stress experienced by patients and relatives fell considerably below the relapse threshold.

FAMILY BURDEN OF MENTAL ILLNESS

With the deinstitutionalization of the severely and chronically mentally ill and the contraction of public mental hospital beds throughout the United States, the burden of caring for the hundreds of thousands of patients with chronic schizophrenic and affective disorders has shifted from hospitals to the family and other community-based agencies. Each year, an estimated one million families receive a mentally ill person back into the home after a psychiatric hospitalization. Approximately 65 percent of discharged mental patients return to their families, either on a full-time or part-time, intermittent basis (Minkoff 1978; Goldman 1982). Since long-term institutional care is becoming rarer, patients tend to spend more time in proximity to their relatives. For example, in the current era of brief, revolving-door hospitalizations for psychotic and other severe disorders, three times as many patients return to live with their relatives than do patients who are hospitalized for six months or longer (Lamb and Goertzel 1977).

Since the 1950s, psychiatric researchers have documented the emotional, physical, and financial strain imposed upon family members who have the responsibility of caring for a mentally ill person. There are a number of elements to this strain, first termed "family burden" by Grad

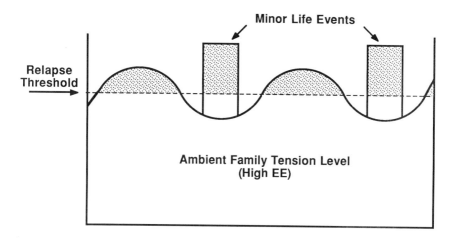

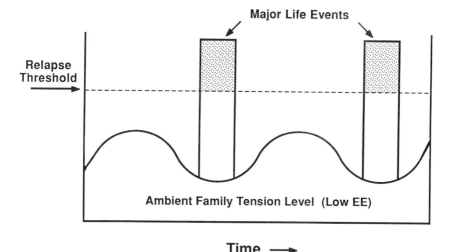

FIGURE 17: How ambient levels of tension and stress within the family of a person with chronic schizophrenia can summate with intercurrent life events to exceed the vulnerability threshold for relapse of the schizophrenic individual. High expressed emotion (EE) consists of relatives whose stress from living with a schizophrenic member leads to maladaptive coping efforts that include emotional overinvolvement with or excessively high expectations and criticism of the schizophrenic member. Low EE consists of emotional attitudes of relatives that are tolerant, supportive, and realistically expectant of the schizophrenic member, thereby providing protection against relapse. The probability of relapse of a person with schizophrenia is three to four times greater in a high EE versus a low EE household.

and Sainsburg (1968). One source of family burden derives from the pervasiveness and severity of the symptoms of mental illness and their associated impairments in most spheres of life. Schizophrenia, for example, presents family members with immense challenges to understand, react to, contain, and cope with—thought disturbances, delusions, hallucinations, and incoherence; in addition, the impairments in work, recreation, affects, habits, activities of daily living, and socializing create even more difficult dilemmas for caring relatives. How are family members to cope with inappropriate or bizarre behavior, tenaciously held false beliefs, extreme social withdrawal, unpredictable moodiness and irritability, and even violence?

Another source of burden comes from the heightened economic responsibility that having a nonworking young adult in the household produces. Not only is it increasingly difficult to obtain Social Security financial assistance, but also there are costs attached to even public mental health care in the current period of fiscal restraints on city, county, state, and federal budgets. For example, in Los Angeles County, county financial support for drug prescriptions for the indigent was recently rescinded, and many psychiatric patients requiring maintenance pharmacotherapy discontinued their medication for lack of funds. Naturally, this was short-sighted, with an upsurge of even costlier inpatient episodes of care. In the long run, however, these constraints on public mental health care have been unloaded onto the family, who are expected to pick up the tab and perform the effort required to connect a patient with an after-care therapist, ambulatory services, medication, and the range of daily living needs.

With the unpredictability of major mental disorders, families assume responsibility for extensive monitoring and supervision of their ill relative. Vacations go by the boards and interruptions in nighttime sleep become commonplace. Patients tend to have reversals in their day and night routines, and many wander from the home and local community to become counted among the thousands of mentally ill homeless individuals. Little wonder, then, that many families coping with a mentally ill relative have their integrity threatened. As conflicts and differences in caregiving between spouses emerge, family separation and divorce may ensue.

Even for families that survive intact, the intrusive impact of harboring a severely and chronically mentally ill person is intrusive and unwieldy. There is a major price to pay beyond dollars and cents. Anxiety and tension, guilt, demoralization and depression, grief, and frustration are great emotional costs on the family members and have inevitable repercussions on the clinical status of the ill relative as well. The stressful experiences reported by relatives of the mentally ill often include psychiatric symptoms; thus, services for the needs of these relatives may result in primary prevention of mental disorder.

> ## LEARNING EXERCISE
>
> Reflect for a moment on your own caseload. Which of your patients are living at home with relatives? Which patients plan to return to home after a current period of hospitalization? Write down the names of at least two such patients and next to the names list the kind of problems that the relatives are likely to face in living with the patient. Finally, place a check mark next to the anticipated problems for which you, as a responsible mental health professional, could provide information and technical advice and assistance, perhaps preventing tension and stress from occurring in the first place. Ask one of your colleagues to share his or her experiences in responding to the problems posed by family burden in the management of chronic mental disorder.

CASE EXAMPLE

Mr. J. and his wife had looked forward to his retirement as a chance to travel and enjoy their many hobbies. They didn't count on their 24-year-old son's developing schizophrenia and forcing them to give up most of their leisure in efforts to care for him. They took turns sleeping to make sure that their son's nocturnal prowling did not result in fires caused by his careless smoking habits. "Even when he's away from home, we're constantly worried and thinking about him. Is he OK? Will he find his way home all right? Will we get a phone call from the police?" This couple exhausted their financial and emotional resources in caring for their adult son. When seen by a psychiatrist in consultation for their son, Mrs. J. was so depressed and anxious that she required treatment for herself.

Stress, Tension, and Guilt

Surveys of family members living with a mentally ill relative have repeatedly revealed significant amounts of stress and tension in the households. It is natural and understandable that relatives living with the erratic and sometimes dangerous behavior of a mentally ill person should themselves experience personal tension and distress that often reaches symptomatic and dysfunctional levels. In one national survey carried out with a sample of 281 relatives of chronically mentally ill persons, over one-third reported such symptoms as sleep disturbances, excessive worry, fear, frustration, grief, depression, anxiety, and a sense of despair. Typically, siblings could not comprehend the patient's acting out on symptoms and tended to blame the patient for misbehaving and the parents for not controlling the behavior.

"We always were on guard, constantly concerned about what would happen next. This produced mental and emotional exhaustion with little patience to cope."

"Our lives have been unbearable at times, since our son became ill. It's been like having an emotional chain around our necks which tie us to feelings of utter defeat."

"With our daughter's unpredictable outbursts and strange behavior, we feel like we're on a knife's edge."

A psychiatrist intoning the diagnosis of "schizophrenia" can evoke reactions as tragic as the news of an incurable, fatal disease; however, the mourning process that follows death and can bring psychological healing often escapes relatives of the mentally ill. Grief over the loss of a once promising child who now seems like a stranger in the home recycles with the remissions and relapses that are often characteristic of schizophrenia and other major mental disorders. No sooner are hopes raised by improvements in symptoms and functioning of the ill family member than they are dashed by a relapse and rehospitalization. Prominent publicity given to new "breakthroughs" in treatment of schizophrenia, which tend to appear on a yearly basis, injects family members with false and unrealistic hopes for cures and sets them up for subsequent disappointment and despair when the prophecy fails.

Guilt is another emotional reaction shared by many family members. Upwards of 50 percent of relatives experience guilt, usually stemming from their felt failure to recognize the early warning signals of the disorder, prevent its occurrence, better manage the illness, or influence the patient to seek and accept treatment. Guilt can be accentuated by the misguided views of professionals who imply that bad parenting played a part in the development of schizophrenia. Even inadvertent comments by professionals about family dynamics can be easily misinterpreted by extrasensitive relatives who are predisposed to hear that they were responsible for their offspring's illness. On the other hand, guilt can be reduced by straightforward explanations by professionals of the unavoidable genetic and biological vulnerability to schizophrenia.

Stress and Relapse

The uncertainty, unpredictability, and mystification that surround a family attempting to adjust and cope with a mentally ill relative readily yield a harvest of helplessness, powerlessness, frustration, and tension. Increased family tension can "corrode the stability of families" (Doll 1976) and bring the normal relatives to the brink of psychiatric symptoms and role impairment (Kreisman and Joy 1974). Stress-related disorders such as hypertension, headaches, insomnia, and depression have been reported by relatives. Some relatives react to ongoing and fluctuating stress

---

LEARNING EXERCISE

Consider a meeting you could arrange with the relatives of a patient in your current caseload. Whether the patient's diagnosis falls within the schizophrenic, affective, or anxiety disorders, make a plan for eliciting and then reducing any guilt experienced by the relatives for the patient's disorder. How will you elicit their possible guilt feelings? You might start by saying, "Many relatives of persons with mental disorders have the impression that somehow they contributed to the person's illness. Have you ever had those thoughts about your son [or daughter]?" In reducing guilt, write an outline to organize your presenting to the relatives a rationale for the stress-vulnerability-coping-competence model of major mental disorders. How can you put into lay terms the idea that schizophrenia and other serious psychiatric disorders are stress-related, biomedical illnesses, not unlike those of rheumatoid arthritis, diabetes, and heart disease?

---

by withdrawing from the situation or by outright rejection of the mentally ill member of the family (Hatfield 1984).

It should not be surprising that some relatives cope with a severe and unremitting mental disorder by attempting to compensate for their sick member's deficits by nurturing and providing solicitous responses. Wanting to minimize disability and overcome the ravages of symptoms on social functioning, well-intentioned parents or spouses can easily take over a patient's life and become emotionally overinvolved in attempts to motivate the patient to higher levels of performance. Overconcern about the patient's whereabouts, dress, grooming, and daily activities can produce an intrusive pattern that has unhappy consequences for patient and relative alike. Other relatives, baffled by the impairments in functioning without any noticeable physical disease, continue to hold previous expectations for performance that were appropriate during the premorbid period but that are translated into criticism and defeatism once an illness has begun. It is clear that in many families, a vicious cycle gets established in which symptoms of mental disorder and dysfunctional family relations have mutually negative effects.

Studies carried out decades apart in London, Los Angeles, Chicago, and India have documented the adverse impact of certain family emotional atmospheres on the course of schizophrenia and depression. As can be seen in Table 26, patients returning to live with relatives who are marked by high stress—expressing criticism, hostility, or emotional overinvolvement toward their ill family member—have a three to four times greater likelihood of relapsing in the nine months following dis-

TABLE 26: Nine-Month Schizophrenic Relapse Rates of Seven Studies: A Comparison of High Expressed Emotion (EE) Families and Low EE Families

	% Relapse Rates	
Study	High EE Families	Low EE Families
Maudsley; London, 1972 (N = 101)	58	16
Maudsley; London, 1976 (N = 37)	48	16
University of California at Los Angeles (UCLA); Anglo-American, 1982 (N = 54)	56	17
UCLA; Mexican-American, 1982 (N = 55)	52	25
Chicago; mixed races, 1984 (N = 24)	91	31
Chandigarh; India, 1984 (N = 70)	30	9
UCLA; recent onset cases, 1986 (N = 29)	37	0

Note. Relapse was conservatively defined by return or exacerbation of psychotic symptoms. High expressed emotion refers to families with excessively high expectation, criticism, or overinvolvement regarding the mentally ill family member.

charge from hospital (Vaughn et al. 1984). In contrast, patients returning to live with relatives who had a better understanding of the illness, and consequently more realistic expectations for performance and a greater tolerance for their sick member's deviance, had a better than expected outcome. Most studies show that approximately 40 percent of patients with schizophrenia will relapse during the first year after discharge from hospital; yet, in the group of patients returning to live with more tolerant and accepting relatives, only 15 percent relapsed. It appeared that tolerance and acceptance of the illness actually conferred protection against relapse to the sick family member.

Interestingly, there are cultural differences in the ways that families respond to a severe mental disorder. In London, approximately 47 percent of the families experienced high stress with criticism and overinvolvement. In Los Angeles, Anglo-Americans tended to more frequently respond with "high expressed emotion" (two-thirds of them were critical or overinvolved). On the other end of the cultural spectrum, in India, where the course of schizophrenia appears to be more benign than in the United States or England, less than 10 percent of relatives were rated as critical or overinvolved. This marked difference in family emotional climates and coping patterns may help to explain why schizophrenia appears to run a smoother course in underdeveloped nations.

The most likely explanation for this strikingly replicated finding on expressed emotion and its impact on relapse is that families are over-stressed by the demands of caring for a seriously mentally ill member. Not having a professional perspective on the nature of mental illness and lacking the skills to cope with a person who has mental illness, family members react with whatever they can muster as overburdened care-givers, including hostility, criticism, or overnurturance.

IMPORTANCE OF CONTACT AND COMMUNICATION WITH PROFESSIONALS

The stress and dysfunctional coping efforts of such a large number of American families are compounded by the indifference of many professionals to the needs of families. Too many professionals continue to ignore relatives, rather than involve them in treatment planning, partly in obeisance to a misguided conception of privacy and confidentiality. Relatives are lucky if they get in to see the professional responsible for the patient's treatment, much less hear of the diagnosis and prognosis. Plainly speaking, relatives are ignored by mental health professionals.

Despite the still prevalent if fallacious views of professionals that families are breeding grounds for schizophrenia and other major mental disorders, and despite the indifference of professionals to the needs of family members for support and counseling, relatives still express a strong desire for contact and communication with professionals, especially the psychiatrist responsible for the patient's care. Because of the great stress and anxiety associated with living with a person suffering from schizophrenia or other severe mental illnesses, relatives regularly articulate a need for information and assistance from professional care-givers. For example, in one survey, (Hatfield 1984), 138 families ranked their needs for professional guidance in the following order of priority: 1) motivating the patient to do more, 2) understanding appropriate expectations for patient, 3) assisting in times of crisis, 4) comprehending the nature of mental illness, 5) accepting the illness, 6) locating housing and financial support resources, and 7) understanding use of medications and their side effects.

The author of this survey, who has also served as President of the National Alliance for the Mentally Ill, pointed out that professionals and family members have profoundly different "world views" of mental disorder that contribute to a harmful schism and to obstacles in developing therapeutic alliances (Hatfield 1984). The professional sees the patient as his or her primary concern and will often try to "protect" the patient from putative harmful family influences by withholding information from the family and hiding behind the cloak of confidentiality. There is a blind spot in the vision of many professionals, who forget that the family directly shares in the caregiving functions. In fact, except for time spent with a therapist, psychiatrist, case manager, or outpatient treatment and rehabilitation facility, the patient with a chronic mental disorder receives the bulk of his or her caregiving from family members. The role of the family with outpatients is similar to the role held by nursing staff when patients are hospitalized. Since modern psychiatry has emphasized interdisciplinary teamwork among hospital caregivers, including high levels of communication and sharing of responsibility, it is both curious, hypocritical, and tragic that professionals have shut out families from active roles in the treatment and rehabilitation of a severely and chronically mentally ill person.

What are the specific needs of relatives for information and contact with professionals? In summary, relatives want to know

- Whether there is a cure for mental illness
- In the absence of a cure, what can be done to limit deterioration and optimize function
- About the nature of mental illness and its treatments
- About practical management techniques
- Whether the patient should live at home or elsewhere
- How to ensure consistency and continuity of treatment
- The diagnosis, prognosis, and changing clinical status of the patient
- How to obtain crisis services and respite from escalating disruptive behavior or symptoms
- About the role of genetics and inheritance in major mental disorder and how this information can be shared with other relatives of the patient who are in the childbearing period

Given the central importance of the family in the care, course, and outcome of major mental disorder, it becomes essential to redress the grievances that relatives have regarding their lack of access and relating to professionals. The scope of these grievances has a basis in the gaps that have grown between professionals and relatives of the mentally ill. For example, one survey of relatives in England found that virtually none of the families had received any advice about the nature of the condition, how to supervise medication, the likely outcome of treatment, or how best to respond to disturbed behavior (Creer 1978). In the United States, one survey of relatives found that over half felt that mental health professionals had "not very adequately at all" helped them to understand the psychiatric illness of their family member. In the same survey, more than 60 percent still expressed desire for greater collaboration with practitioners serving the patient. Despite their frustration and bitterness toward professionals, families continue to see professionals as key resources in their times of need. They want more information, translated to their level of comprehension, so they can grasp the reality of their present and future situation with an ill relative. They want to know how to deal with disturbing behavior, such as withdrawal, aggression, mood swings, and inadequate daily living skills. Until recently, professionals have not been prepared or trained for responding to these needs of families.

LEARNING EXERCISE

To help you, as a mental health professional having contact with relatives of psychiatric patients, improve the quality and amount of communication and information exchange, recently published books on the needs and views of families can serve as a key resource. These books can also be used as a medium of communication between you and the patient's relatives, since you can loan a copy to them and give them reading assignments, quiz them on what they have absorbed, elicit how their situations compare with those presented in the books, and use these discussions as points of departure for family education and management advice. Go to your library or local bookstore and obtain at least one of these volumes:

The Caring Family: Living with Chronic Mental Illness, by Kayla Berneim, Ph.D., Richard Lewine, Ph.D., and Caroline Beale, Ph.D. (New York, Random House, 1982)

Families in Pain, by Phyllis Vine (New York, Pantheon Books, 1982)

Coping With Schizophrenia: A Survival Manual, by Mona Wasow (Palo Alto, CA, Science and Behavior, 1982)

Coping With Mental Illness in the Family, by Agnes Hatfield, Ph.D. (College Park, MD, University of Maryland Press, 1983)

Helping Ourselves: Families and the Human Network, by M. Howell (Boston, Beacon Press, 1973)

Surviving Schizophrenia: A Manual for Families, by E. Fuller Torrey, M.D., Ph.D. (New York, Harper and Row, 1983)

Schizophrenia: Straight Talk for Families and Friends, by Maryellen Walsh (New York, William Morrow, 1985)

How You Can Help: A Guide for Families of Psychiatric Hospital Patients, by Herbert Korpell, M.D. (Washington, DC, American Psychiatric Press, 1984)

After you obtain one or more of the above books, read through some of the material and select a chapter or excerpt that you could review with families of a patient. Make a list of questions that could serve as a focal point for discussing the material after they read it and as a way for you to check on whether they have absorbed and comprehended the information.

FAMILY SELF-HELP AND ADVOCACY GROUPS

Because of the centuries-long stigma toward mental illness, families and patients living with psychiatric disorders took much longer than other groups of medically disabled persons to organize into self-help and advocacy organizations. For decades, families of the mentally retarded have sustained a vigorous advocacy and lobbying organization—the National Association of Retarded Citizens—that has met great success at the national and state levels for promoting services, research, and quality of care for developmentally disabled persons. It wasn't until 1979 that the National Alliance for the Mentally Ill (NAMI) was formed as an umbrella organization for an increasing number of consumer-oriented, advocacy and self-help groups that had spontaneously developed throughout the United States. Several hundred local chapters now exist throughout the country, and the national office, located in Washington, D.C., has become one of the most effective lobbying groups on behalf of the needs of the mentally ill. Over 60,000 persons are members of NAMI, and the organization sponsors a large, education-oriented convention each year that brings the newest research findings to the attention of the family members.

The aims of the National Alliance for the Mentally Ill (NAMI) are a) to engage in cooperative efforts and group action to become informed about mental disorders, b) to learn about the mental health delivery system and its resources, and c) to press for improvements in this system through consumer advocacy and legislative and judicial action. A commitment to grass roots action is a notable feature of local NAMI groups, some of which have already secured influential positions within the advisory bodies to public mental health agencies.

One important benefit of the NAMI groups is self-help and mutual support. Most of the local groups sponsor counseling activities carried out by peers and by professionals as well as support groups that meet on a weekly basis to share coping styles and problem-solving experiences. Although sound professional advice and easy accessibility to professional caregivers are important coping resources for the families of the mentally ill, referral to a local NAMI self-help and support group can also yield tangible reductions in stress and tension in the home with resultant benefits for the relatives and patient alike. Thus, the mental health professional with a working relationship to the self-help family organizations in his or her locale can magnify the impact of educational and informational efforts.

The rapid growth and popularity of NAMI groups in the past five years is both a cause and effect of the reduction in stigma attached to mental illness. Wider public education and more sophisticated media coverage of mental illness has helped to demystify psychiatry and the victims of psychiatric disorders. More citizens view mental illness as a

---

LEARNING EXERCISE

You can work synergistically with NAMI groups in your city or state and thereby promote the coping efforts of relatives of your patients. But it is first necessary that you make contact with such groups, get acquainted with their leadership and membership, and find out ways for mutual assistance. One concrete way to develop a working alliance with these groups is to offer to give a talk or lead an informal coping and support group in a discussion of mental illness. This exercise is a prompt for you to locate at least one NAMI group near your place of professional practice and expose yourself to its activities and members. To locate the nearest group, check your phone book under National Alliance for the Mentally Ill or phone the national headquarters of NAMI in Arlington, Virginia at (703) 378-2353.

---

bona fide medical disorder, not dissimilar from diabetes, kidney disease, or neurological disorders. The promotion of education about mental illness by the NAMI groups has enabled many relatives and patients to "come out of the closet" and openly advocate for improved services for the mentally ill.

A scant fifteen years ago, surveys revealed considerable social stigma among relatives of the mentally ill. However, in a recent survey of 125 families, the large majority of respondents said they did not experience social stigma. Three-fourths indicated that they continued socializing with friends in the presence of the ill relative and were able to speak to co-workers about the illness. Eighty percent said they did not avoid friends or relatives because of embarrassment or shame (Doll 1976).

The acceptance of mental illnesses as stress-related, biomedical disorders will lead to public support for more empirical research on causes and treatments of these illnesses and will serve as a launching pad for increased partnership in treatment and rehabilitation among patients, relatives, and professionals.

FAMILY COPING CAN NEUTRALIZE STRESS AND VULNERABILITY

Individuals with the psychobiological vulnerability to schizophrenia or other major mental disorders are extraordinarily sensitive to stressors, which can provoke an episode of illness or exacerbate existing levels of symptoms and impairments. Stressors may occur as time-limited life events (for example, loss of a job, termination with a valued therapist, death of a loved one, moving to another city) or as longer lasting tensions in the person's day-to-day environment. Stressors external to the family, such as when a patient is denied Social Security benefits, can in turn increase the ambient tensions within the family because of financial pressures.

Ongoing family stress and superimposed challenges to a patient's community functioning may summate until they exceed a threshold of vulnerability above which a relapse or exacerbation of florid symptoms may occur. Very high levels of day-to-day family conflict and tension, as depicted in Figure 17 for families with high expressed emotion (EE), may exceed the threshold for relapse without requiring the added impact of noxious, time-limited life events. On the other hand, if family tension and conflict are at low ebb, as depicted in Figure 17 for families with low EE, the presence of a major stressful life event may be required to trigger a relapse. This theoretical prediction has in fact been supported by studies of families that are high or low on criticism, hostility, and emotional overinvolvement (Leff and Vaughn 1981).

Coping with stressors can be markedly impeded by poor communication and problem-solving efforts among family members. Expressing ideas and feelings and taking big problems in small steps are skills that few families have mastered. The ways in which effective and ineffective communicating and problem solving act upon stress and tension to decrease or increase risk of relapse are shown in Figure 18. I shall return to this conceptualization of stress management later in this chapter when I discuss in detail the behavioral family management treatment modality, which includes training of communication and problem-solving skills as prime elements of working with patients and relatives together.

ARE FAMILIES RESPONSIBLE FOR THE CARE OF THEIR MENTALLY ILL RELATIVE?

Most American families would prefer to see their young adult children develop independence and competence for life on their own. Some cultural and ethnic groups do encourage closer family ties and ongoing extended kin networks. Aside from cultural diversity, almost all parents enjoy the successful transition of their children away from the family home, even if the separation is accompanied at times with sadness, longing, anxieties, and stormy times. Just at the time that independence is occurring, and in part because of the stressful experiences of preparing for and adjusting to independence, individuals who are biologically predisposed to can break down with schizophrenic or major affective disorders. The emergence into independent adulthood is halted and, in many cases, interrupted for long periods of time. The symptoms and associated social and occupational impairments of major mental disorders interfere with the maturational process. As a result, whether they were actively promoting a young person's move toward independence or not, parents find themselves having to care for their sick relative, provide food and room for extended periods, expedite the search for

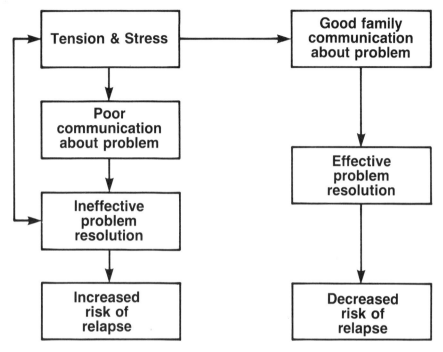

FIGURE 18: Role of the family in protecting a person with schizophrenia or other chronic mental disorder from relapse. Lack of communication and problem-solving skills leads the family and the mentally ill member to cycles of failure in reducing stress and ambient tension in the household. As stress continues to mount, the vulnerability threshold of the mentally ill family member is exceeded and relapse ensues.

treatment and rehabilitation, and undertake a monetarily and emotionally draining commitment.

Sometimes, this labor of love leads parents to neglect other children who may be younger than the patient but who appear to require less attention and nurturance. The dependency foisted on families by major mental disorders also can lead spouses to neglect each other and can thus threaten the integrity and satisfaction of a marriage. Therefore, families need assistance in deciding how much they can invest, emotionally and economically, in the continued care and support of a chronically mentally ill relative. They need to sort out their tangled web of emotions and make realistic decisions about their future and the future of their sick relative. Some families will opt to engage in a major caretaking role for extended periods. Others will be able to engage in caretaking intermittently with periods of respite. Some will decide that support and caretaking are beyond their capacities and means and will benefit from professionals who can assist with making arrangements for public assistance funding, residential care facilities, and other social agency support.

However families ultimately decide on the degree of their involvement in caring for their sick relative, the fact is that scarce and limited resources, personnel, and facilities for mentally ill persons force the caregiving function on most families. According to various reports, approximately one-third of the one million chronically mentally ill persons in the United States live with their families, most often with their parents (Tessler and Goldman 1982). Even when the mentally ill person is not continuously residing with parents or spouse, there is considerable involvement of the family in the form of phone contacts and home visits; transactions with professional caregivers; provision of food, money, clothing, and transportation; and offerings of temporary housing at home during times when fiscal constraints or interpersonal problems make alternative housing untenable.

NEW WAYS OF HELPING FAMILIES COPE WITH MENTAL ILLNESS

For the remainder of this chapter I shall describe a new approach to assisting the family and the patient jointly to improve their coping with severe and chronic mental disorder. The ultimate, long-term aim of this treatment strategy, called behavioral family management, is to strengthen the patient's competencies so that the highest feasible level of independent functioning becomes possible. It is understood, however, that some patients never progress to a point compatible with independence or even semi-independence. For this subgroup, either families or alternate facilities and agencies in the community have to provide support and care. Recent commentary in professional psychiatric circles has pointed to the continued need for long-term hospitals or asylums for this minority of patients with chronic mental disorders. The short-term aim of family management strategies is to provide education and coping abilities to families and patients, and much of this effort does focus on intrafamilial relationships. This does not mean that family management techniques are supportive of the abdication of professional and public responsibility for the care of the seriously mentally ill. It does mean that effective communication and problem solving among members of a family can be a potent first step toward liberating the mentally ill family member for a fuller and more independent role in society.

There are a variety of family management approaches, which comprise different intervention elements, goals, and timing of services. Some approaches, for example, encourage constructive separation between patient and family right from the start. These approaches require the professional to absorb many of the caregiving and case management functions that the family had been providing. To encourage separation of the patient from the family without concomitant provision for a wide range of supportive services would be destructive and possibly unethical. Other family management approaches, with the concordance of the relatives involved, aim to facilitate the family's role in case management. Case management functions that can be assumed, at least in part, by family members include assisting patients' linkages and engagement with needed services, being aware of the comprehensive needs of the patient, monitoring the quality of the services being rendered, helping the patient with meeting daily living needs, being available in times of crisis, and engaging in advocacy efforts to enhance services (Intagliata et al. 1986).

Table 27 lists the kinds of assistance that can be provided by relatives and the things for relatives to avoid. Professional and family caregivers can work in partnership to optimize the quality of services provided to patients with chronic mental disorders. In this partnership, professionals must respect the needs and desires of family members for the type and amount of involvement in the care and management of the patient's illness.

THE WHERE, HOW, AND BY WHOM OF BEHAVIORAL FAMILY MANAGEMENT

While behavioral family management (BFM) requires special training—usually through workshops and supervised, on-the-job practice—a wide

TABLE 27: Ways for Family Members to Assist in the Treatment and Rehabilitation of a Chronically Mentally Ill Relative

Functions to Serve	Traps to Avoid
Assist in locating, linking, and sustaining treatment and rehabilitation services	Overinvolvement with ill relative and trying too hard to help and comfort
Supportive use of medication	Nagging or excessive criticism
Advocate for better services	Isolation from family and friends
Maintain tolerant and low key home atmosphere	Taking for granted small signs of progress
Reduce performance expectations to a realistic level	Expecting too much improvement too quickly
Encourage participation in treatment and low stress activities	Depriving self and other family members of fun, recreation, vacations, and personal activities

variety of mental health professionals have been indoctrinated into leadership roles. These include psychiatrists, psychologists, social workers, nurses, and occupational therapists. The particular disciplinary background is not as important as a directive and assertive style, openness and candid comfort in dispelling myths and mystifications about schizophrenia, and a practical and down-to-earth approach with patients and relatives. Previous experience working with people having chronic mental disorders is very important. Adherence to complex and sophisticated conceptualizations of mental disorders may interfere with learning BFM techniques.

Behavioral family management can be offered to patients together with their relatives or can be offered separately. Both separate and conjoint sessions together can be offered as well. Some professionals feel that it is best to start the educational process shortly after the patient is admitted to a hospital in relapse, whereas others wait until the patient has stabilized on medication as an outpatient. Some educational programs are offered as "mini-marathons" lasting up to a full day, whereas others are spread out in two-hour weekly programs. It does seem important to give relatives a chance to ventilate and abreact their strong feelings about the stress and strain of harboring a mentally ill person at home, and this may be best done without the patient present. Unless such abreaction is given vent, stored-up feelings can interfere with the later work aimed at more constructive goals and communication.

Behavioral family management sessions have been conducted in the home, in the hospital, in clinics and mental health centers, and in storefronts in shopping malls. Multimedia aids are helpful in the teaching process: Videotapes have been produced that convey educational material and highlight coping strategies, and flip-charts and blackboards are the constant companions of professionals plying the family management approach.

COMBINING MEDICATION AND BEHAVIORAL FAMILY MANAGEMENT

Clinicians who work with schizophrenic persons and their families have left the old ideological battlefields where advocates of drug therapy versus psychotherapeutic approaches once jousted. We have outgrown the "either drugs or psychotherapy" dialectic. Modern, effective treatment of schizophrenic patients requires both, depending on the patient's characteristics, the point in the patient's course of disorder, the characteristics of the family emotional climate, the intensity of treatment environments, the pharmacokinetics and dose-response of neuroleptic drugs, and the availability of psychosocial interventions (such as BFM) that are more specific and practical than the psychotherapies of decades

---

LEARNING EXERCISE

Are you convinced of the value of BFM in the care of schizophrenia and other chronic mental disorders? If not, read on. If yes, here's a homework assignment: Find a colleague tomorrow at work and initiate a discussion of BFM and how it might fit into your clinical setting. Where would you offer it? Who among your colleagues would you invite to assist in the educational sessions? What personal and professional resources could you draw on to create a dazzling and captivating educational workshop?

---

ago. It is time for contemporary treatment of schizophrenia to catch up with current concepts of the nature of the disorder, which include both biological and psychosocial determinants.

Here are some guidelines for appropriate use of drug therapy and BFM.

1. Antipsychotic drugs should be used with most schizophrenic individuals to control and stabilize the florid symptoms of psychosis prior to introducing the patient into BFM sessions. Medication facilitates cognitive functions and improves the patient's ability to learn from his or her treatment environment.

2. Whether conducted in groups or with individual family units, BFM is most effective when containing practical suggestions for coping with everyday challenges and specific goal setting for engaging in attainable tasks.

3. A continuing positive relationship is central in the overall management of a patient with schizophrenia and improves the patient's constructive engagement in the therapeutic enterprise, whether it be drug or psychosocial treatment. Medication is never given in a vacuum, and its effects can be facilitated or impeded by the nature of the patient-therapist and family relationships.

4. Medication needs to be titrated to the changing needs of the patient for protection against stress. For example, stress can rise when, after successful psychosocial treatment, the patient takes on new social and vocational challenges. Stress can also increase when a patient and family agree to separate and the patient attempts independent living. Medication needs may decrease when the patient is involved in a supportive and constructive rehabilitation program, such as BFM. If small steps are taken and liberal use of positive reinforcement is made, stress is reduced and so may the patient's need for antipsychotic drugs.

5. Psychosocial rehabilitation such as BFM should be placed in a time frame of years. When the initial goals of BFM have been achieved (that is, reduction of stress and burden within the family, stabilization of the patient's symptoms, engagement of the patient and family members in a working alliance with professionals), it may be desirable to increase the scope of rehabilitation efforts to include vocational training, job placement, and friendship building. These psychosocial goals are ambitious and require lengthy periods of gradual progress to attain. It is likely that indefinite, if not lifelong, psychosocial support and guidance are optimal for most persons with schizophrenia. Just as neuroleptic drugs are most effective in maintaining symptomatic improvement when continued indefinitely, it should not come as a surprise that psychosocial interventions are similarly optimized by continuity.

WHAT IS DISTINCTIVE ABOUT BEHAVIORAL FAMILY MANAGEMENT?

Several variants of family management approaches have been developed and found effective. All have in common an educational and supportive effort with relatives, teaching them about the nature of schizophrenia (or other severe mental disorders) and how to cope with the disorder. One particular variant mixes families from high- and low-stress households in a group with the aim to promote mutual sharing of coping methods. In this mixed group, it is hoped that a learning process develops through which relatives under great stress can acquire coping skills and strategies from their counterparts who are successful in managing stress. Another variation on the family management theme encourages networking among families, facilitating their joining together in self-help and social support activities.

While educational programs, social support, empathic outreach, practical advice grounded on current best knowledge of schizophrenia, and accessible and responsive professionals are hallmarks of all family management approaches, BFM also emphasizes systematic skill building through behavioral training techniques. The structured behavioral methods of skill building are the major distinctiveness of BFM.

It is too early to say whether the additional elements of structured training of communication and problem-solving skills found in BFM also yields superior outcomes; clinical research is required to answer that question. It does appear from studies to date, however, that structured training is not required to achieve marked reductions in symptomatic relapse. All programs tested thus far have cut relapse rates to below 10 percent in nine months following discharge from the hospital. Still in question is whether the skill-building techniques integral to BFM produce better social and vocational outcomes, better quality of life,

---

LEARNING EXERCISE

Now that you have gotten a glimpse of BFM and its effectiveness, think of a patient living at home with his or her family who might benefit from this modality. Write that person's name down on a piece of paper and then list the types of additional services, beyond BFM, that the patient and relatives would need for successful community adaptation.

---

greater improvement in negative symptoms, and more independence and autonomy for the individual afflicted with schizophrenia.

It should be clearly understood that the three major elements or modules of BFM—family education, training in communication skills, and training in problem solving—are not sufficient in themselves for the effective management of schizophrenia. These elements must be embedded in a comprehensive array of services that can meet the wide-ranging needs of chronic mental patients. Services such as crisis intervention, case management, advocacy, psychoactive medications, medical care, supportive psychotherapy, vocational rehabilitation, and social skills training are all needed at some time or another in the optimal treatment and rehabilitation of the chronic mental patient. These services can be provided by the same person or by a team that delivers the BFM, or can be offered by other service providers who are closely linked and coordinated with the BFM professionals.

THE BASIC COMPONENTS OF BEHAVIORAL FAMILY MANAGEMENT

It is instructional to learn about BFM in modular fashion since it is possible to disassemble and reassemble the BFM components to fit the prevailing resources and constraints of any one clinical site. The components of BFM are as follows:

1. Behavioral or functional assessment of each individual and the family as a whole.
2. Education on the nature of mental disorders and their modern treatment.
3. Training in communication skills, including expressing and acknowledging positive feelings; actively listening; making positive requests; and expressing negative feelings directly.
4. Training in systematic and structured problem solving.
5. Special behavioral techniques used to help individual family members or the family group to overcome distress, dysphoria, symptoms or

motivational problems that do not respond readily to the educational strategies noted above in components 2, 3, or 4.

Each of the components of behavioral family management will be described and highlighted with clinical examples and learning exercises. It should be understood that one or more of the components can be used with any given patient and family. Some families and patients might only be able to accept or manage the educational components, while others would have time and resources for engaging in the skill-building components as well. The components can be given in a variety of formats, including multiple family groups, seminars, or workshops, and with patients together with or separate from family members. Flexibility is desirable in considering how best to apply the components of BFM—in module fashion—with the exigencies of families and clinical facilities determining the service delivery.

BEHAVIORAL ASSESSMENT OF THE FAMILY

The specific nature of the patient's and relatives' problems and goals should shape the scope and focus of BFM. Therefore, it is essential to begin with a comprehensive and sensitive assessment of each person's needs in the family as well as the strengths and deficits of the family as a whole. The process of behavioral assessment and analysis is inextricably interwoven with the process of therapy and behavior change; accordingly, it continues throughout the duration of BFM rather than being limited to the initial sessions. Analyzing and pinpointing problems, setting goals and priorities, and selecting interventions go hand in hand with monitoring of progress.

Since the patient and relatives may come to a therapist for family intervention with little or no previous contact, it is essential to have a method for collecting and sorting information efficiently. Each individual member of the family should be assessed for his or her behavioral assets and deficits, self-defined problems and goals, reinforcers, and motivation for change. These assessments can be carried out using a variety of questionnaires, interview formats, therapist observation, or self-monitoring by the individual. Meeting individually for at least one session with each member of the family, or for a portion of a session, helps the rapid assembly of these data and fortifies the development of the therapeutic alliance.

Meeting with the family as a whole permits assessment and analysis of family strengths and deficits, their problem-solving styles and their ability to communicate. The power structure (for example, who makes the decisions), status, and role of the family members can be assessed through questionnaires, role-plays, structured family interaction tasks, and naturalistic observation of the family process. For example, family questionnaires are available that inquire about the patterns of decision making and the degree of satisfaction that members of the family have about the existing mechanisms for allocating family resources (Stuart 1980).

CASE EXAMPLE

Paul, a 29-year-old, single, unemployed clerk, was discharged from his fourth hospitalization in a psychiatric unit of a general hospital after an exacerbation of his schizophrenic disorder. He had been ill for six years, but functioned reasonably well living at home with his parents between relapses. Recently however, his relapses had become more frequent despite good compliance with his neuroleptic maintenance medication.

Questionnaires and interviews with Paul and his parents revealed a clear pattern of decision making: They were made by default by his mother, who tended to ignore or emotionally withdraw from entreaties made by Paul and his father for family action or family activities. For example, it was decided that Paul would return to live at home with his parents after his most recent hospitalization when suggestions by Paul and his father that he obtain his own apartment went unresponded to by his mother, who also kept the checkbook and would have had to have written out a check for the first month's rent. Further observation of the family together revealed that there was little mutual acknowledgment of feelings and opinions expressed by one or another of the family members. Each member of the family would reliably fail to receive feedback for ideas or emotional expression. To obtain a better grasp of how the family members perceived problems, the therapist asked each individual to describe something that happened during the past week that was a source of tension or distress. This was followed by determining the extent to which each person shared the feelings and the way concern and coping were expressed by others.

As a result of this assessment, a goal was set to focus on the importance of a shared approach to decision making for matters that affected everyone in the family, like where Paul might live. Moreover, among the communication skills that would have to be trained, prime among them would be active listening and making a positive request.

Besides the training of communication skills, the family assessment leads to the identification of problems that one or more of the family members are struggling with and that can become grist for the BFM mill. These problems can be stressors within the family system—such as parents trying to cope with the negativism and social withdrawal of a young adult offspring who has schizophrenia—as well as those emanating from outside the family, such as financial or housing problems.

Interview instruments or questionnaires are available to assess the quality of the emotional relationships among patient and relatives (Snyder and Liberman 1981). Questions center around the patient's and relatives' perception of the development of the mental disorder; their understanding and views about the disorder; conflicts, quarrels, and irritability; the family time budget; management of household tasks and responsibilities; and subjective attitudes expressed by each member of the family about each other. In evaluating the family interaction relationships, the therapist looks for signs of unrealistic expectation for improvement and functioning, criticism, intrusiveness, and emotional overinvolvement.

Are there deficits in communication between parents and a young adult schizophrenic son who secludes himself in his room? How well do the family members deal with a major problem, such as unexpected denial of Social Security benefits to the sick relative? Are the family members spending excessive time together, to the exclusion of their own, independent needs for recreation and socialization? Are relatives inadvertently reinforcing maladaptive or symptomatic behavior in their sick family member through overprotectiveness and oversolicitousness? A major aim of the family assessment and behavior analysis is to take the "temperature" of the family emotional climate and specify the individual and interpersonal problems, deficits, and assets that contribute to the "fever."

A highly productive way of gaining an assessment of the abilities of a family to engage in constructive communicating and problem solving is to identify a problem or issue that each member has endorsed as being current and marked by disagreement. The therapist then can ask the family, who are being observed in a session, to spend five minutes attempting to solve the problem or reach a consensus. What unfolds in front of the therapist's eyes are the capabilities and deficiencies of the communication and problem-solving style of each family member and of the family as a whole. More detailed descriptions of how to conduct behavioral assessment and analysis are available (Taylor et al. 1982; Patterson et al. 1975; Falloon et al. 1984).

Whatever the problems are, the assumption of the therapist, shared with the family, is that the family is coping with the problems as best they can, given their present resources and capabilities. The aim of BFM and the responsibility of the therapist are to enhance the family's capacities through goal setting, education about the nature of the disorder and how to obtain needed treatment and rehabilitation, communication, and problem-solving skills training.

LEARNING EXERCISE

Reinforcers are people, places, things, and activities that are enjoyed, preferred, selectively chosen, and interacted with frequently. Reinforcers serve to motivate behavior by strengthening the attitudes and actions of an individual that immediately precede them and elicit their occurrence. For example, going to a movie or a sporting event after a productive day at work tends to increase future productivity. The most common reinforcers are social in nature, such as praise, warmth, friendliness, and acknowledgment from friends, co-workers, teachers, supervisors, and relatives.

It is important, in family management of chronic mental disorders, to identify reinforcers for each member of the family, especially for the patient with the disorder since loss of intrinsic motivation and interests is often a core characteristic of the disorder. One way to identify reinforcers that can be used to selectively strengthen desired behavior and progress toward goals is to survey each member of the family for his or her current preferences for people, places, and objects. With one of your current patients, ask the following questions to elicit that person's idiosyncratic reinforcers.

1. Among your personal contacts each week, who do you spend most of your time with? With whom would you like to spend more time?
2. Where do you spend most of your time? In which room of your home? What activities do you prefer to engage in? What would you like to do more often?
3. What would you like to have more of? What foods, drinks, possessions, hobbies, clothes? When you have money, what do you spend it on?

EDUCATING THE FAMILY ABOUT SCHIZOPHRENIA

The element common to all of the newer forms of family intervention with chronic mental disorders is education about the nature and treatment of the disorder. This education can be given in many different ways; for example, some therapists and clinics offer half-day or full-day "survival skills workshops" to relatives and patients with serious mental disabilities. The aims of the workshop are to give information; familiarize families with available treatment, rehabilitation, and social services; connect the patient and relatives to the clinicians and the agency for continuing care; and promote social support among the families. Other formats are equally effective in accomplishing these aims, such as meeting with relatives and patient separately for education; providing the education in brief increments as part of an ongoing family therapy program; conveying education through self-help and advocacy organizations like the Alliance for the Mentally Ill; and providing educational seminars for multifamily groups.

Educational efforts are facilitated by high-quality media for translation of technical information to a layperson's level of comprehension. This is particularly important for families with limited education or in cases in which literacy is marginal. Videotape productions on schizophrenia have been produced (Backer and Liberman 1986), and diagrams, brochures, and informational handouts are useful supplements to verbally transmitted information (National Institute of Mental Health 1986). The content of the education focuses on what is currently known about the disorder in question and its causes, course, and treatment. In Tables 28 and 29 are shown a selection of information provided to patients and relatives through lecture, discussion, and brochures.

TABLE 28: Examples of Information on Schizophrenia Provided to Families in Educational Sessions

1. Schizophrenia is a major mental illness that affects 1 in 100 people.
2. The symptoms include delusions—false beliefs; hallucinations—false perceptions, usually voices; difficulties of thinking, feeling, and behavior.
3. The exact cause is not known, but appears to produce an imbalance of the brain chemistry.
4. Stress and tension make the symptoms worse and possibly trigger the illness.
5. People who develop schizophrenia possibly have a weakness, which may run in families, that increases their risk of getting schizophrenia.
6. Some people recover from schizophrenia completely, but most have some difficulties and may suffer relapses.
7. Although there are no complete cures available, relapses can be prevented and life difficulties overcome.
8. Family members and friends can be most helpful by encouraging the person suffering from this illness to gradually regain his or her former skills and cope with stress more effectively.

TABLE 29: Information on Antipsychotic Drugs Presented to Families During Educational Sessions on Schizophrenia

1. Regular tablet taking is the mainstay of treatment of schizophrenia. Motivating techniques for adherence.
2. Major tranquilizers are very effective medicine for the treatment of schizophrenia.
3. In low doses, they also protect a person from relapse of symptoms.
4. Side effects are usually mild and can be coped with.
5. Street drugs make schizophrenia worse.
6. Other therapies and rehabilitation facilitate drug effects.

CASE EXAMPLES

John is a 24-year-old who dropped out of college at age 19 because of a psychotic episode and who had never achieved a full remission of his delusions and hallucinations. Despite adequate trials and various doses of neuroleptics, he remained actively psychotic and severely disabled. At first he refused to attend the family education sessions with his parents; however, when he noted that they came regularly to the seminars offered by the local mental health center, he also joined in. Gradually, he gave up his denial of having a mental illness and accepted a referral to a rehabilitation program that was offered during the educational session that centered on local resources for the chronically mentally disabled.

Vivian had languished at home for four years, with little or no psychiatric attention for her extreme social withdrawal, suspiciousness, and incoherent speech. Her parents' attendance at regular meetings of the Alliance for the Mentally Ill led them to the decision to locate an alternative living arrangement for their daughter. With added confidence from encouragement and examples of other families at the meetings, Vivian's parents insisted that she obtain psychiatric consultation and medication. Shortly after beginning a regimen of antipsychotic medication, which reduced some of her symptoms, Vivian joined a transitional employment and housing program directed by a nonprofit corporation in her community.

Paul and his parents came weekly for three sessions on education about schizophrenia. When the symptoms of the disorder were discussed, he spoke openly about the fear and dread he had of his "voices"; surprisingly, his mother confided that she had had a "nervous breakdown" many years before that had required a brief psychiatric hospitalization. The therapist encouraged Paul and his mother to "compare notes" and discover the similarities and differences in their symptoms. Paul's father, who had been aloof and distant from Paul's illness heretofore, took a more active interest as he learned about the biobehavioral roots of schizophrenia. In particular, he seemed to grasp the biological basis of schizophrenia from the diagrams of synapses and neurotransmitter receptors offered during the educational sessions.

During the educational sessions, the therapist turns the patient and the relatives into the real "experts," by soliciting their experiences and personalizing the learning experience. When the symptoms of the disorder are described, each person in the family gives his or her own perspective on the specific symptoms of the patient in the family. Some patients are surprised that anyone would want to know about how they coped with the distressing and fearsome symptoms. Relatives show gratitude that a professional would spend time going over the basics of knowledge of the disorder or even explain the rudimentary facts of mental illness, its genetics, and how it is diagnosed. Many of these educational sessions have a cathartic effect, and families learning the material together often form spontaneous mutual help and support groups that long transcend the end of the family educational program.

TRAINING IN COMMUNICATION SKILLS

While psychoeducational approaches to family management can give information, promote cognitive mastery and demystification of mental disorders, permit emotional abreaction, and facilitate social support, a more active effort at inculcating skills to patients and relatives is necessary for enduring effects on stress reduction, relapse prevention, and social adjustment. Behavioral family management represents a skills development approach to patients and relatives alike.

Two of the skills required by patients and relatives who are coping with a chronic and severe mental disorder are effective means of communication and constructive problem-solving techniques. As was noted above in the section of this chapter on stress and relapse, the tensions and conflicts that embroil patients and relatives in high expressed emotion households can have deleterious effects on both. Since communication and problem-solving skills are not taught in schools, it is only through incidental learning from influential models that anyone learns such skills for use in human relations. The aim of BFM is to provide training in these interactional skills so that stress and relapse may be reduced while social adjustment and quality of life may be enhanced. The flow chart depicted in Figure 18 (discussed earlier) highlights the mechanism involved in reducing relapse through training in these skills.

KEY COMMUNICATION SKILLS

In almost all areas of human relations, the interactions between individuals are mediated by generic skills for expressing emotions and obtaining instrumental and affiliative needs. These skills are

- Initiating positive statements and suggestions
- Acknowledging positive actions of others
- Making positive requests of others
- Active listening and empathic responsiveness
- Expressing negative feelings constructively

If the discrete verbal and nonverbal behavioral components of these skills can be pinpointed, it would be far easier to teach them to patients and relatives. The assumption of BFM is that by building behavioral competencies in communication through repeated practice, the subjective, internalized emotional congruence experienced by the individual will gradually develop. As an example of the specific verbal and nonverbal components inherent in communication skills, those relevant for "making a positive request" are listed in Table 30. Since a core deficit in many chronic mental patients is lack of initiative and motivation, learning how to effectively request actions and responses can be helpful for relatives' overcoming obstacles induced by the patient's behavioral inertia and apathy.

TABLE 30: The Verbal and Nonverbal Components of the Communication Skill "Making a Positive Request."

MAKING A POSITIVE REQUEST

- LOOK AT THE PERSON
- USE PLEASANT FACIAL EXPRESSION AND TONE OF VOICE
- SAY EXACTLY WHAT YOU WOULD LIKE THEM TO DO
- TELL HOW IT WOULD MAKE YOU FEEL

IN MAKING POSITIVE REQUESTS, USE PHRASES LIKE:

- "I WOULD LIKE YOU TO _____ "
- "I WOULD REALLY APPRECIATE IT IF YOU WOULD DO _____ "
- "IT'S VERY IMPORTANT TO ME THAT YOU HELP ME WITH THE _____ "

CASE EXAMPLE _____

After 4 sessions of education on schizophrenia, Paul and his parents were ready to begin training in communication skills. Because it is better for family morale and builds good feelings for later training in managing anger, irritation, and frustration, training began for the skill, "acknowledging positive actions in others." Each person in the family group was given a chance to practice—under the direct supervision of the therapist—the correct use of verbal and nonverbal elements in this communication. For example, Paul was coached to make better eye contact and to say with more vocal emphasis, "Dad, when you let me use your car last night to drive to the movie, I really felt good. It gave me a boost with my friends to be able to offer them a ride instead of bumming a ride from them."

Paul's father chose to compliment his wife on her cooking and home redecorating, but needed some modeling from the therapist in coming to the point quickly and in being specific about what he liked. Paul's mother had a knack for this particular skill and required very little instruction. During the next weeks, Paul and his parents practiced this communication skill daily through a homework assignment called, "Catch A Person Pleasing You." The diary or log used to prompt and record the homework on this communication skill is shown in Figure 19, with the particular entries made during the course of one week by Paul's mother included. It should be noted that in practicing communication, family members are encouraged to use the skills with a variety of people, both inside and outside the family. This widespread use of the communication skill aids its durability and generality.

FAMILY THERAPIST AS TEACHER AND TRAINER

Behavioral family management is a highly structured, relatively brief treatment requiring an active, directive therapist. In many ways, the behavioral competencies of the therapist more resemble those of athletic or drama coaches than they do the skills of a traditional psychotherapist. Structuring the session is key if the goals of BFM are to be met. Pacing the session—almost like an orchestra conductor—as well as setting rules and guidelines that determine the behavior and interactions of family members as well as the therapist provide structure. The BFM therapist actively intervenes to prompt and shape adherence to the agenda set for a particular session. For example, if family members violate the rule, "no blaming is allowed," the therapist must consistently interrupt and redirect any blaming statement.

Behavioral family management also places a heavy emphasis on instigating behavior change in the home environment. Effective instigation involves the induction and maintenance of collaboration between

CATCH A PERSON PLEASING YOU

DAY	PERSON WHO PLEASED YOU	WHAT EXACTLY DID THEY DO THAT PLEASED YOU?	WHAT DID YOU SAY TO THEM?
MON	Paul	Washed the family car	Told him how nice the car looked.
TUES	Husband	Complimented my hairdo	Gave him a kiss!
WED	Neighbor	Loaned me some butter	Thanked her.
THURS	Paul	Went to the State Dept. of Rehabilitation	Told him how pleased I was that he was interested.
FRI	Paul	Took his medication without a reminder	Said it relieved me of worry
SAT	Husband	Went grocery shopping for me	Let him know it gave me some free time
SUN	Sister	Phoned me long distance	Showed excitement in my voice.

Examples:

Looking good	Work in yard	Going to work	Being considerate	Attending treatment
Being on time	Being pleasant	Offering to help	Going out	Making phone call
Helping at home	Having chat	Tidying up	Showing interest	
Cooking meals	Making a suggestion	Making bed	Taking medicine	

FIGURE 19: Diary form used in behavioral family management to encourage and reinforce all family members to practice the communication skill "Acknowledging pleasing and positive actions." Each day, Paul's mother noted at least one pleasing event or comment initiated by another family member and acknowledged verbally how that positive action made her feel.

therapist and family members, compliance with homework assignments, and positive changes in the family interactions made quickly and early in the series of sessions. Compliance with homework is abetted by the therapist's emphasizing the importance of the task, gaining commitment from the family members to do the assignment, anticipating potential excuses or obstacles in the completion of the assignment, and providing adequate prompts for doing the assignment in the home itself.

Failure to complete homework assignments should not be reinforced by a "business as usual" response or by supportive understanding from the therapist. If necessary, family members should be required to complete their homework assignments during a therapy session.

A good behavioral family therapist is a good teacher. In explaining principles and guidelines to patients and relatives, therapists frequently overestimate their capacity for processing information. Even highly educated patients and relatives, because of the stress they are experiencing and other intrinsic learning disabilities, need information that is transmitted simply and clearly in their own language. Frequent repetition is required, along with inquiries that ascertain how well the therapist's communications are being decoded by family members. In addition, the therapist must make sure that patients and relatives are learning principles rather than simply enacting new behaviors in response to the expectations of the therapy program.

LEARNING EXERCISE

To expose yourself to the active and directive skills required in effective behavioral rehabilitation with chronic mental patients, try out the following steps in a therapy session with one of your current patients or families. Adapt the methods to your own comfortable style and to the nuances of the therapeutic relationship; however, be prepared to feel some discomfort and awkwardness in being a behavior therapist if your past clinical work has been primarily nondirective and nonpsychodynamic.

1. Start by giving the patient and/or family members a rationale for learning one of the communication skills, for example, "acknowledging positive actions by others." Explain how this communication skill will reduce stress and tension in relationships, reinforce the positive features of others, and just make others feel good about themselves.

2. Ask the patient and/or relatives to repeat, in their own words, the rationale you've just given and to embellish the rationale from

continued

Learning Exercise *continued*

their own experiences in giving or receiving positive acknowledgment from others.

3. Demonstrate the skill by taking the role of the patient and/or one of the relatives who needs to learn the proper way of expressing this communication. For example, you might say (if taking the role of a relative of a person with schizophrenia), "It really made me relax and feel more optimistic when I noticed that you had taken your medication without any reminders last week."

4. Instigate a behavioral rehearsal in which the patient and/or the family member emulates your demonstrated or modeled expression of positive acknowledgement. Encourage the person to incorporate the behaviors that had been modeled into his or her own inimitable style.

5. Prompt and coach the person who is going through the behavioral rehearsal. This will require you to get out of your seat and position yourself close to the person performing the behavioral rehearsal. Coaching may involve using hand signals or gestures, giving verbal cues (such as, "Good, keep up the eye contact"), and kneeling or standing close to the person to provide emotional support.

6. When the rehearsal is finished (and, incidentally, keep it brief—not longer than a few minutes at most), provide abundant positive feedback for the person's efforts in using the communication skill. The feedback you give should be specifically focused on the component behaviors that were well communicated: For example, you might say to your patient or family member, "You made good eye contact and spoke with a warm tone of voice when you complimented his attire."

7. Adopt a "shaping" attitude, which means looking for and responding to small signs of improvement in the patient's or family member's ability to express feelings and needs. The awkward and halting efforts seen initially will give rise to greater fluency in patients and relatives as repeated rehearsal and positive feedback are provided in the course of skills training.

Keeping the patient and relatives on track during structured sessions can be facilitated by the therapist who evokes a positive climate at the start of each session and who clears away distracting and intrusive preoccupations of the family members. For example, the compleat behavior therapist starts each session by effusively greeting the patient and relatives, acknowledging positively their attendance, smiling, and putting them at ease with small talk. The therapist solicits information regarding any crisis facing the family since the last meeting and specifies how and

LEARNING EXERCISE

You may do this exercise through self-observation or by observing one of your colleagues who is attempting to practice behavioral rehabilitation techniques. Check each of the competencies listed below if you observe it being done.

☐ Actively helps the patient and family in moving from global problems toward setting and eliciting specific goals.

☐ Assists the patient and family in building possible scenes for behavioral rehearsal in terms of "What emotion, problem, or communication?"; "Who is the interpersonal target?"; and "Where and when?"

☐ Orients and instructs patient and family to promote favorable expectations from BFM before role-playing begins.

☐ Structures role-playing by setting the scene and roles to client and family members.

☐ Engages the patient and family members in behavioral rehearsal—gets the client and family to role-play with each other.

☐ Models for the patient and family appropriate and alternative modes of communication and problem solving.

☐ Prompts, coaches, and cues the patient and family during the role-playing, being out of a seat and providing close support.

☐ Gives patient and family positive feedback for specific behaviors.

☐ Gives patient and family corrective feedback for specific deficits and suggests alternative behaviors.

☐ Ignores or suppresses inappropriate behavior.

☐ Gets physically within one foot of the patient and family during role-playing.

☐ Suggests an alternative behavior, communication skill, or strategy for a problem situation that can be used and practiced during the behavioral rehearsal or role-playing.

when attention will be given to it. If the family group is expected to complete homework assignments, then they must be reinforced for doing so by having the homework focused on as soon as possible in the therapy session. Review of the quality and quantity of completed homework provides an opportunity to reinforce approximations to successful in vivo use of the communication skills being taught and to determine which family members will require attention to remediate deficiencies implicit in the evaluation of the homework. Just as it begins each session, homework ends the session as well.

TRAINING IN PROBLEM SOLVING

Once the family unit has gained some experience and skill in communicating using the verbal and nonverbal elements described above, the therapist can proceed to teaching them systematic problem solving. The communication skills serve as building blocks for subsequent efforts at problem solving: Without the ability to listen to each other, acknowledge positive efforts, make positive requests of each other, and express unpleasant feelings noncritically, family members will not be able to engage in constructive problem solving.

What are the problems that face patients and relatives who are dealing with a chronic mental disorder? They include all the stressors and painful events of everyday life plus the special burdens added by a pervasive and unrelenting illness, marked by symptoms and disability. The following problems are particularly common in families harboring a chronically mentally ill relative. It should be noted that each problem affects all members of the family, albeit to different degrees and in different ways.

- Social withdrawal, irritability, suspiciousness, erratic eating and sleeping patterns, mood swings, and aggression.
- Excessive supervision, nagging, and monitoring of the patient.
- Poor grooming and self-care, lack of initiative or desire to participate in activities.
- Frustration in obtaining needed help from professionals in a timely and sufficient manner.
- Stigma of mental illness felt with friends, siblings, relatives, co-workers, and others in the local community.
- Lack of appropriate housing and vocational alternatives for the person with the mental disorder.
- Frustration and obstacles in obtaining disability benefits through Social Security Administration and state vocational rehabilitation agencies.

While elements of the problem-solving sequence, depicted in Table 31, are implicitly used by everyone, a highly structured and systematic teaching of the entire sequence is felt to be important with the chronically mentally ill, for two reasons. First, unless the training is thorough, with overlearning of the steps and sequence, the information-processing deficits of persons with schizophrenia and the stress experienced by relatives of the mentally ill will inevitably interfere with effective problem solving.

Second, the problem-solving strategy taught in this phase of BFM will serve as the principal vehicle for generalization and durability of clinical gains beyond the direct intervention period itself. Thus, the careful and systematic training of problem-solving skills—built upon previously learned communication skills—becomes the single most important component in the BFM approach to chronic mental disorders. The key role of the problem-solving phase in the overall BFM approach is depicted in Figure 18.

In the actual training of problem-solving skills, each session begins with the therapist soliciting the report of previous problem-solving (the homework assigned from the last session) efforts by the family unit. If the problem previously pinpointed has not been adequately dealt with, the family is asked to consider continued work on that problem before proceeding to another one. In all cases, however, the family members are given the responsibility to designate problems and their priority for solution. Using a worksheet similar to the outline depicted in Table 31, the family works through each of the problem-solving steps. One member of the family takes a turn at being the "scribe" for the family unit and fills in the spaces on the worksheet as the family generates alternatives, weighs pros and cons of each alternative, and works toward an implementation plan.

CASE EXAMPLE

Paul and his parents presented the problem of Paul's lack of privacy as the problem they wished to work on. Paul described it first as coming from the smallness of their home and the presence of a nephew who lived with them and tended to tease and provoke Paul. In addition, Paul complained that his parents' dissension and arguments would invariably draw him into their conflict, heightening his stress and exacerbating his symptoms. Paul's father conceded that Paul did lack privacy and felt that the nephew was a major source of the difficulty. Once all family members had a chance to reflect on the problem and to contribute to its clarity and specificity, the therapist asked Paul to serve as scribe and began to generate alternatives for solving the problem.

Paul's mother suggested soundproofing Paul's room; his father suggested jogging or puttering around with house chores to get his mind off the stress. Paul countered with an idea for renovating a old spare room in an unattached section of the home that would place him further away from others in the family. He also thought that listening to music through headphones might help. Paul's father indicated that Paul could visit his aunt for periods of respite, as she lived nearby. Several other alternatives were presented before the family evaluated each alternative.

TABLE 31: Form Used to Guide Families in Six-Step Process of Problem Solving During Weekly Family Meetings

STEP 1: WHAT IS THE PROBLEM?

Talk about the problem, listen carefully, ask questions, get everybody's opinion, then write down <u>exactly</u> what the problem is.

_____

_____

STEP 2: LIST ALL POSSIBLE SOLUTIONS.

Put down <u>all</u> ideas, even bad ones. Get everybody to come up with at least one possible solution.

1) _____

2) _____

3) _____

4) _____

5) _____

6) _____

STEP 3: DISCUSS EACH POSSIBLE SOLUTION.

Go down the list of possible solutions and discuss the advantages and disadvantages of each one.

STEP 4: CHOOSE THE BEST SOLUTION OR COMBINATION OF SOLUTIONS:

_____

_____

STEP 5: PLAN HOW TO CARRY OUT THE BEST SOLUTION.

Step 1 _____

Step 2 _____

Step 3 _____

Step 4 _____

STEP 6: REVIEW IMPLEMENTATION AND PRAISE <u>ALL</u> EFFORTS.

A consensus was reached on the desirability of renovating the spare room and it was implemented during the next month. Paul's father was a handyman with tools and Paul launched the renovation by making a positive request for his father's assistance in the project.

LEARNING EXERCISE

Using a problem from your own clinical or personal domain, go through the problem-solving sequence. Choose a problem that has been relatively refractory to resolution in the past. See if you can make the problem-solving sequence work for you. When you generate alternatives, it is important to suspend judgment and evaluation of consequences—simply brainstorm any and all options that come to mind. Later, when you move to the evaluation stage, you can introduce feasibility, realism, and appropriateness to each alternative.

SPECIAL BEHAVIORAL TECHNIQUES

Professionals experienced in the use of behavior analysis and therapy are able to interpolate these methods into the BFM approach. Specific problems faced by one or another family member may not be remediable through the modules listed above; they may require more focused and definitive interventions drawn from the repertoire of a skilled behavior therapist. Examples of problems that have responded to behavioral techniques include phobias, psychogenic pain, enuresis, extreme social withdrawal, and aggression. Social skills training techniques, elaborated in Chapter 5, are frequently employed by professionals in the course of BFM to improve the social functioning and role skills of individual family members.

CASE EXAMPLE ————————————————————————

Paul was stabilized on fluphenazine and attending BFM with his mother and father when he complained about his difficulty in meeting peers at the local community college he had enrolled in. He was making good progress in learning communication skills in the family sessions, so the therapist decided to set aside some time at the end of one session to offer social skills training on meeting fellow students. Paul readily agreed to role-play approaching a female student after class. He received coaching and modeling from the therapist on how to initiate a greeting and an invitation to study together over coffee in the school cafeteria. After repeating the role-play twice, Paul felt ready to carry out an assignment to approach the young woman the next day in class. He was given a small assignment card by the therapist to remind him to make good eye contact, speak with a firm tone of voice, and use gestures.

LEARNING EXERCISE

Do you have a patient or client who might be suitable for BFM? Even patients with disorders other than schizophrenia can benefit from this modality. Once you've selected a potential patient in your mind, consider the value of offering that patient social skills training in the context of the BFM. One major advantage of linking social skills training with BFM is the promotion of autonomy and individuation. It has been shown in families containing a schizophrenic member, where stress and strain are at high levels, that less than 35 hours per week of face-to-face contact between the patient and his or her relatives can reduce the likelihood of relapse. So, social skills training can have a dual benefit—moving the young adult patient toward greater independence while at the same time reducing stress within the family environment.

For the patient you've chosen, what interpersonal scene would you formulate for use in social skills training? With whom would the patient interact? Over what social or instrumental need? What would the patient's short- and long-term goals be in that situation? What additional consultation and training would you require before initiating social skills training with that patient?

SUMMARY

Families of patients with chronic mental disorders are ill equipped to manage the primary caretaking responsibilities that have fallen to them because of deinstitutionalization. Practitioners in hospital and community-based facilities for the severely and chronically psychiatrically disabled are only beginning to educate families about the nature of illnesses such as schizophrenia, to train them in specific skills that are helpful in coping with the long-term management of the mentally ill, and to provide support for the families burdened by the stress and tension of chronic illness.

For those handicapped mentally ill persons who live with or near their families, the importance of the family can scarcely be overstated. Family members often represent the patient's primary source of companionship, involvement in activities, and assistance in coping with day-to-day problems.

The responsibilities for providing case management for their mentally ill relatives often creates stress and conflict within the family unit. Relatives can become overinvolved with a mentally ill family member who appears to be helpless to fend for himself. Without support and education from professionals, relatives can also lack the understanding of the nature of chronic schizophrenia that enables them to lower their performance expectations of the patient to a more realistic level.

Schizophrenia can be considered to be a stress-related illness, and tension in the home with frustration, disappointment, criticism, intrusiveness, and demoralization can contribute to an emotional climate that fosters relapse. An increase or reappearance of psychotic symptoms in a person who is biologically vulnerable to schizophrenia can be an outcome of the precarious balance between the amount of life stressors and the problem-solving skills of the individual and his or her family system. Too much stress—such as criticism or overinvolvement with a relative—or too few coping and problem-solving skills can lead to symptomatic exacerbations.

The goals of BFM are to reduce tension and stress in the family system by transmitting to the patient and his or her relatives a clear understanding of schizophrenia or other major mental disorders in lay terms; to teach problem-solving and communication skills; and to increase the patient's adherence to antipsychotic medication and psychosocial rehabilitation programs. A further aim of BFM is to enhance the social adjustment and quality of life of the patient and relatives through teaching them the functional skills for meeting their needs and obtaining required mental health and social services.

Behavioral family therapy is highly structured and systematically employs principles of learning and behavior change. However, it is conducted in a nurturing manner by therapists who aim to maintain a warm and encouraging learning environment for the patient and relatives. The therapist's firm and directive, yet gentle and supportive, style keeps the family on track through the various educational objectives inherent in the therapy. In the initial phase of BFM, information is presented to families through a didactic format, using visual aids and handouts on the nature, course, and treatment of schizophrenia. Family members are asked to share their perceptions and experiences, and the patient is encouraged to discuss symptoms as the "expert" in that area. Schizophrenia is presented by the therapist as a disorder marked by severe problems in living—working, self-care, socializing, thinking, and feeling. Education on the etiology and treatment of the disorder is tailored to the level of sophistication of each family. The educational process, offered in a supportive manner, helps families to lighten their burden of guilt, overresponsibility, confusion, and helplessness. Relatives become less judgmental, intrusive, and critical of the patient's behavior and learn to set more realistic goals for themselves and the mentally ill family member.

Since the stress of chronic mental disorders poses continuing challenges for problem solving over the long haul, patient and relatives alike are helped to learn how to communicate effectively with each other and the world around them. Effective coping, communicating, and problem solving together have the potential for reducing impairments and disabilities of major mental disorders, reducing the burden of illness on the family, and maximizing social and instrumental role functioning. Communication and problem-solving skills are taught systematically by providing a rationale for each targeted skill, step-by-step instruction in the use of the skill, demonstrations and practice through behavioral rehearsal, and homework assignments aimed at generalization and overlearning. Unqualified praise for each step taken toward acquiring and using the skills and knowledge imparted in BFM reinforces the learning process.

Results from well-designed and controlled-outcome studies suggest that BFM and its analogues can reduce family stress, burden, and relapse. Marked improvements in social functioning can accrue to patients and relatives alike. Optimism can be gained from the impact of family-based approaches to psychiatric rehabilitation when therapies harness available principles of learning and methods for facilitating interpersonal relationship skills. Much progress can be expected by expanding family involvement in the community management of schizophrenia and other chronic mental disorders. It is obvious that family members having extended contact with a patient have the potential for magnifying the impact of mental health services. By teaching patients and relatives a conceptual and factual understanding of mental illness and how to better cope, communicate, and solve problems, mental health professionals can increase their efficacy in a manner that will prove cost-effective.

REFERENCES

Backer T, Liberman RP: Living on The Edge [videocassette with discussion guide], 1986. Available from R. Liberman, Camarillo-UCLA Research Center, Box A, Camarillo, CA 93011

Backer T, Liberman RP: What is Schizophrenia? [videocassette with discussion guide], 1986. Available from R. Liberman, Camarillo-UCLA Research Center, Box A, Camarillo, CA 93011

Creer C: Social work with patients and their families, in Schizophrenia: Towards a New Synthesis. Edited by Wing JR. London, Academic Press, 1978

Doll, W: Family coping with the mentally ill: an unanticipated problem of deinstitutionalization. Hosp Community Psychiatry 27:183–185, 1976

Falloon IRH: Family Management of Schizophrenia. Baltimore, MD, Johns Hopkins University Press, 1985

Falloon IRH, Liberman RP: Behavioral family interventions in the management of chronic schizophrenia, in Family Therapy in Schizophrenia. Edited by McFarlane WR. New York, Guilford Press, 1983

Falloon IRH, Boyd JL, McGill CW, et al: Family management in the prevention of exacerbation of schizophrenia. N Engl J Med 306:1437–1440, 1982

Falloon IRH, Boyd JL, McGill CW: Family Care of Schizophrenia. New York, Guilford Press, 1984

Falloon IRH, Boyd JL, McGill CW, et al: Family management in the prevention of morbidity of schizophrenia. Arch Gen Psychiatry 42:887–896, 1985

Grad J, Sainsbury P: The effects that patients have on their families in a community care and control psychiatric service. Br J Psychiatry 114:265–278, 1968

Goldman HH: Mental illness and family burden: a public health perspective. Hosp Community Psychiatry 33:557–560, 1982

Hatfield A: The family, in The Chronic Mental Patient: Five Years Later. Edited by Talbott J. Orlando, Grune and Stratton, 1984

Intagliata J, Willer B, Egri G: Role of the family in case management of the mentally ill. Schizophr Bull 12:699–708, 1986

Kreisman DE, Joy VD: Family response to the mental illness of a relative. Schizophr Bull 10:34–57, 1974

Lamb HR, Goertzel V: The long-term patient in the era of community treatment. Arch Gen Psychiatry 34:679–682, 1977

Leff JP, Vaughn CE: The role of maintenance therapy and relatives' expressed emotion in relapse of schizophrenia: A two year follow-up. Br J Psychiatry 139:102–104, 1981

Minkoff K: A map of chronic mental patients, in The Chronic Mental Patient. Edited by Talbott J. Washington, American Psychiatric Association, 1978

National Institute of Mental Health: Schizophrenia and the Role of the Family [brochures], 1986. Available from Schizophrenia Research Branch, National Institute of Mental Health, 5600 Fishers Lane, Rockville, MD 20857

Patterson GR, Reid JB, Jones RR, et al: A Social Learning Approach to Family Intervention. Eugene, OR, Castalia, 1975

Snyder KS, Liberman RP: Family assessment and intervention with schizophrenics at risk for relapse, in New Directions in Mental Health Services: New Developments in Interventions with Families of Schizophrenics. Edited by Goldstein MJ. San Francisco, Jossey-Bass, 1981

Stuart RB: Helping Couples Change. New York, Guilford Press, 1980

Taylor CB, Liberman RP, Agras WS: Treatment evaluation amd behavior therapy, in Treatment Planning in Psychiatry. Edited by Lewis JM, Usdin G. Washington, DC, American Psychiatric Association, 1982

Tessler RC, Goldman HH: The chronically mentally ill in community support systems. Hosp Community Psychiatry 33:208–211, 1982

Vaughn CE, Snyder KS, Freeman W, et al: Family factors in schizophrenic relapse. Arch Gen Psychiatry 41:1169–1177, 1984

CHAPTER 7

VOCATIONAL REHABILITATION

HARVEY E. JACOBS, Ph.D.

Far and away the best prize that life offers
is the chance to work hard at work worth doing.

Theodore Roosevelt
Labor Day Address
Syracuse, New York (1903)

One of the saddest things is that the thing a man can do for eight
hours a day, day after day, is work. You can't eat eight hours a
day nor drink for eight hours a day nor make love for eight
hours—all you can do for eight hours is work.

John Faulkner

Work plays a number of important roles in human behavior. As a central element of adult life, work provides a basic structure for social behavior. In most cultures, work activities are significant in determining status and influence among group members (Weiss and Reisman 1961). This, in turn, dramatically affects individual opportunities for socialization, productivity, consumption, quality of life, marriage, and child-rearing. The importance of work on well-being has also been noted in research on the effects of unemployment among workers during economic downturns and plant closings (Catalano et al. 1981; Dooley and Catalano 1980; Jahoda et al. 1960). Each study noted an increase in the incidence of physical and mental illness, asocial behavior, marital problems, and other distress following job loss. These problems were typically rectified when employment opportunities increased.

Consonant with the stress-vulnerability-coping-competence model of chronic mental disorders, the ability to work is an important indicator of psychiatric rehabilitation. To find and keep a job, a person with a mental disorder must be able to execute a broad range of social, community, vocational, coping, and symptom management skills that ensure stable patterns of behavior. Deficits or lapses in any of these areas can result in job loss. In this manner, work is not only a test of the patient's vocational competence, but of his or her overall coping skills and competence. Generally, more favorable vocational outcomes can be expected for individuals with mental disorders who are protected from stress and vulnerability by previous success in family, peer, school, and work experiences.

Other factors in the stress-vulnerability-coping-competence model also contribute to vocational outcome. For example, psychotropic medication, when given in optimal doses, can promote job retention. On the other hand, side effects of drugs can impede job functioning and motivation to seek employment. At the environmental level, the presence or absence of protectors (for example, practical and supportive psychotherapeutic interventions) and stressors (for example, major life events or high expressed emotion in families) interacts with a person's psychobiological vulnerability to determine success or failure in job search and job retention.

Work is both an outcome and a determinant of the course of chronic mental disorder; for example, having a job can serve as a protective factor against symptomatic relapse by buffering or neutralizing stressors. Possession of a job can ameliorate other stressful life events and promote coping through the structure, mastery experiences, and social networks that work provides. Studies have shown that holding a job—even a voluntary or sheltered job—is a significant predictor of sustained remission and community tenure for chronic mental patients (Stein and Test 1980). Moreover, many patients report a decrease in psychiatric symptoms when they are actively engaged in productive work activities (Strauss and Hafez 1981). The interpersonal relations inherent in a work environment can also provide a social support network and source of leisure and recreational contacts. Finally, the income provided by a job is often the only way that the patient can cover the costs involved in community life, helping the patient transform his or her social status from that of a dependent to that of a contributor.

HISTORY OF PSYCHIATRIC WORK REHABILITATION

Work has long been recognized as an important tool for facilitating psychiatric rehabilitation. Crucial components of Pinel's moral treatment in the early 1800s focused on "prayer, good manners and occupied hands and minds" as key elements for rehabilitation. Idleness was considered a contributing factor to psychiatric disability, and a full complement of activities was a leading prescription for patients with major mental disorders of the time. Noted authorities such as Rush, Freud, and Kraepelin provided support for the role of work in treatment and rehabilitation.

With the advent of large state hospitals in the late 1800s, work therapy programs declined in favor of treatment under an institutional model. Work for patients, when it occurred, was typically tailored to the needs of the hospital instead of the needs of patients. Work therapy programs subsequently began to reattract professional attention in the mid-twentieth century, on the basis of results in Great Britain that indicated that work programs could improve patient management, reduce the effects of psychotic symptoms, and serve as a productive and time-consuming activity (Bennett 1983). These programs received a substantial boost from advances in psychopharmacology during the 1950s that helped patients control florid symptoms of psychosis. Control of symptoms resulted in a greater number of patients who were eligible for rehabilitative services and a need for more programs. By 1967, it was estimated that one half of all psychiatric hospitals in the United States had work therapy programs in operation and that 72 percent of all discharged patients had some kind of work therapy experience while in the hospital (Hartlage 1967).

One of the biggest changes accompanying the rediscovery of work therapy was the development of a wider range of treatment options. Although earlier programs were designed to occupy patient time through structured activity, newer programs emphasized returning the individual to competitive community employment or sheltered work environments. This, in turn, changed work therapy from makework to a comprehensive system of work evaluation, training, guidance, and placement that was similar to vocational rehabilitation programs offered to other disabled populations (Anthony 1979). The reformulation of work therapy also placed more responsibility on the psychiatric treatment team for each patient's posthospitalization outcome.

DOES VOCATIONAL REHABILITATION WORK?

Despite the increased interest in work rehabilitation, there is substantial controversy about its overall effectiveness (Bond and Boyer 1978). Over the past decade, a number of investigators have concluded that in-hospital work therapy programs have little or no effect on posthospitalization employment of persons with psychiatric disorders (Anthony 1979; Anthony et al. 1972, 1978, 1984; Kunce 1970). Less than 30 percent of all discharged psychiatric patients obtain employment, and less than 25 percent of this select group maintain full-time jobs one to five years later. In a series of studies designed to identify factors related to vocational outcome among persons with schizophrenia, Strauss and Carpenter (1974, 1977) concluded that the best predictor of posthospitalization employment was prehospitalization work history, which also questioned the role and effectiveness of vocational rehabilitation interventions.

Contrary to these findings, other programs such as Fountain House (Beard et al. 1978), the Community Lodge (Fairweather et al. 1969), and the Brentwood Job Club (Jacobs et al. 1984) have reported high placement and job maintenance results with chronic psychiatric patients. Both the Community Lodge and Fountain House are community-based psychosocial rehabilitation programs that use work as a central theme in helping former inpatients adjust to community life. Though not exclusively work restoration programs, they emphasize work competence as a prime requisite for community survival and in preventing relapse. The Brentwood Job Club is a hospital-based program that initially emphasizes assessment and training in job-seeking skills and then focuses directly on job finding, using a variety of behavior analysis, skill-building, and goal-setting procedures.

The controversy over the value of vocational rehabilitation suggests that there is a wide range of factors to consider when evaluating the potential of work restoration programs. Not only does the specific vocational program assume importance, but also each patient's vocational skills and history, history of psychiatric disability, current level of psychopathology, social and family support system, social skills, ability to handle stress, adequacy of coping mechanisms, and treatment options that are available all interact to determine vocational outcome.

Typically, these variables interact, requiring individualized assessment and intervention for each patient. Hence, even patients with similar job histories and social skills may react differently to stress and require different vocational goals. One patient may be suitable for competitive community employment, while another may be ready only for sheltered employment. Factors extrinsic to vocational rehabilitation programs, such as the availability of jobs in society, can also affect employment outcomes. Hence, patients in good remission may find that the labor market has changed since their last job and may have to consider training in a new occupation before finding employment. Other patients' expectations may exceed their abilities.

CASE EXAMPLE

Joe had been originally diagnosed as having schizophrenia 15 years earlier and appeared to follow cycles of symptom remission and exacerbation. Although he had been able to secure employment between psychotic episodes, he had rarely held a position longer then eight months. Now ready to leave the hospital once again, he was interested in stepping out into a secure and promising future by learning how to program computers. He secured a government loan for a programming course that would last for 18 months.

Will Joe succeed or fail in his efforts to become a computer programmer? In answering this question one may consider Joe's past history and cycles of psychopathology relative to his sincerity and initiative toward the new vocational goal. Will Joe's motivation to learn a new skill and help from his treatment team be able to overcome his vulnerability to stress? What will the consequences of failure be if he attempts his new objective, compared with the failure if he never has the chance to try? There are no easy or prescribed answers to these questions.

CONTINUUM OF REHABILITATION SERVICES

Perhaps the best way to promote effective vocational rehabilitation and work restoration is to view the process as a continuum of services. Each patient has a unique profile of assets, deficits, vulnerability to stress, and severity of symptoms that will require an individually tailored prescription for intervention along the continuum. As noted in Figure 20, this continuum can be divided into seven steps: a) assessment of vocational skills, b) adjustment to work, c) job skill training, d) sheltered employment, e) transitional employment, f) finding a job, and g) job maintenance.

Most psychiatric patients do not move directly from the hospital to a job, but rather progress through a sequence of steps according to their personal needs and abilities. In some cases the patient may be able to progress through all of the steps and find a job in the community. If the patient is severely disabled, he or she may be most secure and productive at an intermediate level, such as a sheltered workshop or transitional employment program. Although not vocationally independent, this person still has been able to reach his or her vocational potential.

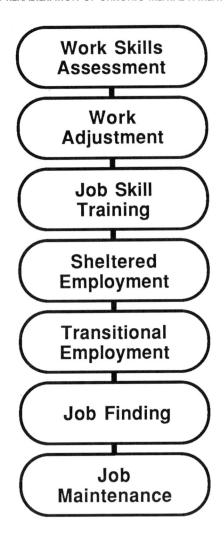

FIGURE 20: Vocational rehabilitation comprises an interlocking continuum of assessment and intervention phases. Restoration of work functioning in a chronic mental patient may begin or end at any point along the continuum. The patient's progress through the continuum may skip phases, depending on vocational opportunities and support available from rehabilitation agencies.

Some patients who possess strong skills may begin work restoration activities at the middle or end of the continuum, while other patients who experience cycles of psychopathology may have to move along the continuum as symptom remission permits. The primary idea of the vocational rehabilitation continuum is that each step is related to an overall goal of work restoration that is unique to each patient. By breaking long-term goals into a sequence of short-term steps, it is possible to develop effective assessment and training programs for vocational rehabilitation and coordinate these programs with other elements of comprehensive care for the person with chronic psychiatric disabilities.

While not all patients will progress through the full continuum of services, the sequence can be conveniently conceptualized in the seven steps listed above. The first step is the assessment of vocational skills, which includes evaluation of both the premorbid and the current vocational skills available to the patient. The assessment can be conducted by either direct observation of patient skills, reports from work supervisors and significant others, patient self-report, or a combination of these procedures.

Second, it is necessary to assess the patient's adjustment to work, that is, the ability to be at work on time, to handle equipment, to get along with fellow workers and supervisors, and to manage his or her time while at work. These skills, often termed *prevocational*, are as important as the technical skills of specific occupations and can be assessed using observation, in vivo ratings, and informants familiar with the patient.

The third step is training in a specific job, trade, or skill. Training can be provided in hospital settings, trade schools, or on the job, depending on skill requirements and available programs.

In sheltered employment settings, which is the fourth step, patients can experience simulated vocational opportunities in a therapeutic environment within the hospital or community. Any problems the patient may experience in adjusting to work demands can be monitored by program staff and addressed through selected interventions. This setting is also excellent for promoting work adjustment skills, vocational skills, and social skills such as interacting with co-workers during work and break periods.

Patients who are successful in the sheltered employment setting or who have substantial prevocational skills may progress to the fifth step, transitional employment. Receiving payment for gainful jobs, patients work under the supervision of a mental health or rehabilitation professional in an industrial or commercial establishment. By moving outside the hospital setting, patients learn how to adjust to natural workday requirements while still receiving the prosthetic support of therapeutic staff.

In order to enter full competitive employment, the sixth step in the continuum, it is necessary to first find a job, a task that has been traditionally difficult for people with chronic psychiatric disabilities. Recent developments in job placement programming, such as the Job Club, have helped to significantly increase the number of competitive employment opportunities for psychiatric patients.

Finally, finding a job and maintaining a job are two different challenges, requiring different skills and support mechanisms. The patient who can successfully master this seventh step of keeping a job has reached the goal of maximum vocational rehabilitation and may be fully integrated into the community.

The following sections present a closer look at each of the seven elements of service that are involved in the vocational rehabilitation continuum.

ASSESSMENT OF VOCATIONAL SKILLS

Because research and clinical experience clearly demonstrate that vocational history is one of the best predictors of future vocational success, assessment of vocational skills is an important prerequisite for effective work restoration. The skills assessment should evaluate both the technical competencies of the patient and how the patient applied or used these skills in previous work settings. This provides important diagnostic information about future training that may be required for the patient to enter employment at his or her highest functional level.

CASE EXAMPLE _____

Larry had been out of work for one year because of a severe depressive episode. He was now ready to return to work as a quality assurance engineer at a major aerospace manufacturing firm. During his intake assessment, the vocational counselor wanted to learn about Larry's past work history in terms of number of jobs he had held since school, specific tasks performed at each job, reasons for leaving each job, and how he got along with other people on the job. The vocational counselor was especially interested in learning what types of skills Larry had used in previous positions. This would help the counselor decide at what vocational level Larry should attempt to reenter his profession. Learning about specific skill abilities, rather than just general occupational interests, also provided the counselor with information to help present other types of jobs Larry could consider if he was not able to reenter his previous profession.

There are a variety of assessment methods that are relatively accessible and inexpensive. Most frequently a combination of the following procedures will provide a clear understanding of the work skills the patient brings into the rehabilitation setting and what additional training is needed.

Vocational History

Past vocational experience is a good source of information about a patient's skills, competency, and ability to work. A job history also indicates the typical job longevity for the patient, consistency of employment over time, type of positions held, and potential long-term vocational problems, such as being fired or frequently laid off. This information can often be obtained through patient self-report or via interviews with significant others and former employers. Because verbal recall may not always be accurate and vocational skills may deteriorate over time as a function of prolonged illness or lack of work, it is often helpful to substantiate reported skills through a second party, vocational testing, or direct observation in a real or simulated work setting.

Work Assessment Instruments

A number of standardized vocational and work sample instruments are available for assessing specific work skill abilities. These instruments range in their complexity, cost, administration time, and diagnostic clarity. Because most instruments were designed for assessing physically disabled persons or the general population, they require careful interpretation when evaluating the work abilities of the psychiatrically disabled. Typically, these tests evaluate physical work capacity and specific occupational skills. As previously noted, since both technical and work adjustment competencies are necessary adjuncts to successful work restoration, standardized instruments may offer only a limited view of a patient's vocational status.

Some instruments such as the Strong-Campbell Vocational Interest Inventory and the Kuder Occupational Interest Survey are paper-and-pencil tests that are designed to evaluate vocational interests. They are especially useful when helping a patient with little work experience decide on areas of vocational interest. Other tests, such as the Otis Employment Tests, the Singer System, and VALPAR evaluate work skills by requiring the patient to perform representative skills or work samples in a laboratory setting. Although these tests allow direct observation of some work skills, they are often incomplete measures since they test only portions of skills and evaluate performance under sterile laboratory conditions instead of in a regular workday setting. This provides little opportunity to evaluate how well the patient can integrate his or her skills into the daily work environment. However, the tests take on added effectiveness with patients who have little previous work experience by allowing a preliminary analysis of the person's inherent skills that can be subsequently drawn upon in job training.

In Vivo Observation

Evaluation of the patient performing vocational skills in a regular work environment is typically the most useful and informative assessment procedure to conduct, but it is also the most costly, time consuming, and difficult. Generally this requires one-on-one evaluation for an extended period of time. However, by observing the patient in vivo, the evaluator can assess technical proficiency as well as the work adjustment skills required by the job.

CASE EXAMPLE _____

Albert wanted to return to his previous position of electronic assembler after suffering a psychotic episode. However, before his former employer would consider him for his old job, he wanted to be assured that he could still do the work and function in the factory environment. A two-week work evaluation period was set up at the factory during which Albert's work was carefully monitored by both the production supervisor and a vocational therapist from the state rehabilitation department. Using a form similar to the one in Table 32, Albert's rate of production across each task in the assembly process was monitored on a half-hourly basis. The quality of his assembly work was also monitored in terms of number of acceptable circuits and number of rejects.

By the end of the two-week trial period, Albert's former employer was satisfied that he remained technically proficient in his job and allowed Albert to rejoin the company.

_____

Obviously, it is not necessary to use all of these methods, nor are all assessment procedures always useful or relevant. It is therefore important to identify what procedures are available to assess vocational skills, in addition to what information you may need and can expect to receive from each procedure. For example, take the case of Mike, a 28-year-old person with chronic schizophrenia who never worked before. The absence of any vocational history tells us that major deficits are likely to exist, but provides little specific information about what these deficits are or, more important, what strengths we can build upon. In such a situation, we even have to consider the questions that we are going to ask. Think this is easy? Well, let's try the following exercise.

ADJUSTMENT TO THE WORK EXPERIENCE

The patient's ability to work with others and deal with the day-to-day pressures of holding a job are just as important as competent technical

TABLE 32: In Vivo Assessment of Work Performance

Scoring Criteria

5 = Excellent	Meets or exceeds competitive employment standards in unskilled or semiskilled jobs.
4 = Good	Above-average sheltered employment performance, but does not fully meet competitive employment standards.
3 = Fair	Average sheltered workshop performance.
2 = Poor	Below-average sheltered workshop performance. Needs assistance to improve skills.
1 = Inappropriate	Notable problems such as behavior, exacerbated symptoms, medical problems, withdrawal, etc. require specialized assistance beyond the scope of workshop staff.

Please rate each behavior below as noted.

Date:_____   Time of Rating

_____ _____ _____ _____ _____

Morning Arrival Time
Takes Breaks on Schedule
Follows Lunch Schedule
Leaves at Proper Time

Body Odor and Hygiene
Personal Dress and Grooming

Production Speed
Production Quality
Care of Equipment
Concentration to Task
Following Instructions
Problem Solving Skills
Ability to Work Independently
Ability to Change Tasks

Acceptance of Supervision
Relationship to Supervisor
Work Interaction with Co-workers
Social Interaction with Co-workers
Acceptance of Criticism
Ability to Work with Others

Please note comments on individual skills and summary of work day on the back of this sheet. Thank you.

> **LEARNING EXERCISE**
>
> Develop a list of criteria that you would use in evaluating the range and quality of your own vocational skills. What types of behaviors and skills would be of interest to a vocational evaluator who was assessing your skill competencies? What behaviors would be sampled, and how would the skill be rated? Would you still keep your job?

performance. Often referred to as work adjustment or prevocational skills, the presence or absence of these abilities can substantially affect the individual's tenure in a job.

Although the specific work adjustment skills required vary from job to job, the following list includes some of the basic skills that are required in almost any work setting.

- Attendance and punctuality
- Personal hygiene and grooming
- Use of leisure time on the job (breaks and lunch)
- Accepting job-related compliments
- Accepting job-related criticism
- Following specific instructions
- Helping co-workers
- Prioritizing tasks
- Requesting help from co-workers
- Following general workshop rules
- Responding to conversation
- Initiating conversation with co-workers
- Initiating requests for special needs
- Interacting with supervisors, customers, and other authority figures

As with vocational skills, there are many ways to assess work adjustment skills. Attitudinal or projective tests are often used by large corporations to try and identify traits within prospective employees that the company thinks are essential to productivity and good work habits. Unfortunately, these types of instruments are not very reliable when used alone in the corporate world and are even more problematic when used with mentally restored patients. A major problem is trying to measure attitudes: These instruments assume that the people being tested already have the basic work adjustment skills needed for the job and that the motivation to display these traits is the important issue. Clinical experience has shown that quite the opposite is true. Most patients display exceptionally positive attitudes about getting back to work but have trouble with many of the previously noted work adjustment skills. For example, in our own Brentwood Job Finding Club we frequently run into the following situation.

Patient: I know that I have been out of work for five years but I really want to go back and pick up my career as a computer operator.

Counselor: Do you really feel that you can jump back into your work? You know, the field has changed a lot in the last five years.

Patient: Oh, but I really want to work and I am very excited about going back to work.

Counselor: But you don't even show up for your appointments here. How can an employer expect you to be punctual on the job?

Patient: Hey! Don't hassle me . . .

Accordingly, functional in vivo assessments of the specific work adjustment skills required on the job are preferred. This can be accomplished in several ways, and a combination of the following procedures is frequently used.

When possible, it is preferable to assess work adjustment skills on the job or in a structured setting that is as close as possible to a regular job. When an actual job site is not available, the assessment is frequently conducted in sheltered workshops, industrial therapy placements, volunteer jobs, ward assignments, or even day programs where there are structured activities. Ultimately, performance should be evaluated using the same industrial standards that the patient would be expected to adhere to on the job. This does not mean that patients who fail to meet these criteria during their initial assessment should be excluded from vocational rehabilitation. Good work habits take time to develop, and the initial assessment simply allows both the counselor and the patient to assess the magnitude of any deficits. This, in turn, can help both the patient and the counselor to work together to set reasonable therapeutic goals.

In the absence of a bona fide work setting, prevocational assessment can also be conducted via role-play situations and scenarios, as described in Chapter 5. Although these procedures allow observation of actual behavior samples, the contrived conditions of the role-play often differ from actual job conditions. Both patients and evaluators may be sensitive to even subtle differences between reality and simulations, leading to invalid assessments. For example, patients may not try as hard knowing that the role-play is a simulated condition, or evaluators may be more lenient in their assessment than work supervisors would be. The timing, presentation, or latency of performance feedback may also differ in the role-play as compared with the job site. Accordingly, it is important to understand these limitations when interpreting patient performance in a role-play or confederate assessment.

Finally, when work site and role-play assessments are not available, paper-and-pencil tests or structured interviews may be used to ask the patient about his or her work adjustment skills. In these assessment modes, the patients may be asked how punctual they are, what they would do if confronted by their boss or co-worker about a shoddy job, what would happen if they observed a co-worker stealing, and so on. As previously noted, verbal reports alone yield information of questionable validity regarding the person's actual abilities. In addition, patients who are eager to get back to work may inadvertently overestimate their skills or underestimate the stressful demands of the work environment. However, in the absence of other assessment procedures, the patient's self-report of his or her work adjustment skills may be all the information that is available for assessment.

Ideally, a mixture of methods should be used to assess work adjustment, depending upon the available resources, time, and information that are needed to make a proper judgment. Consider the assessment protocol presented in the learning exercise below that we have put together for Sally, a 33-year-old married career woman who had a brief psychiatric hospitalization for an acute major depressive episode superimposed on a more chronic state of dysthymia. Prior to her hospitalization, Sally had worked as a bookkeeper at a major bank in the Los Angeles area where she was required to respond to customer inquiries about bank balances, delinquent bills, and mortgage rates. This high-level position required assiduous attendance, meticulous attention to details, and good interpersonal interaction skills. Accordingly, performance standards for assessing Sally's grooming, attendance, and responses to criticism were set at the high levels that her employer would expect on the job. Note that the vocational assessment was carried out by the mental health staff on the psychiatric inpatient unit, using naturally occurring situations that simulated vocational expectations relevant to Sally's job. The question that the criterion-based assessment protocol attempted to answer was, "Is Sally ready to return to work?"

JOB TRAINING

Once vocational and work adjustment assessments are completed, job training would be the next logical step in the work restoration process for individuals lacking previous job experience or desiring a change in occupation. The type of job training required will vary according to the career interests and existing skills of the patient, the type of job that the

LEARNING EXERCISE
Sally's Work Adjustment Assessment Protocol

Behavior	Method of Assessment	Minimum Acceptable Criteria
Arriving to work on time	Direct observation: Punctuality at therapy sessions	98% punctuality at therapy sessions
Attendance	Direct observation: Attendance at all ward events	95% attendance of all ward events
Personal hygiene and grooming	Direct Observation: Free of detectable body odor and neatly dressed as determined by staff at morning, noon, evening checks	No detection of body odor at any of the checks; neatly dressed at 95% of checks
Responding to positive criticism	Role-play test: Staff member will provide Sally with corrective feedback regarding her housekeeping duties on the ward	Accepts criticism from staff member; applies it to the task
Responding to negative criticism	Role-play test: Staff member will "hassle" Sally for not doing a task on the ward that she obviously did do	Accepts criticism without getting angry; explains that she has already completed the task

Complete Sally's work adjustment assessment protocol for the following prevocational skills:

> Initiating conversation
> Use of leisure time
> Prioritizing tasks
> Following general rules
> Requesting help from co-worker

Now, let's turn the tables on you. There are numerous work adjustment skills that you engage in every day whether you are a student or a professional. They include getting up every morning; engaging in appropriate social behaviors with colleagues, faculty, and patients; and assuring that you have the proper financial support to continue your studies or maintain your practice. Make a list of at least 10 primary work adjustment behaviors that you must engage in each day and how you could measure each. Then write down the adverse effects that might occur if you were not capable of performing each of these behaviors on a consistent and competent basis.

patient is capable of filling, training programs available, and the amount of time and resources that the patient has to participate in a job training program.

In many cases, the final decision about what type of job training to pursue, if any, will be a compromise of the above noted issues. In a few cases, patients may already possess credible job skills and require no additional training. The patient with no job skills who is interested in a position that requires years of preparation is at the other end of the spectrum. In such situations it may be possible to convince the patient to approach a less educationally demanding position as an interim goal with the opportunity to pursue more advanced training after he or she demonstrates the ability to handle the lesser position. For example:

CASE EXAMPLE

Wilbur was interested in becoming a diesel truck mechanic although he had little experience in the area. Before his most recent hospitalization, however, he did work in a small gas engine repair shop and was very successful, but he was not interested in that type of work anymore. Because he could not afford mechanic's school, he decided to work as a mechanic's assistant in a local truck stop to both gain more experience and save money for school.

Even after the patient has decided to develop new job skills, it is still important to find a training program to meet the special needs of a mentally restored patient. This includes competent technical training that is presented in a comprehensible manner to the participant, training in work adjustment skills (or liaison with such a training program) when needed, and counseling to help the patient manage the daily affairs and problems that arise in the training program. Tables 33 and 34 provide an example of a systematic curriculum in job skills training that is used with persons with psychiatric disabilities. A stepwise curriculum with incremental educational objectives and liberal use of reinforcement for goal attainment will be more effective for the chronic mental patient.

In some cases, comprehensive training programs will be available within existing hospital and mental health facilities. Due to the diversity of skills and positions that patients may pursue, however, it is unlikely that any one vocational rehabilitation program can offer effective training programs across many areas of patient interests. It is therefore often necessary for rehabilitation practitioners or mental health therapists to collaborate with job training programs in the community to meet these continuing needs. Most frequently this requires close liaison between

TABLE 33: Example of a Systematic Curriculum in Job Skills Training for Persons With Psychiatric Disabilities

TASK ANALYSIS FOR CLEANING THE SINK

1. Take spray cleaner from container.
2. Shake spray cleaner.
3. Spray entire sink with back-and-forth sweeping motions.
4. Replace cleaner in container.
5. Reach over to towel dispenser.
6. Pick up two paper towels.
7. Put paper towels together.
8. Wipe sink sides and edges with back-and-forth strokes.
9. Wipe between faucets with back-and-forth strokes.
10. Wipe faucets by lightly grasping them with towel and twisting them back-and-forth.
11. Wipe sink bowl with circular and back-and-forth motions.
12. Turn on cold water.
13. Swish water around bowl with towel.
14. Turn off cold water.
15. Wipe sink bowl again with towel, using circular and back-and-forth motions.
16. Bend over wastebasket, which is located under sink.
17. Throw dirty towels in wastebasket.

From Cuvo AJ, Leaf FB, Borakove LS: Teaching janitorial skills to the mentally retarded: acquisition, generalization and maintenance. Journal of Applied Behavior Analysis 11:345–355, 1978

programs, with the mental health or rehabilitation program taking responsibility for providing specialized counseling and reinforcement that the job training program does not offer.

The degree of contact, support, and cooperation required between programs will depend upon the "fit" of each program. Many businesses that offer transitional work sites have supervisors who have little knowledge about the needs of persons with psychiatric disabilities; thus, supervisory personnel will need training and guidance on these issues from mental health or rehabilitation agencies. In other cases, rehabilitation and mental health programs may be run under the auspices of different government or private agencies, requiring close liaison to ensure that the patient does not get squeezed between conflicting policies and procedures. Different philosophies between mental health treatment teams and rehabilitation professionals may also have to be addressed to assure consistency in the patient's continuing rehabilitation program. In each

TABLE 34: Example of Systematic Curriculum in Job Skills Training for Persons With Psychiatric Disability

FURNITURE REFINISHING PROGRAM

1. AIM: To develop the skills necessary to work as a furniture refinisher in local industry.

2. PRINCIPLE DUTIES AND AREAS OF INSTRUCTION: The participant receives instruction and practical training to enable him to successfully refinish furniture-grade materials at a professional level of quality. Training progresses from basic skills to more complex skills according to the demonstrated performance of the participant. The following skill areas are covered over an average duration of 12 months:

> A. Safety and preparation of the work environment.
> B. Removal of old finishes and cleaning of the furniture.
> C. Repair and reconstruction of the furniture.
> D. Sanding and preparation of the furniture for refinishing.
> E. Staining.
> F. Painting.
> G. Applying clear finishes such as varnish, lacquer, and plasti-cote.
> H. Re-assembly of furniture.
> I. Customer relations.

case, it is incumbent upon the psychiatrist, psychologist, or other person who is designated as the primary caregiver to assure that adequate liaison and training is provided. This can be done most effectively through a combination of clinical conferences, on-site visits, and telephone consultation.

Depending on each patient's overall vocational abilities following training, the newly graduated patient may directly enter competitive employment from the training program or may require additional work experience through sheltered workshops and transitional employment programs before final job placement can be secured. Now let's see how you would assess the following job situation.

SHELTERED EMPLOYMENT

Sheltered employment programs, also known as sheltered workshops or compensated work therapy programs, can provide important work opportunities for individuals who are not ready for the rigors of competitive employment. The reduction of daily on-the-job pressures, the decrease

---

LEARNING EXERCISE

Joe is a 38-year-old male with little work experience. Originally diagnosed with schizophrenia when he was 18, he has been in and out of hospitals for the past 20 years. Over the past year, Joe's symptoms have stabilized to the point at which both he and his treatment team feel that it may be possible for him to consider employment. Joe is enthusiastic and expresses an interest in a job as a computer programmer. Because the hospital doesn't have a computer training program, Joe will have to enroll at the local university for four years of courses to learn the profession before getting a job.

Identify the pros and cons of Joe's pursuing his interest, relating his prospects to his work history and abilities. Why should he pursue his interests, and why should he not pursue them? If you decide that he should not pursue this goal, give some alternatives and explain how you might negotiate these options with Joe.

---

in the length of the work day, the simplification of tasks, and the structured, positive work environment enable patients to engage in productive and profitable activity for extended periods of time. Some programs are housed and operated by psychiatric treatment facilities who contract with outside businesses and vendors for work. More typically, sheltered workshops are managed by independent, nonprofit agencies such as Goodwill Industries or Jewish Vocational Services. Work is brought to the workshop where patients earn either piece-work pay or hourly pay according to their abilities and the specific contract. Liaison is desirable between the patient's responsible psychiatrist or treatment team and the workshop to promote a modicum of work opportunities for even a severely disabled patient. In this manner, the sheltered workshop can offer viable and productive long-term placements for patients consistent with the severity of their impairments.

For patients who are less severely impaired, sheltered employment programs offer other types of opportunities. The rich diversity of social interactions that occurs in the structured workshop setting makes it a functional environment for patients to practice the social skills that they may be concurrently learning or to develop work adjustment skills that are needed to enter competitive employment. In situations where sheltered workshop activities parallel the technical vocational skills that the patient has just recently learned, he or she may be able to practice and further develop these abilities in the workshop before assuming a competitive job. Because sheltered workshop programs emulate working environments, they can also be used as a base for vocational or work adjustment evaluation by carefully observing patients' participation over the course of a prolonged evaluation period. By combining social skills, prevocational, and vocational assessment procedures, the sheltered work setting can offer a very flexible and "holistic" environment in which to observe and train complex work behaviors that are not frequently seen by psychiatric practitioners.

CASE EXAMPLE

Mary got along fine with everyone on the ward, including the staff, and it appeared that it was time to consider discharging her. Because she had no job before entering the hospital, she was referred to a vocational rehabilitation counselor who placed her in a sheltered workshop program to assess her vocational and social skills. Initially Mary was very shaky, did not complete her tasks at the required level of proficiency, and remained isolated from the other workers. Gradually, with the help of shop staff and co-workers, Mary began to adapt to these new surroundings and gain vocational proficiency. Her behavior on the ward was also noted to be much more animated, and she was soon ready for transfer into a community program. The sheltered workshop experience not only helped Mary gain important vocational experience, but also helped her learn that she could successfully adapt to new and oftentimes foreign environments.

Although sheltered employment offers many benefits to work restoration, it can also threaten the momentum of progress through the rehabilitation continuum when used as an exclusive agent for vocational rehabilitation. In places where the community support system lacks the other components required for comprehensive rehabilitation, the workshop itself can easily revert to a make-work rather than a skill-training environment. When this occurs, it is highly unlikely that any patients, except those with strong vocational and work adjustment skills, will be able to attain competitive employment. Unfortunately, the limitations of the spectrum of rehabilitation options within communities has resulted in some experts questioning the utility of sheltered employment in the rehabilitation continuum (Anthony et al. 1984). It is our opinion, however, that a properly designed sheltered workshop can be a vital component in the rehabilitation process.

TRANSITIONAL EMPLOYMENT

Transitional employment positions are real-work jobs within industrial or commercial establishments that are supervised by mental health or rehabilitation professionals. The concept is credited to Mr. John Beard, who was interested in developing intermediate work environments for

---

LEARNING EXERCISE

Sheltered workshops are often criticized as providing only make-work opportunities for patients or, even worse, of "enslaving" patients to the needs of the workshop or hospital. This occurs when patients are placed in positions that benefit the hospital or program, and the decisions to retain or advance patients are made on the basis of hospital needs rather than patients' therapeutic needs. This problem was pervasive during the first half of the 20th century and was responsible for the closing of many sheltered work programs across the country. List the steps that could be taken to prevent this problem in your locality.

Fountain House members who were more advanced than those in sheltered workshop settings but who were not yet ready for independent competitive employment.

According to the program design, the vocational rehabilitation program contracts with local businesses for the jobs and assumes responsibility for their completion. The rehabilitation program assigns each position to one or more patients who are then responsible for executing the job to industrial standards. Patients earn the same pay as those in the regular position in proportion to their work and effort. Hence, if two patients assume the same job, each working half-time, each patient will receive one half the normal salary for the position. For example, in the Fountain House program with a Sears department store, Fountain House assumed responsibility for a custodial position within Sears that had previously been filled by a regular employee. The position was vacant at the time and the company had problems keeping it filled. In assuming responsibility for the position, Sears agreed to let Fountain House complete the work using as many patients as appropriate, and Fountain House assured Sears that the job would be completed to industrial standards, even if Fountain House staff had to do the work themselves. The remuneration for the job to Fountain House was exactly the same as for any one person who had previously worked in the position.

Originally, Fountain House split the position between two patients, each of whom received half of the position's full salary. Each patient worked a half day at Sears under supervision of a Fountain House therapist who provided assistance with vocational, social, and other challenges that the patient faced on the job. Initially, patients remained on the job for three or four months to gain experience in a competitive position before moving on to their own nonsupervised job so that another patient could move into the position. Over time, additional positions have been added to the program, and long-term placements have also been developed for those who are capable of working effectively in a professionally supervised position but who cannot cope with the demands of a regular competitive position. In one transitional employment program, linked to the Thresholds psychosocial club in Chicago, methods were successfully developed and implemented to accelerate the rates of placement of psychiatric patients into jobs (Bond and Dincin 1986). Methods included use of screening and evaluation instruments that accurately predicted employability of ex-patients as well as more intensive methods of counseling and on-the-job supervision.

Transitional employment programs appear to offer a variety of benefits for patients as well as businesses. Transitional employment positions offer the patient the opportunity to experience a competitive position while still having accessibility to therapeutic staff. Unlike the impoverished pay given in most sheltered workshops, the transitional employment position pays a normal wage. Many of the positions that are best suited for patients in transitional employment programs are basic jobs that the business often has problems keeping filled. By working with a transitional employment program, the business is assured that the positions will be filled, that the work will be completed, and that they are contributing to their public service image. At the Thresholds psychosocial club, one transitional employment program was so successful that when the collaborating employer decided to expand his factory, he did so by enhancing the size of the "contract" for ex-patients' jobs with Thresholds. At a later time, when business contracted and the employer had to reduce the size of his workforce, he laid off regular employees and kept on the ex-patients who were participating in the transitional employment program.

On the other hand, businesses that are solicited for establishing a transitional employment program are taking the risk of contracting jobs with an unknown and possibly unreliable source of manpower, and of offending customers who do not understand psychiatric disability. Some firms simply prefer to avoid having to deal with psychiatric patients and having to get involved in rehabilitation issues that they do not understand. Thus it is often difficult to convince a business (especially a small business) to enter into a transitional employment contract. Consider some of these issues in the learning exercise on the next page.

CASE EXAMPLE ───

Eden Express, Inc. is a nonprofit corporation that runs a restaurant-based, vocational training program for the mentally disabled. Located in a Northern California community, the restaurant offers full-service

---

LEARNING EXERCISE

Operating a transitional employment program involves convincing a business to turn over one or more jobs and let you place your patients in the position. Remember: To a businessman, "time is money" and "the road to hell is paved with good intentions."

First, select a potential firm in your community that might be willing to consider accepting a transitional employment program. Next, make a list of all the pros and cons that a business might consider in determining whether to open up a position for transitional employment. Think of as many economic, political, prejudicial, social, and other reasons you can.

Next, come up with good supporting evidence for the positive reasons and good arguments against the negative reasons.

Finally, develop a balance sheet of the benefits and costs to employers who participate in transitional programs. If you owned a business, would you be willing to cooperate with such a program?

---

lunches and dinners to the general public and has received numerous awards and recognition for its outstanding menu and service.

Eden Express is specifically structured to help persons recovering from mental disabilities accomplish the following rehabilitation goals:

- to cope with their illness and compensate for their disability
- to deal comfortably with the public and become appropriately assertive with citizens in the community
- to function capably in competitive employment
- to become economically independent

Eden Express teaches confidence and job skills in an actual restaurant that is open to the public. A potential trainee fills out an application, tours Eden Express, and has an interview to determine his or her appropriateness for the program. When an applicant is determined to be appropriate, he or she is referred to the State Department of Rehabilitation for assistance with financing the costs of the training, transportation, and uniforms. The trainee's strengths and weaknesses in academic, communication, and work skills are identified by using information obtained from the trainee as well as observations by staff members. After evaluation and acceptance into the program, a trainee progresses through four levels of training: 1) Work Adjustment, 2) Job Skill Training, 3) Vocational Planning, and 4) Job Search.

The Work Adjustment phase takes from two weeks to one month to complete. During this phase trainees participate in back-room activities such as washing dishes, laundering, cleaning, and preparing food. Trainees are assessed on punctuality, cleanliness, response to direction, ability to follow directions, and relationships with co-workers. When a trainee appears to be motivated and desirous of learning job skills, has appropriate personal grooming and the ability to complete tasks, and follows directions and attends regularly, he or she is deemed ready for the next phase.

Job Skill Training focuses on learning the actual job skills, refining certain behaviors, increasing speed in completing tasks, and using appropriate etiquette. Trainees learn skills for positions including beverage bar worker, waitress/waiter, hostess, and cashier. Trainees are rotated through as many of the positions as they are appropriate for (for example, some patients are not able to calculate money and thus they are not trained for the cashier position). When sufficient skill and speed are maintained for at least one week, the trainee begins the vocational planning phase.

Vocational Planning continues the Job Skill Training with the emphasis on trainees' taking total responsibility for their assigned job stations. An adult education teacher evaluates their academic level and teaches the skills they require (for example, the patient may be taught to use a calculator or how to use a bank account). At this point the patient develops a résumé and identifies what he or she wants to do.

The Job Search phase can be started whenever the individual has sufficient job skills, confidence, and stamina to handle the regular working world. The trainee still remains in the work experience program but works fewer hours. He or she practices interviewing skills and develops a job contract, planning the steps for securing a job. During this time, the trainee goes out on several job interviews a week until a job is secured.

All facets of Eden Express have a wide variety of community volunteers and business groups that support the program. These volunteers are used as waiters/waitresses and serve as role models. They also participate on committees and serve on the restaurant advisory board. Many have commercial experience in running restaurants and provide input accordingly. The restaurant employs one social worker, one rehabilitation counselor, one administrator, one bookkeeper, five restaurant workers, and eight nonpaid consultants. They collectively contribute approximately 400 person-hours per week.

Although Eden Express is only one program within the larger community support system, it provides psychosocial rehabilitation services in vocational rehabilitation; supportive work opportunities; back-up support to families, friends, and community members; the involvement of community members; protection of patients' rights; and case management services.

The average training time is five months. After three years of operation, 133 people had entered the program for training or work evaluation. Of those who graduated, 62 percent obtained jobs, 26 percent went on to school or further training, and 12 percent discontinued the program.

JOB PLACEMENT

Because few patients have jobs waiting when they are ready to assume competitive employment, job placement is a crucial linchpin in successful work restoration. There are generally several different approaches to job placement including counselor-based referral systems and job club programs. Unfortunately, most mentally restored persons have little access to job placement services and must fend for themselves with advocacy and assistance from a responsible psychiatrist and case manager or therapist.

"Traditional" counselor-based referral systems usually involve one-on-one services between a vocational counselor and the patient. Most of these services are provided by state, vocational rehabilitation agencies, and employment development services, although some private agencies do exist on a fee-for-service basis. Once an individual is either referred to a state department of rehabilitation by a mental health professional or goes there him- or herself, it becomes the responsibility of the agency's vocational counselor to assess the patient's motivation, interests, abilities, and limitations; provide vocational counseling; find a job or a job training option for the patient; and assure his or her placement in the position. Because most vocational counselors are under placement quotas and persons with chronic psychiatric disabilities are difficult to place, the latter are often the last to receive rehabilitation services from state agencies. In some cases, the counselor cannot provide the extended time and effort necessary to facilitate a successful outcome; in other cases, counselors lack the knowledge and skills for working competently with the psychiatrically disabled. These factors contribute to the disproportionately low acceptance and placement rates for persons with psychiatric disabilities that are noted in many vocational rehabilitation agencies.

CASE EXAMPLE ―――――――――――――――――――――――――――

Acceptance of mentally ill persons by vocational rehabilitation counselors working for state agencies is fraught with obstacles and difficulties. Stigma of mental illness, unfamiliarity with the mentally ill person and his problems, lack of training of counselors in mental disorders and their modern treatment, and counselors' concern over poor employment outcomes traditionally associated with mental disorders combine to restrict services and rehabilitation opportunities. Thus, it is crucial for the referring psychiatrist and mental health team to make a clear and strong case for the referral.

To assure that appropriate services are provided to the patient, the referring psychiatrist or other mental health service provider should write a letter that describes the diagnosis; the patient's current functional capacity and readiness for work; the patient's motivation and desire for work; and the clinical indications for the patient's appropriateness for vocational rehabilitation, work training, or job placement activities. A letter should be accompanied by phone and in-person consultations by the psychiatrist with the vocational rehabilitation counselor to further advocate for the patient's receipt of counseling services and to assist the counselor in dealing with problems. A consulting, collaborative relationship between the referring psychiatrist and the counselor working for the state rehabilitation agency is a necessity to ensure follow-through and continuity in the rehabilitation plan. For example, if the patient verbalizes symptoms of his or her disorder to the counselor or shows signs of exacerbation of symptoms or stress, the psychiatrist and mental health treatment team must be available to respond in a constructive way to the counselor's concerns.

The following letter is an example of the first step in a successful referral. The referral letter was followed by phone consultation, which led to the patient's receiving a subsidy from the state department of rehabilitation for a vocational training course in automobile repair.

To the California Department of Rehabilitation:

I am referring a patient of mine, Mr. G.C., for vocational rehabilitation services. Mr. C. has significant medical and psychiatric impairments and disabilities that have been effectively treated. He is now considered ready for vocational training and subsequent job placement services.

Mr. C. suffered knee trauma during a skiing accident some years ago which required reparative surgery. Subsequent to that time, he experienced post-traumatic arthritis in that left knee that has been successfully treated with anti-inflammatory agents. His knee is currently functional and his arthritis is under good control with maintenance medication. In addition, Mr. C. has suffered from a schizophrenic disorder since the age of 25. The impairments from this disorder have included problems concentrating on tasks of an academic nature, resulting in his having to discontinue graduate studies in law. He also has experienced occasional delusions and hallucinations. Fortunately, Mr. C. has responded well to treatment of these symptoms with ongoing antipsychotic drug therapy and has been in good remission for over one year. He reliably takes maintenance, low-dose antipsychotic medication as a prophylactic measure, once daily at bedtime.

While his disorder and its impairments have disabled him from pursuing a law career, the patient and I believe he can become successfully employed in another field that does not tax or stress his cognitive capacities. Because of his lifelong interest in cars and auto repair (he has serviced and repaired his own car and those of friends and relatives for many years), we believe that participation in a formal course of automobile mechanics will be an effective rehabilitation plan.

Mr. C. had an excellent work history before his disability began 3 years ago. He had several long-term, albeit part-time, positions during high school and college and worked each summer on a full-time basis. He has held positions as a paralegal and has performed well in those jobs. Despite his psychiatric disorder, Mr. C. has continued to work in volunteer and part-time positions, more recently in a transitional employment position at a local department store.

I would appreciate your careful evaluation of Mr. C.'s potential for vocational training in auto mechanics, which appears to be an occupation that would capitalize on his assets and interests and would not pose excessive stress on him. Participation in a vocational training program would markedly improve Mr. C.'s self-esteem and be the first step back to a productive life. I would appreciate your considering him for such services as vocational evaluation testing, aptitude testing, tuition for auto mechanics school, reimbursement for travel and books to school, and payment for uniforms. Please call upon me should any questions or concerns arise. I will phone your office in two weeks to consult with you on Mr. C.'s progress.

Sincerely yours,
[name of referring psychiatrist]

JOB CLUB

Even when a patient has been accepted into a state vocational rehabilitation program and has been successfully placed in a job, the patient has not learned how to independently find a job and would be dependent upon the counselor in the future when a new job is needed. The Job Club program, initially developed by Dr. Nathan Azrin and his associates (Azrin and Besalel 1980; Azrin et al. 1975; Azrin and Phillip 1979), takes an alternative approach that places the responsibility of finding a job on the patient, with the assistance of rehabilitation staff. Emphasis is placed on the use of skill building, goal setting, and structured environments that are designed to help patients find their own jobs. A basic tenet of the program is that finding a job is a full-time job, and patients are expected to participate in the program on a full-time daily basis. In addition, by learning job-seeking skills and taking responsibility for the job search, patients learn independent employment-seeking skills that may be needed in finding other jobs later.

During the first week of the program, patients learn basic job-seeking skills such as how to locate sources of job leads, how to look for a job, how to fill out job applications and résumés, effective use of the telephone, appropriate grooming and dressing skills, and how to participate in interviews. In the second week of the program, patients begin a full-time job search and remain in the program until they find a job or leave the program unemployed.

To facilitate the job-finding process, the Job Club provides the basic resources needed to conduct a job search, including telephones, desks, fresh job leads, secretarial support, and counselors to help patients set and adhere to their occupational goals. Motivational systems are also used to encourage morale and persistence. Participants are teamed in pairs to aid and support each other through the job search. Monetary or token reinforcement systems, in conjunction with counselor encouragement, supplement peer support. For example, in the Brentwood Job Finding Club (Jacobs et al. 1984) patients earned $0.50 per hour for participation; they received frequent monitoring and social support by program staff as well.

Daily goal-setting exercises were also used to help each participant more effectively manage the many responsibilities and demands of a job search. In this manner they were able to break down large and seemingly unattainable tasks into more attainable objectives. In Table 35 is presented a sample of the daily goals for one participant in the program.

The role of the Job Club counselor is also structured to help maximize patient contact hours. Hence, paperwork and other administrative functions are reduced to a minimum, meetings are arranged outside of normal working hours, and assistance to patients in pursuing job finding becomes the most important part of the counselor's job.

To date, Job Club results across a wide range of populations have been impressive. One study (Azrin and Phillip 1979) revealed that Job Club members started work an average of 14 days after beginning the program, whereas clients randomly assigned to a traditional, counselor-mediated placement program took an average of 53 days to find employment. The starting salary for Job Club members was 36 percent greater than that of non-Club members, and it cost an average of $20 to place a participant in the Job Club, compared to $300 per placed patient in the control group. As noted in Figure 21, the Brentwood Job Finding Club has reported similar results. Approximately 65 percent of

TABLE 35: Job Club Daily Log Form

NAME: JOHN SMITH   DATE: 6 / 20 / 86   8:15 Meeting YES: NO:

ACTIVITIES I WILL TRY TO ACCOMPLISH TODAY: (see examples)

(1) Telephone Canvass Burbank
(2) Mail Application to ABC, Inc.
(3) Review Want Ads
(4) Call Rehabilitation Department

Time	Job Lead Source	Activity: in person or phone contact, résumé, interview, EDD, etc.	Company: Name and Address Phone Number	Name of Person Contacted	Type of Job	Results of Contact	Follow-Up
9:00 A.M.	Yellow pages	Telephone contact	Acme Auto Body Repair 14000 Wilshire Boulevard Tel: (213) 888-5555	Mr. Jones, Owner	Mechanic	Come in and fill out application	Yes
	Job Club Group Meeting	Telephone contact	Help Temporary Services 11100 Wilshire Boulevard Tel: (213) 788-8883	Susan, Employment Rep.	Photocopy operator	No job, call back tomorrow	Yes
	N/A	In Person	Job Club Office Tel: ( ) -	Don, Job Club Counselor	N/A	Help with Job Application	N/A
			Tel: ( ) -				
10:00 A.M.	N/A	By Self	Job Club Office Tel: ( ) -	N/A	N/A	Continued filling out application	N/A
	Previous Contact	Telephone Call	Burbank Motors 876 Victory Boulevard Tel: (818) 237-4900	Alvin Rosen, Service Manager	Mechanic	Come in for Interview	Yes
	Previous Contact	Travel Time and Interview	Burbank Motors 876 Victory Boulevard Tel: (818) 237-4900	Alvin Rosen, Service Manager	Mechanic	To call back tomorrow for results	Yes

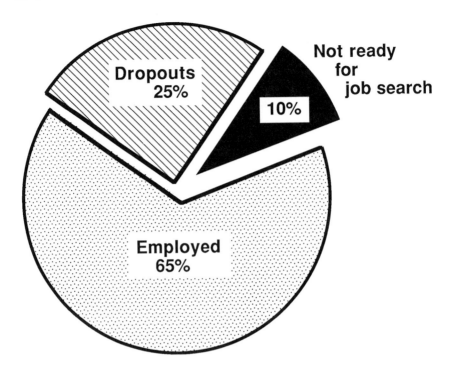

FIGURE 21: Outcomes from 200 consecutive psychiatric patients who participated in the Brentwood VA Job Finding Club. Ten percent of the patients were returned to their wards or clinics because their level of psychopathology was too great for embarking on the rigors of a job search. Twenty-five percent of the patients completed at least three days of the Job Club but discontinued the program before finding work.

all patients entering the program began full-time employment or vocational training following an average of 23 days of participation. These data compare favorably to other Job Club reports, in which 65 percent to 85 percent of all participants entered employment, and are vastly superior to the 10 percent to 30 percent placement rates noted for traditional psychiatric work restoration programs.

One of the most impressive findings in the Brentwood program has been that chronic psychiatric impairment alone does not detract from the likelihood of finding employment. A study of over 200 psychiatric patients in the Brentwood Job Finding Club indicated that length of disability or diagnosis did not predict vocational placement; for example over 50 percent of the participants suffered from schizophrenic disorders. Program participation appeared to be the most important determinant of employment outcome, with increasing age and severity of psychopathology also having an influence.

CASE EXAMPLE

Tony joined the Brentwood Job Finding Club following two months of hospitalization for symptoms of acute paranoid schizophrenia. His work history consisted of a series of transient jobs, which he held after receiving a psychiatric discharge from the military. He had been receiving antipsychotic medication intermittently during the past ten years. As part of his delusional system he was convinced that he "contracted" schizophrenia at the time when he had volunteered to give a pint of blood at a Red Cross drive. He felt the doctor had purposely taken out two pints of blood instead. His motive for joining the Job Club was to be able to save up enough money to hire a lawyer to sue the doctor and get his missing pint of blood back.

Although he entered the Job Club with staff members' reservations, he quickly picked up the daily routine and began searching for a job as a bookkeeper's assistant or bank teller. He was able to remain discreet about his symptoms and had well-developed interpersonal skills. The first two months were rough, and he was rejected after a number of job interviews. Tony persisted, however, and subsequently did find a position as a bank teller, remaining on the job for a full year.

CASE EXAMPLE

Mildred was a 28-year-old woman with multiple psychiatric hospitalizations over the past six years for schizophrenia. Some of her problems appeared to be job related. She worked in more than 16 positions during her career as a secretary/clerk, with no position lasting more than three months. Frequently, problems on the job and symptom exacerbation occurred at the same time, resulting in rehospitalization. Accordingly, evaluation and treatment for her current hospital admission included extensive vocational and social assessment in a series of structured work settings.

Mildred was first assigned to a sheltered workshop where her work and social behavior patterns could be observed in a simulated job setting. Initial observations indicated that Mildred repetitively nagged her supervisor about tiny details of the job. He noted, "She is an extremely insecure person in terms of her job duties and wants to make sure that she is doing everything right. Even the simplest of tasks assigned to her results in her asking me if she is doing it right, or how to do it, or clarification of the assignment. It is not unusual for her to ask me questions every ten minutes or so. She is driving me crazy." In addition, the supervisor noted that she socially isolated herself from co-workers. Hence,

LEARNING EXERCISE

The Job Finding Club is obviously a complex program that cannot be easily simulated in a textbook exercise. Instead, consider two of the components of the program—finding job leads and presenting job histories.

1. Job Leads. To find a job you have to have effective job leads to locate potential positions. For most of us with good social skills and contacts in the community, this is fairly easy. For the psychiatrically impaired person who has few friends and resources, it is a different story.

Make a list of all of the different types of job leads that you can think of that you might use in a job search. Be creative. Then indicate which of these sources of job leads would be available for a chronic psychiatric patient who hasn't functioned effectively in the community for years. Can you think of other leads that this person could use?

2. Job Histories. One issue that keeps popping up regarding job interviews and employment applications is what to do about major gaps in employment. Should the patient be honest about such periods of unemployment or should he try to "cosmetically" alter such problems? On the one hand, if he tells the truth, he may not get the job. On the other hand, if he lies and is caught later, he may be fired. The individual also has to live with a guilty conscience while on the job. Of course this is not an absolute issue, and it is ultimately up to the patient to decide upon his or her ultimate course of action. Still, patients will come to you for your advice. What would you tell them? Under what conditions would you change your position? Would your advice be different for a patient applying for a job with a firm that has an affirmative action program that gives priority to hiring the handicapped? How would you feel or react if they followed your advice with disastrous consequences? Discuss your reactions with a colleague.

Mildred's initial work-related problems were pinpointed as deficient identification of work role requirements, need of excessive supervision, poor communication with supervisors, deficits in problem solving and decision making, and deficient social skills with peers.

These problems were subsequently remediated through coaching and feedback both in the workshop and in her social skills training classes over the next three months. By integrating rehabilitation goals across therapies, it was possible to help Mildred quickly acquire new skills and apply them to practical situations. Soon Mildred was ready to look for her own competitive community employment through the Job Club program.

Mildred was prompt for the Job Club orientation meeting and related well to the staff and other participating patients. The following day she was the first person at the initial Job Club training session. While less extreme than before, Mildred betrayed her insecurity by asking many questions. However, the Job Club staff was prepared and worked with Mildred to be more succinct and to the point. For example, during job interview training sessions, a great deal of emphasis was placed on her asking only pertinent questions. Positive and negative feedback was differentially provided to her on the basis of her verbalizations. She was coached on how to ask only those questions that directly related to the job.

Although Mildred made considerable progress in the Job Club and sought employment with a feverish pace, her high level of social anxiety appeared to prevent her from obtaining a job. To provide more real world experience to ensure a successful vocational outcome, both Mildred and the Job Club staff decided to find a transitional employment setting where she could further hone her skills while serving as a productive employee. The Job Club staff helped Mildred develop a "marketing strategy" that emphasized her considerable skills and the fact that an employer who hired Mildred and helped her adapt to the workplace would have an outstanding and dedicated employee.

Several weeks later, Mildred found an office job with a supervisor who was willing to work with both her and the Job Club staff. The supervisor was briefed on Mildred's skills, deficits, and vocational interests and was given assistance in setting up a conducive work environment. Because of Mildred's clerical skills and her interest in computers, her initial assignment was for straight typing at a computer console that was isolated from other staff. This helped reduce work distractions and allowed her to integrate into the social environment at her own pace.

Gradually, as Mildred gained more confidence in her duties, more responsibilities were given to her, and she began to learn word processing. Other office staff also began to give her social support, making sure that she was invited to coffee breaks and included in office conversations according to her comfort level. Job Club staff also made follow-up visits to the office to encourage and help Mildred with the demands of the position. Initially, these visits were made weekly, but over time they were reduced to periodic telephone calls to Mildred or her supervisor.

Six months after beginning the job, Mildred received a promotion to word processing specialist. Although she is still somewhat more sensitive to workday pressures than most of her co-workers, she has found the support and the skills necessary to cope and remain employed.

JOB MAINTENANCE

Finding a job is no promise of keeping a job, and a wide range of problems may preclude job tenure. Frequently, technical competence is a relatively minor obstacle to job maintenance compared with other problems that the newly employed worker may face. For example, many patients find that they have to start at the bottom of the ladder in transitory or unskilled positions that are in constant risk of being closed out. Other patients face the syndrome of being the last-hired and thus the first-fired during economic recessions. Those with relatively stable jobs may face other problems such as adjustment to the new worksite or adjusting to changes in life-style that come with employment status. The latter includes finding a new place to live, locating transportation, managing a budget, meeting new people, and integrating the demands of work with the demands of daily living. Each of these issues represents a potential stressor that may exacerbate symptoms, decrease stability, and threaten job longevity. Finally, changes in medication and the variable course of mental illness may also affect job productivity and stability. Take our previous example, Tony, who, as you will recall, found a job as a bank teller.

CASE EXAMPLE ⸻

Tony had to leave the job after one year due to symptom exacerbation. Tony's employers were pleased with his work, but he discontinued his neuroleptic medication and became increasingly paranoid about the standard security systems that the bank employed. He finally walked off the job brimming over with delusional fears for his safety. He was able to avert a rehospitalization because of rapid neuroleptization by his psychiatrist, who also referred him back to the Job Club. The vocational counselors contacted Tony's bank employer and worked out an Employee Assistance Program that required Tony to meet monthly with his psychiatrist and remain on low doses of maintenance antipsychotic medication.

Entry into competitive community employment does not signify the termination of rehabilitation services, since many patients will still require continuing clinical support with on-the-job problems. In fact, the stressors faced by mentally restored persons who begin employment often demand increases in the level of rehabilitative and psychiatric intervention. Ultimately, effective follow-up depends upon the program resources that are available for such services, the needs of individual patients and cooperation from both employers and patients. Frequently, mentally restored individuals choose to disassociate themselves from the hospital in order to remove the social stigma associated with psychiatric care, making follow-up and job maintenance proportionately more difficult.

At a minimum, good job maintenance services require both periodic and as-needed contact with employed patients to assess their progress, with one-on-one counseling, program referral, and other interventions as necessary to address new and developing problems. Weekly, monthly, or even daily contacts may initially be required to help the patient adjust to the demands of the new environment, but these contacts can be reduced as time passes and the patient adapts. Ultimately, the frequency of contact for each patient will vary as changes in symptoms, stressors, medication, and other factors affect job performance.

From a basic level of monitoring and supportive interventions, more intensive programs can also be developed, including on-the-job visits by rehabilitation staff, alumni clubs through which employed patients can meet for mutual support, and individualized social skills and work adjustment training that further patients' coping abilities. Although more intensive job maintenance programs cost more money, they are usually more effective in helping patients stay on the job and in the community, and are ultimately less expensive than relapse and inpatient hospitalization.

CASE EXAMPLE

Fred was 28 years old and had been able to hold only temporary jobs as a truck driver and shipping clerk during the five years since being discharged from the Marines. He suffered from chronic depression and symptoms of posttraumatic stress disorder resulting from his combat experiences in the Vietnam War. He was fired from most jobs because of poor attendance, substance abuse, and explosive anger and fights with co-workers and supervisors.

Following successful treatment of his psychiatric disorders in a Veterans Hospital, Fred enrolled in a typewriter-repair training program and completed the vocational training in 13 months. His first job required him to interact with customers when he made visits to offices to repair typewriters. His supervisor had received numerous complaints from customers regarding Fred's rudeness and temper and was on the verge of firing Fred when his vocational rehabilitation counselor undertook a series of training sessions with Fred to improve his interpersonal relations on the job.

Thirteen scenes were constructed involving interactions with customers, security guards, co-workers, and his supervisor. Five target skills were identified for training, based on assessments made of Fred's role-playing these scenes: 1) nonverbal behaviors such as voice volume, affect, and eye contact; 2) acknowledging and responding to customers' feelings; 3) eliciting suggestions to solve problems; 4) requesting clarification when criticized by others; and 5) making appropriate self-assertions when criticized unjustly.

Training was provided in 90-minute sessions with the counselor, who role-played customers, supervisor, and security guards in buildings that Fred visited on his repair jobs. Instructions, modeling, praise for signs of improvement, and homework assignments were used as the training methods. Fred readily responded to the training and transferred the skills learned in the office sessions with the counselor to his work in the field. Indeed, at 9 months' follow-up, the supervisor reported no further complaints about Fred's relations with customers and co-workers and indicated complete satisfaction with Fred's performance on the job. The improvement in Fred's target goals for training is shown in Figure 22, where training was introduced at different times sequentially to document the causal linkage between the intervention and its impact on Fred's behavioral skills.

Some patients, as in Tony's case, will lose their jobs or relapse, despite the most heroic efforts at rehabilitation, for reasons beyond programmatic control. Such cases do not represent a failure of vocational rehabilitation; rather, they underscore the need to reintegrate the patient back into the appropriate level of services within the vocational rehabilitation continuum. In this manner, vocational rehabilitation remains a fluid and dynamic process, adapted to the changing needs of its patients. However, be ready to defend the vocational rehabilitation continuum in the eyes of your agency's administration, as in the following learning exercise.

LEARNING EXERCISE

Although most administrators ascribe to the benefits of job maintenance programs as a means of helping patients stay out of the hospital, these types of services are usually the last to be organized and the first to go when budgets are cut. Develop an effective argument supporting the establishment of a job maintenance program within your facility. Try to find and incorporate both clinical and financial resources and cost-benefit data to support your position.

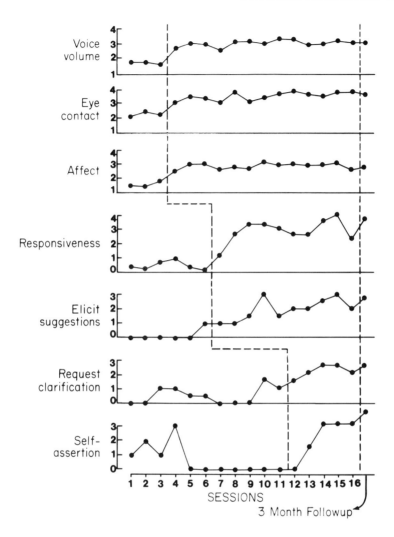

FIGURE 22: Acquisition and maintenance of work-related social skills in a patient with a chronic depressive and anxiety disorder. Skills training was provided during a four-month period. The broken line on the left denotes the initiation of training for each skill. Voice volume, eye contact, and affect are based on the sum of scores of 4-point scales, with higher numbers indicating better performance. Other behavioral skills were scored on a frequency-of-occurrence basis during role-play assessment. Reprinted with permission from Mueser KT, Foy DW, Carter MJ: Social skills training for job maintenance in a psychiatric patient. Journal of Counseling Psychology 33:360–362, 1986.

SUMMARY

By now it should be evident that vocational rehabilitation is a comprehensive and dynamic effort that encompasses much more than just finding jobs for the mentally restored. Accordingly, this chapter has presented a continuum of services that represents a model for comprehensive work restoration. Although individual practitioners or mental health facilities may not be able to provide all of the noted services, it is still possible to provide a spectrum of rehabilitation by joining ranks with other mental health workers and rehabilitation agencies to combine elements that together may compose the work restoration continuum.

There is an expansion in the growth and specialization of rehabilitation disciplines responsible for serving disabled and handicapped individuals throughout the continuum of rehabilitation programs. Vocational rehabilitation counselors are trained in baccalaureate, master's and doctoral degree programs in many universities; in addition, other individuals are being trained in vocational assessment and evaluation techniques. A half-dozen professional organizations and over 10 journals support the professional identities and subspecialization of these practitioners. Unfortunately, the linkages and communication channels between rehabilitation and mental health professionals are often unwieldy and rife with misunderstanding of one another's philosophy, goals, and methods. In coming years, it will be essential for the mental health disciplines to become more familiar with the conceptual base and specific techniques used by rehabilitation workers, and vice versa. Unless close collaboration is forged among psychiatrists, case managers, and other primary therapists of chronic psychiatric patients, patient care and rehabilitation outcomes will suffer.

As with any dynamic process, not everybody will follow the same course of rehabilitation. Some patients may progress through each of the steps that have been outlined sequentially and secure stable competitive employment. Other patients, due to various limitations, may be able to progress only to sheltered workshop status, while still others may need very little retraining and can enter job placement directly. Finally, some patients will reverberate through the different levels as new skills develop or new needs arise.

Although this chapter presents the vocational rehabilitation process as a rational, orderly sequence of steps, most individuals obtain jobs or other vocational experiences more opportunistically. Job leads pop up unexpectedly and are often taken, even when the individual may not be fully prepared for the rigors of work. In such cases, the psychiatric practitioner can raise his or her level of intervention and provide more liaison and supportive counseling with the patient and employer. In that manner, the job itself may become the venue for some of the missing elements of work adjustment and work "hardening." Opportunities and timing, as well as skills, are important to career development, making it important to maintain a flexible and adaptive system. The mark of an efficient and effective system is how well it adapts to prevailing patient needs for productive engagement in work, rather than how well people adapt to its operation.

Ultimately, a successful vocational outcome transcends job skills alone to the overall social competence of a mentally restored individual. Finding and keeping a job requires effective social skills, strategies for coping with daily stressors, judicious pharmacotherapy, community support, family education, problem-solving abilities, effective symptom management, and an ability to integrate these protective factors into an effective whole (Liberman et al. 1986). Deficiencies in any one of these can result in job loss and vocational failure. Thus, perhaps more than in any other area, the significance of integrating the various elements of comprehensive psychiatric rehabilitation is highly evident in vocational rehabilitation. The other chapters of this book highlight the protective factors required for comprehensive and successful rehabilitation of mentally restored persons in jobs and their communities.

REFERENCES

Anthony WA: Principles of Psychiatric Rehabilitation. Baltimore, MD, University Park Press, 1979

Anthony WA, Buell GJ, Sharratt S, et al: Efficacy of psychiatric rehabilitation. Psychol Bull 78:447–456, 1972

Anthony WA, Cohen MR, Vitalo R: The measurement of rehabilitation outcome. Schizophr Bull 4:365–383, 1978

Azrin NH: The job-finding club as a method for obtaining eligible clients: demonstration, evaluation and counselor training [Final Report #51-17-76104]. Washington, DC, U.S. Department of Labor, 1978

Azrin NH, Besalel VA: Job Club Counselors Manual: A Behavioral Approach to Vocational Counseling. Baltimore, MD, University Park Press, 1980

Azrin NH, Flores T, Kaplan SJ: Job finding club: a group-assisted program for obtaining employment. Behav Res Ther 13:17–27, 1975

Azrin NH, Phillip RA: The job club method for the job handicapped: a comparative outcome study. Rehabilitation Counseling Bulletin 23:144–155, 1979

Beard JH, Malmud TJ, Rossman E: Psychiatric rehabilitation and long-term rehospitalization rates: the findings of two research studies. Schizophr Bull 4:622–635, 1978

Bennett DH: The historical development of rehabilitation services, in Theory and Practice of Psychiatric Rehabilitation. Edited by Watts FN, Bennett DH. New York, Wiley, 1983

Bond, GR, Boyer SL: The evaluation of vocational programs for the mentally ill: a review, in Vocational Rehabilitation of Persons with Prolonged Mental Illness. Edited by Ciardiello JA, Bell MD. Baltimore, MD, Johns Hopkins University Press, 1978

Bond GR, Dincin J: Accelerating entry into transitional employment in a psychosocial rehabilitation agency. Rehabilitation Psychology 31:143–155, 1986

Catalano R, Dooley D, Jackson R: Economic predictors of admissions to mental health facilities in non-metropolitan areas. J Health Soc Behav 22:284–297, 1981

Dooley D, Catalano R: Economic change as a cause of behavioral disorder. Psychol Bull 87:450–468, 1980

Fairweather GW, Sanders DH, Maynard H, et al: Community life for the mentally ill: an alternative to institutional care. Chicago, Adeline, 1969

Hartlage A: Hospitals and patients' view of industrial therapy. Psychiatr Q 41:264–267, 1967

Jacobs HE, Kardashian S, Kreinbring RK, et al: A skills-oriented model for facilitating employment among psychiatrically disabled persons. Rehabilitation Counseling Bulletin 28:87–96, 1984

Jahoda M, Lazarsfeld PF, Ziesel H: The Sociography of an Unemployed Community. Chicago, Aldine and Atherton, 1971

Kunce JT: Is work therapy really therapeutic? Rehabil Lit 31:297–320, 1970

Liberman RP, Jacobs HE, Boone S, et al: New methods for rehabilitating chronic mental patients, in Our Patients' Future in a Changing World. Edited by Talbott JA. Washington, DC, American Psychiatric Press, 1986

Stein L, Test MA: An alternative to mental hospital treatment: I. Conceptual model, treatment program, and clinical evaluation. Arch Gen Psychiatry 37:392–399, 1980

Strauss JS, Carpenter WT: The prediction of outcome in schizophrenia. Arch Gen Psychiatry 31:37–42, 1974

Strauss JS, Carpenter WT: Prediction of outcome in schizophrenia. III. Five-year outcome and its predictors. Arch Gen Psychiatry 34:159–163, 1977

Strauss JS, Hafez H: Clinical questions and "real" research. Am J Psychiatry 138:1592–1597, 1981

Weiss RS, Reisman D: Social problems and disorganization in the world of work, in Contemporary Social Problems. Edited by Merton RK, Nisbet RA. New York, Harcourt, Brace and World, 1961

CHAPTER 8

COMMUNITY SUPPORT

CATHERINE PHIPPS, M.S.
ROBERT PAUL LIBERMAN, M.D.

No one ever touches me.
My skin is cold, old, I am turning to stone.
No one ever listens to me.
There's nothing to hear, but fear, I am alone.
No one ever looks at me.
There's nothing to see, but me, an old crone.
No one knows what's inside of me.
A soul whole Unknown.

Eugenia G. Wheeler
"The Bag Lady"

Deinstitutionalization, which began in the 1950s, has resulted in the release of many persons with long-term mental illness from state hospitals. In 1955, the number of hospitalized mental patients was 558,992; twenty years later, the number was 193,436, a reduction of 65 percent (National Institute of Mental Health [NIMH] Division of Biometry and Epidemiology 1979). These patients were not cured; rather, their locus was switched from back wards of large hospitals to "back streets" of communities. In 1981 an estimated 800,000 chronic mental patients with severe disabilities were residing in the community; an additional 700,000 individuals had a partial disability due to a mental condition (Goldman et al. 1981). Responsibility for their care has been placed on the communities into which they have been released.

New service delivery models and methods for the care and treatment of the severely psychiatrically disabled in the community have been developed during the past two decades and have been termed *community support programs*. Prime among the attributes of a community support program is comprehensiveness of service elements. This means that the full spectrum of the psychiatrically disabled person's needs must be met within the context of an agency or community mental health center that coordinates the provision of services by a range of other agencies in such areas as medical and psychiatric care, housing, social and financial benefits and pensions, vocational rehabilitation, advocacy, and recreational activities. Usually, the coordination of services is carried out through a system of case management. Case management duties include patient identification and outreach, individual assessment, service planning, linkage with requisite services, monitoring of service delivery, and patient advocacy.

The development of comprehensive and effective community support programs in the various states has been stimulated through conferences, provision of technical assistance, and the granting of funds for start-up efforts by the NIMH.

The stress-vulnerability-coping-competence model, described fully in Chapter 1, highlights the role of community support programs in the rehabilitation effort. Community programs serve as environmental "protectors" that can reduce the noxious effects of critical, nonsupportive, emotionally overinvolved, and/or overstimulating social environments on biologically vulnerable individuals. In addition, community support programs can strengthen the "protective" effects of skills training on chronic psychiatric patients. Learning problem-solving skills, conversational skills, and vocational, leisure, and self-care skills within the context of a community support program promotes the chronic patient's attainment of realistic goals and improved clinical and social outcomes. Goal attainment, in turn, increases the patient's self-efficacy. Chronically mentally ill individuals who participate in community support programs, therefore, are more likely to obtain their needs as they learn to meet the challenges and solve the problems of every-day life. Given the personal and environmental protectors present in community support programs, it is not surprising that patients enrolled in these programs have fewer relapses and improved social and vocational adjustment (Stein and Test 1980).

NEEDS OF PSYCHIATRIC PATIENTS IN THE COMMUNITY

Unfortunately, communities across the United States that have deinstitutionalized their chronically mentally ill have not adequately replaced state hospital services with community services; most communities have not provided appropriate and comprehensive treatment. Fifty to sixty percent of all discharged psychiatric patients cannot sustain life in the community for two years, and there has been a thirty percent increase in the annual rate of readmission of schizophrenic patients in recent years (Liberman et al. 1984). Moreover, deinstitutionalization has led to the dumping of thousands of patients into custodial care in nursing or boarding homes or, worse, into homeless existences in our cities' skid rows (Bachrach 1984; Lamb 1979).

While in the community, patients may experience a host of problems related to inadequate and/or unavailable treatment (Lamb 1976). For example,

- Many chronically mentally ill persons are denied emergency treatment because hospital beds are not available.
- Many mentally ill persons receive little or no treatment in board and care homes.
- Many mentally ill persons are placed in jails because more appropriate placements are lacking.
- Many mentally ill individuals live on the streets without receiving any services.
- The burden of caretaking in many cases has fallen upon the relatives of the mentally ill.

These problems and inadequacies in service delivery are compounded by the oft-documented inability of patients to function adequately in the community (Kuehnel et al. 1984). For example,

- Chronic mental patients frequently need assistance in bathing, dressing, and grooming.
- Although most patients receive psychoactive medication, few follow a prescribed medication regimen.
- Most chronically mentally ill persons are unable to maintain a home or apartment, keep appointments, or hold a paying job.

- Few psychiatrically disabled persons are able to manage money appropriately.
- Many schizophrenic persons have low self-initiative, low sociability, high depression, numerous maladaptive habits, and psychotic symptoms.
- Most chronically mentally ill persons exhibit vulnerability to stress, deficits in coping skills, extreme dependency, difficulties in interpersonal relationships, and vocational deficiencies.

In addition to inadequate treatment and the deficits in patient functioning, lack of a social support network may also affect a patient's tenure in the community. Psychiatric hospitals provide only a temporary and highly artificial social network that is rarely maintained upon release. In addition, the patient's social network, utilized prior to hospitalization, may weaken or dissipate completely during hospitalization. Even for mentally ill individuals who do not get hospitalized for longer than brief periods, the disabilities and behavioral abnormalities imposed by their illness often leave them far behind their peers in maturation and life development, a further cause of isolation and loneliness.

Social support networks are vital to successful community tenure. Social network characteristics are significantly associated with degree of psychiatric illness. Severely ill patients have smaller networks, highly dominated by family members, with only a few friends. While the circle of supportive individuals is smaller, these individuals are used with greater frequency, often leading to burnout and alienation of family members (Heller and Swindle 1983). The stress and tension that build between a mentally ill person and relatives can produce the high expressed emotion of families, described in Chapter 6, that has been found to be a powerful predictor of relapse.

Other studies on social networks have found that chronically disordered individuals who have strong connections with family, friends, and fellow workers enjoy increased community tenure. When relapse does occur, it is often preceded by a disruption in the patient's social network (Hammer 1963, 1964). Further, the strength of the patient's network has been shown to have an inverse relationship with severity of psychiatric symptoms; thus, smaller networks predispose patients' likelihood of returning to the hospital (Sokolovsky et al. 1978).

One form of community mental health service that has attempted to compensate for the lack of social support networks among the chronically mentally ill is the social club. Emerging from the psychosocial rehabilitation approach of normalizing the lives of ex-patients residing in the community, the first social club was opened in the 1940s in New York City and was called "Fountain House." It was located in a homelike setting and has provided a meeting place for ex-patients. Fountain

House encourages a sense of belonging, of being needed, of involvement in a community of caring people. It helps strengthen the patient's support network.

CASE EXAMPLE _____

Ronald Peterson, a rehabilitated ex-patient who had the social support of the Fountain House Social Club, describes what he feels are the chronic mental patient needs:

> Maybe if all of us patients who are chronic and need help in the community could become little again, it would be easier for everyone to solve the problem . . . I'm thinking of a family and what seems to go on there. . . . Your life seems real, and most of the time almost everything that happens to you, you talk about it. Sometimes you have good news; sometimes you have bad news. But most of the time it's just talking about what is going on.
>
> It's a place you go from—to the doctor or to the hospital or the dentist, or school, or to the movies or to a job, but it's a place where you belong, where you somehow learn a lot. You change, I'm sure, but usually without knowing it. And you certainly are not looked at as a patient or one who is being rehabilitated. You don't get discharged or terminated; and even when you grow up and get a job of your own and move away, it's a place you keep in touch with and visit. There's always an interest, and that's what makes the difference. I think this is what we need for the chronic mental patient.

ELEMENTS OF A COMMUNITY SUPPORT PROGRAM

The NIMH began the Community Support Program (CSP) in 1977 to assist states and localities in developing community-based services. The first overall goal of the Community Support Program is to instigate improved treatment and rehabilitation for the most severely mentally ill and handicapped, a population often ignored by traditional mental health facilities and practitioners. The second goal is to promote broad-based community participation in all aspects, thus assuring local ownership of the system. The final goal is to periodically reassess changing circumstances and needs and to modify the program accordingly.

The Community Support Program achieves these goals by encouraging localities to develop a system of services within their community. A CSP provides comprehensive services to chronically mentally ill persons on a local level. These services usually are provided by local, independent programs that are coordinated by a designated, responsible agency. An effective CSP helps establish and/or strengthen the individual's support network as well as provides treatment of a person's delusions or anxiety. There are 10 necessary services to be provided by an adequate CSP:

1. Identify the population in the hospital and the community and reach out to offer appropriate services.
2. Provide assistance in applying for entitlements.
3. Provide crisis stabilization services in the least restrictive setting possible.
4. Provide "psychosocial rehabilitation services" such as goal-direction, rehabilitation, evaluation, transitional living arrangements, and vocational rehabilitation.
5. Provide supportive services of indefinite duration, such as living arrangements, work opportunities, and age and culturally appropriate daytime and evening activities.
6. Provide medical and mental health care.
7. Provide backup support to families, friends, and community members.
8. Involve concerned community members in planning, volunteering, and offering housing or work opportunities.
9. Protect patient rights, both in the hospital and the community.
10. Provide case-management services to assure continuous availability of appropriate forms of assistance.

Assuming that these services are available, the following conditions must be met by the CSP:

- The comprehensive needs of the population at risk must be assessed.
- There must be legislative, administrative, and financial arrangements to guarantee that appropriate forms of assistance are available to meet these needs.
- There must be a core services agency within the community that is committed to helping severely mentally disabled people improve their lives.
- There must be a single person for teams at the client level responsible for remaining in touch with the client on a continuing basis, regardless of how many agencies get involved.

CASE EXAMPLE ━━━━━━━━━━━━━━━━━━━━━━━━━━━━━━━━━━━━━━
Donald's case clearly illustrates how clients can benefit from participation in a CSP.

Donald is a 31-year-old resident of Clackamas County, Oregon. Over the past five years, he has been hospitalized 20 to 25 times, including at least 10 times at the state hospital, and is considered by his case managers to be chronically disabled. Donald is now well integrated into a web of services, activities, and social networks in Clackamas County. Since entering the Clackamas County CSP, he has been able to remain in the community for 18 months—a major success.

Donald is enrolled in the Community Support Unit of the Clackamas County Community Mental Health Center. He currently lives in one of the public housing units operated by the Center. He shares his two-bedroom apartment with three roommates and pays only $50.00 a month in rent and utilities.

All of Donald's income comes from Supplemental Social Security (SSI) payments. Although he now receives SSI, his application for benefits was denied on three occasions in the past. Except for an occasional odd job, he has been virtually unable to work for the past two years. He is currently becoming involved with the vocational rehabilitation agency and hopes to begin an educational or training program.

Donald was referred to the Clackamas Community Support Unit following his last stay at the state hospital, which lasted nine months. He is enrolled in the unit's case management program and the Gladstone Day Treatment Center and has been an active participant for 18 months. He participates regularly in outpatient therapy, a drug and alcohol group, a medication group, relaxation therapy and recreation therapy. On the advice of his therapist, he and his family are beginning family conferences at the Gladstone Center. He seeks out the therapists at Gladstone for informal one-to-one counseling and support. In addition, he does other things at the Center such as helping with lunch, taking out the garbage, and socializing with other patients. Donald takes antipsychotic medications that are monitored closely by a nurse practitioner in a medication group.

He is integrated into a circle of friends, and he prefers the company of friends to being alone. He has a "lady friend" and another former patient who is his confidante.

Donald is well integrated into the network of services available to the mentally disabled, and has an active social life. He receives income support, housing, extensive mental health services, vocational rehabilitation and socialization opportunities. Donald feels that the resources he needs are there, and he is generally satisfied with the services he is receiving. He has, he notes, been able to avoid the state hospital for a significant period of time for the first time in years.

Four of the key services provided in a CSP are case management, residential alternatives, crisis intervention, and psychosocial clubs. These service areas will be described in the next sections of the chapter. A final section will describe a model program of community support that integrates all the elements required by persons with chronic mental illness.

LEARNING EXERCISE

Through contacting your state and local mental health program officials, identify the Directors or Coordinators of the state and local CSPs. Write down their names, addresses, agency affiliations, and phone numbers for future reference. Then place a phone call to one of these officials and obtain the names and phone numbers of the local agencies that participate as components in your local CSP. These people represent informants that can be contacted to identify existing programs or services in your area to provide needed services to the chronically mentally ill.

This program has been documented in research studies to be more cost-effective than traditional methods of delivering mental health services (Stein and Test 1980).

CASE MANAGEMENT

Deinstitutionalization has left thousands of chronic mental patients to fend for themselves in community systems that are complex and fragmented. Community-based care for the severely psychiatrically disabled patient is often of questionable value:

> In most treatment settings the question is not whether intensive psychotherapy, or even brief psychotherapy, is of value for schizophrenics, but rather, whether the schizophrenic patient will have time to brush his teeth and take a shower before being discharged through the hospital's "revolving door" with fluphenazine in his butt, a prescription in his hand, and an appointment to see a well-meaning but harassed aftercare worker two or three weeks later. This is the current practice and professional reality that must be confronted by those who are developing, evaluating and justifying psychosocial approaches for the treatment of schizophrenia. (Liberman et al. 1980, p. 49)

Persons who are discharged from psychiatric hospitals, as well as those who are diverted from institutions because of more stringent admission criteria, require services in the community. These individuals are frequently resistant to treatment, incapable of securing entitlements for which they are eligible, and unable to mobilize and use potential supports. They are therefore largely invisible to the public service agencies on whom they theoretically depend for care (Bachrach 1984a).

Furthermore, an adequate system of community supports is frequently not available even if the patient seeks treatment. There has traditionally been resistance among mental health professionals to working with the long-term mentally ill patient (Lamb 1976). Agencies not specifically designed to work with the mentally ill, such as housing and social services, are especially reluctant to get involved. In addition, the complex and diverse needs of the chronically mentally ill exceed the resources that are available. Community resistance and stigma have also created barriers to the allocation of funds to develop the needed services. In actuality, the decentralized and fragmented system of community care has become a labyrinth that is functionally inaccessible to chronically mentally ill patients (NIMH 1977).

Although case management cannot, in and of itself, remediate an inadequate system, it can assist chronic mental patients in maximizing their use of existing resources, thereby increasing their independence and quality of life. Case management is designed to coordinate the range of services needed by the chronically mentally ill. A carefully organized system of case management helps to assure accountability, continuity of care, accessibility, and efficiency. Case management includes the following functions:

- patient identification and outreach
- individual assessment
- service planning
- linkage with requisite services
- monitoring of service delivery
- patient advocacy

Although all these areas are necessary in an effective case management system, the relative emphasis of each function, the organization, and the number of personnel required varies according to the needs of the patients served and the service system itself (Kemp 1981).

Identification of patients to be served is a prerequisite to other case management services. In many cases patients are identified through referrals from mental health professionals and agencies, friends, family, and the patient him- or herself. Unfortunately, many chronically mentally ill persons do not independently seek out assistance, they are not in contact with mental health agencies, and they do not have a social support network to refer them, thus necessitating creative attempts at outreach on the part of the case manager.

Patient assessment ideally is initiated immediately following referral and should include a detailed assessment of the patient's strengths, deficits, and potential for independent living. The patient's current level of functioning as well as his or her highest level of functioning prior to hospitalization need to be considered. A detailed description of functional assessment is provided in Chapter 2. The outcome of the assessment provides information for making judgments about the patient's needs for specialized resources that need to be included in the service plan.

The service plan should be based upon the information obtained from the functional assessment of a patient. The plan needs to be a comprehensive written document that can be updated as necessary. It is imperative that the patient be involved in the planning. Service plans usually include

- clearly defined priority areas for needed services,
- short- and long-term measurable objectives within each of the areas that can be used to evaluate patient progress,
- specific actions that must be taken to meet the goals,
- agencies to which the patient is referred,
- realistic time frames for completing activities, and
- identification of potential barriers to service utilization and delivery and proposed solutions to these problems.

The next step involves linking the patient to the necessary services. This involves not only referring the patient, but doing whatever is necessary to get him or her to the service. This may include providing transportation, establishing interagency agreements, or following up on referrals.

After services have been secured, the case manager needs to monitor the services to assure that the patient receives what is expected and that the services remain appropriate to the patient's needs. The case manager therefore needs to maintain ongoing contact with both the patient and all service providers. Ideally, the case manager is occasionally present to observe while services are being delivered. The patient, in conjunction with the case manager, evaluates the quality and appropriateness of the services rendered by local agencies.

The final responsibility of the case manager is advocacy. Typically, long-term mentally ill persons have not been seen as a priority population, yet they require a multiplicity of services, thus making advocacy a necessity. Advocacy needs to occur both at the patient level and the systems level. At the patient level, the case manager needs to assist the patient in receiving all benefits to which he or she is entitled. At the systems level, the advocacy requires applying pressure to the system in order to make modifications and improvements. Often, the family needs to be linked with the case manager to enhance the impact of advocacy (Intagliata 1986).

The National Alliance for the Mentally Ill (NAMI) is a voluntary organization including relatives and friends of those with severe long-term mental illnesses. This organization has been highly effective in advocating for the needs of the chronically mentally ill. In coalition with other groups, NAMI has had an impact on public policy and legislation

---

LEARNING EXERCISE

Different agencies or facilities utilize various systems for providing case management services. It is important to identify the people within your facility that provide these services. If you needed to refer a patient to a different facility, who would you contact? Who provides case management services for the patients you serve? Who conducts functional assessments for chronic mental patients in your facility or agency? How often? Which people are involved in developing the treatment plan? What advocacy agencies are available in your area? What are their phone numbers? Once a patient leaves your facility, what type of contacts are made? How often?

---

in 1) maintaining funding for the CSP, 2) promoting increased flexibility in the use of funds for community mental health centers to include psychosocial services, 3) stopping the Social Security Administration from removing the mentally ill from their rolls and the passage of Social Security disability reform legislation, and 4) helping to pass a Fair Housing Law to protect the mentally ill against discrimination.

Although case management serves all of the above functions, the specific roles of case managers vary depending on the objectives of the case management system, the functions assigned to case managers, and the nature of the case management model that is implemented. The following roles are served by case managers: diagnostician, counselor, planner, advocate, procurer/broker, expediter, record keeper, community organizer, and consultant (Kemp 1981).

RESIDENTIAL TREATMENT

Chronically mentally ill patients in the community require indefinite residential support. To meet the variety of needs of chronic mental patients, a continuum of residential alternatives is necessary.

The residential continuum ideally provides the least restrictive housing for a patient by including all of the following alternatives:

- Hospital
- Group home
- Halfway house
- Board and care homes
- Supervised apartment
- Satellite apartment

Unfortunately, the least restrictive housing alternative does not necessarily yield more independence for a patient. Patients may reside in a setting that does not restrict their movements, but they may not be taught skills for independent living. Living freely but without access to training in social and independent living skills does not produce autonomy in a patient. In fact, a patient who lives in a halfway house may engage in fewer activities of daily living than when he or she was in the hospital. Further, not all housing alternatives are suitable for all patients: Some patients may be able to live in a supervised apartment immediately upon release from the hospital, while other patients may never be able to live without daily supervision.

A description of each of the residential alternatives follows, along with a list of skills that the patient could potentially acquire in that setting. Within each of these alternatives there is room for variability from program to program to accommodate the differences among residents, staffing, programming, and financing.

Hospital

The hospital theoretically represents the most restrictive residential setting. Within the hospital, patients may be placed on a locked or an unlocked ward. Both types of wards frequently do not permit the independent practice of home care and self-care skills. Cooking and cleaning are the duties of hospital personnel, and patients are usually not involved in these areas. Self-care skills are usually initiated by staff, and patients are often prompted to complete the tasks. In addition, community outings occur only with staff escort and supervision.

Hospitals can, however, teach many skills necessary for independent living. Some of the skills that have been successfully taught within a hospital setting include social skills, independent leisure skills, independent grooming, medication self-management, money management, and food preparation (Wallace et al. 1985).

Group Home

Group homes are the most restrictive placement within the community. Usually, several patients live within the same house under 24-hour supervision. Skills required to live in the community are taught. Patients receive hourly staff monitoring, active stabilization efforts, and staff assistance and participation in carrying out activities of daily living. Responsibilities for group home residents include

- taking medication as prescribed;
- attending two social program activities per week;
- attending daily activities as assigned, 80 percent of the time without prompting (for example, Day Treatment program);
- performing bedroom chores with assistance;
- performing personal hygiene duties as needed with instruction;

LEARNING EXERCISE

Patients in the community are frequently unaware of the programs and services that are available. Meet with one of the patients in your facility. Ask him or her to identify three agencies that provide leisure/ recreation activities (for example, Department of Parks and Recreation). Call the agencies and ask for a schedule of activities for the coming month.

Identify the specific programs and facilities available in your community that fit into the residential continuum:

Hospital
Group home
Halfway house
Board and care homes
Supervised apartments
Satellite apartments

- performing assigned group home chores with prompting;
- engaging in some form of physical exercise twice a week;
- attending all required house and community meetings;
- attending all medication and counseling appointments with assistance;
- using the city transit system with assistance.

Halfway House

Halfway houses focus on further acquisition of community skills in a less structured and less intensively supervised setting than group homes. As in group homes, several patients live in the same house with 24-hour supervision. Interpersonal skills and self-control are encouraged as well as the active development of a patient's home maintenance skills. Patients still receive daily staff monitoring, crisis support, and some staff assistance in carrying out activities of daily living. In the ideal halfway house, residents are encouraged by staff to

- take medication without prompting;
- attend all prescribed social program activities;
- attend daily activities 90 percent of the time without prompting;
- perform bedroom chores without assistance and only occasional prompting;
- perform personal hygiene duties as needed with minimal prompting;
- perform assigned home chores with minimal prompting;
- record all appointments on a monthly calendar and attend them with minimal prompting;

- use the city transit system without assistance;
- eat nutritional and balanced meals;
- develop and submit a written budget;
- arbitrate conflicts.

Board and Care Homes

Board and care homes is a term that describes a variety of facilities. The number of residents ranges from one to more than a hundred. Common characteristics of these homes include the following: They are unlocked, patients share rooms, three meals a day are served, medications are dispensed, and minimal staff supervision is provided. Board and care homes should make social and vocational rehabilitation, recreational activities, and mental health treatment available to their residents.

Supervised Apartments

Patients live in several apartments within the same apartment complex. Supervision is maintained by a staff member who also occupies an apartment in the complex. Usually, two patients share an apartment. The focus is on social skills development and independence in supervised apartments. Patients should have already acquired the basic skills before they move into the supervised apartments. The development of problem-solving skills is a major focus at this step. Patients receive daily staff monitoring in the beginning, and this gradually decreases to weekly staff monitoring. Social and independent living skills that patients learn in a supervised apartment include the following:

- keep medications and take them as prescribed;
- attend and participate in social programs twice weekly and participate in one outside community activity;
- keep apartment clean and pass daily inspection;
- attend and participate in apartment meetings at least twice a week;
- meet with staff twice a week to discuss progress;
- submit one sample menu using good nutrition and cooking skills;
- write and stick to monthly budget with staff supervision;
- keep all appointments and record on own calendar and submit to staff;
- display good negotiation skills with roommate and others;
- begin to do own grocery shopping;
- decide on goals for future living situation.

Satellite Apartments

In satellite apartments, patients are taught to live independently in their own community apartment. Minimal staff monitoring (once monthly) is provided. Many of the activities focused upon at this level are the securing of items that will be needed for independent apartment living. Residents' goals in satellite apartments include the following:

- obtaining a stable income to live upon;
- accumulating enough money for the initial move to the community;
- finding a place to live;
- getting access to adequate transportation;
- finding and building meaningful relationships;
- participating in a social network;
- assuming responsibility for taking own medications.

CASE EXAMPLE

The Mental Health Residential Program transitions severely psychiatrically disabled individuals from the state hospital into the most appropriate, least restrictive community-based living environment available. This program is a component of Alternatives Unlimited in Massachusetts.

At entry into the Mental Health Residential Program, individual functional assessments are completed with each patient. These assessments develop the overall rehabilitation goals of the patient for his or her chosen living environment. The goals are stated in terms of stabilizing in a particular residential environment or transitioning to another environment. The functional assessment identifies specific skill and resources strengths and deficits relative to the specific demands of the living environment of choice.

The residential programs have been developed on a three-tiered continuum. The first level, supervised apartment living units, has a high staff-to-patient ratio to provide more comprehensive programming for those patients who have significant basic activities of daily living skills deficits. This increased ratio helps to stabilize them within the community.

The residence program, the next level, has fewer staff, and focuses on developing patients' social and community skills which are necessary for successful integration into the community. The highest level in the continuum is the cooperative apartment program, in which the residents apply skills for maintaining themselves independently in the community with minimal direct program support. As the individual moves through the continuum toward the least restrictive level, the patients increasingly rely on and utilize generic, community-based supports and resources.

Deficits in critical activities of daily living skills are assessed in the following functional areas or domains using a five-level ordinal scale: public transportation, meal preparation, personal hygiene, use of time, physical health care, personal development, self-medication, budget planning, telephone use, response to emergencies, household maintenance, social development, and community integration. Both the residential staff and the patient rate performance in each of these areas.

Rehabilitation problems are pinpointed, reinforcers are identified, and the intervener is specified. Each individual patient develops with staff a unique rehabilitation plan, documenting the interventions that will occur so that the patient can reach his or her overall goal of stabilizing successfully in the present environment or transitioning to the next environment in the continuum. Individual and group direct skill teaching for acquisition, programming, and monitoring for the application of skills occurs for each resident within the residential environment and the community.

Independent Living

At this level, patients are living on their own. They must choose a residence, pay for it, and maintain it. The patient's case manager still contacts the patient periodically to ensure that things are running smoothly and to provide occasional assistance when needed.

LEARNING EXERCISE

Patients need to be competent in a variety of independent living skills to live successfully in the community. What independent living skills do you help your patients to develop? What scheduled activities and learning programs are available to teach patients skills in your facility? What types of skills that are not being taught at your facility should be added to the program?

CRISIS INTERVENTION

Persons afflicted with severe and long-term psychiatric disorders are highly vulnerable to stressful life events that challenge their limited coping abilities. A change of therapist, moving from one home to another, temporary loss of Social Security pensions, and tension in family relationship can easily provoke social and symptomatic decompensation— or crisis—in chronic mental patients. Crises can be defined as a significant increase in psychopathology and/or decrement in social functioning and support, usually in response to an internal or external threat or stressor. Any CSP that aims to work effectively with chronic mental patients must include flexible forms of crisis intervention.

Crisis intervention has as its goal rapid restabilization of a patient's symptoms and social adjustment. Ordinarily, both medication and psychosocial interventions are required to assist the patient and his or her social support system to reconstitute from a crisis and to regain the ability to function in the community. Crisis services are often hospital based because of their emergency nature and their need for medical resources. Because it has been well documented that expanded treatment of crises has the adverse effect of inducing dependency in patients and their support system, crisis intervention has been organized as short-term and time-limited in focus.

People who are dangerous to themselves or others or who are incapable of taking care of themselves and have concurrent psychiatric symptoms are considered to be in a psychiatric crisis. Many patients with a history of chronicity require crisis services without reaching the point of being a danger to themselves or others. Interventions with these patients frequently only result in a restoration of precrisis functioning. The patient generally still will require continued community support services following the crisis.

There are a variety of crisis services that patients may need, depending on the severity of the crisis. These services may be delivered in the patient's home or in a designated place outside the home. The patient may, for example, remain at home with either daily phone contact or daily visits by a mobile emergency or home treatment team, receive crisis care in a hospital or clinic emergency room, or leave his or her home to live in a respite home or in crisis lodging.

Initially, when a patient is referred, it is important to conduct a thorough assessment. The assessment should determine the nature of the presenting problem, the patient's strengths and weaknesses, the extent of natural support and agency support available, the presence of delusions and hallucinations, and the severity of the crisis. From this information the appropriate services, both medical and psychosocial, can be determined and provided.

Telephone support is the least restrictive form of intervention. The patient remains in his or her own home and has the opportunity to deal with the crisis in the same environment in which it occurred. Daily contact via the telephone is made by the crisis intervention program to see how the person is doing and to monitor his or her progress in coping with the presenting problem.

In home support, the patient still remains at home, but services provided include visits, phone support, and meetings with the patient and his or her family. The home visits encourage 1) progress in coping with the problem, 2) obtaining other needed services that are available, 3) resolution of psychiatric symptoms, and 4) developing plans for achieving the short-term social recompensation of patient and family.

Homes in the community are used if the patient is not able to remain in his or her own home. Patients are placed in these homes in which the family and/or staff is trained to work with chronic mental patients in

---

LEARNING EXERCISE

Crisis intervention services vary from one community to another. When a patient of yours is in crisis, whom should the patient or family call? Who provides transportation for patients who need crisis intervention in your area? Develop a list of crisis services that are available in your community. Write down the name of the program, a contact person, and the phone number. Pass this list out to your patients.

---

crisis. Typically, these homes ensure that the patient takes his or her medications, is fed properly, attends ongoing programs, and is not in danger. These homes are not appropriate for persons who are so much at risk that they require 24-hour supervision. Average tenure in these homes is approximately two weeks.

Crisis lodging may be used if the patient requires a) constant supervision because of being a danger to self or others or because of major changes in medication, b) brief separation from the living situation to regain control of psychiatric symptoms, or c) temporary management and supervision pending an available bed in a psychiatric hospital or less restrictive residential alternative. These programs frequently use rapid tranquilization or neuroleptization procedures to reduce hallucinations, incoherence, delusions, and agitation. Patients may stay in crisis lodging for up to five days in most programs. At that time the patient may return home; however, follow-up calls or home visits should be made to help ensure a smooth transition even if the crisis situation has been resolved and stabilization of symptoms and functioning has occurred.

PSYCHOSOCIAL CLUB MODEL

The psychosocial club model had its origin in the early 1940s, when patients who had been discharged from the Rockland State Hospital in New York began meeting on the steps of the New York City Public Library. The group named itself We Are Not Alone. The club's emphasis was on providing a meeting place for ex-patients. They did not receive any professional or financial backing and used only a few nonprofessional volunteers. The informal meetings gradually grew into a social club for mutual aid and emotional support, which eventually found a building for its activities, which became Fountain House.

The primary intent of the clubhouse is to assist mentally ill persons (called members) to increase their level of effective personal participation. Every member is viewed as having something to contribute and the clubhouse provides a setting for channeling and structuring members' personal and social contributions. Members experience a strong sense of ownership in the running of the clubhouse, have a sense of being actively needed by the clubhouse, and recognize that their contributions are critical to the effective functioning of the clubhouse.

Psychosocial clubs have common characteristics in that they typically focus on vocational and social rehabilitation and provide some type of residential programming. Fountain House has become the prototype and has disseminated its model program to over a hundred other sites in the United States and continues to effectively serve over 300 ex-patients each day. Members who attend Fountain House are usually unemployed and have histories of multiple psychiatric hospitalizations. The social atmosphere of Fountain House is best shown in the following description by Cora, a member.

CASE EXAMPLE

I'm a dictaphone secretary at a big textile company in Manhattan. I make $185 a week. I go to school two nights a week and I'm studying to be a court reporter. I have my own apartment, I have a cat, and I have a boy friend. I have a driver's license, and a new piano. Most of what I have in my life is due to Fountain House. If Fountain House had not existed at the time I came out of the hospital, giving me all the moral support, I would be back in the hospital. Even now, as a member, I feel like I came to visit a very wonderful relative when I came here tonight. You know I really don't think I could have made it, because I did not have that much health or that much strength at that time, ten years ago, when I was discharged from the hospital. I wouldn't have been able to talk myself through depressions or feelings of fear and disappointment. A big part of my success are the friends that I made here at Fountain House.

Members at Fountain House work side by side with staff in activities that range from the simple to the complicated. A few activities carried out by members are

- Writing, editing, printing and collating a daily newspaper that is distributed throughout the clubhouse.
- Doing the menu planning, shopping and preparing for luncheon, and cleaning up afterwards for 250 members.
- Greeting visitors and giving them a tour of the facility.
- Making visits to members who have been hospitalized or have withdrawn from the program and encouraging their return to the program.

- Spending time helping to refurbish apartments leased by Fountain House in which members reside.
- Helping members secure income from public assistance and Social Security for which they are eligible.
- Operating and teaching others to operate the Xerox machine.

Outcome studies conducted at Fountain House (Beard 1978; Malamud 1985) found that regularly attending club members had lower rehospitalization rates than did members who did not attend.

MODEL PROGRAMS MUST BE COMPREHENSIVE

The elements of service that compose a CSP, such as the ones described above, are essential in their own right. Each element of service has reverberating effects beyond its own goal area; for example, the availability of a spectrum of housing alternatives for the severely psychiatrically disabled reduces the burden on families and can significantly reduce relapse and rehospitalization because it permits a toning down of the tension and stress that exists so often within families containing a mentally ill person. Crisis stabilization services permit the maintenance of mentally ill persons in the community and out of hospitals because these services fit the needs of the young adult chronic patients who refuse treatment but accept "rescue" by professionals.

The comprehensiveness of service elements, however, is the key attribute to the few truly effective CSPs that have been developed in American cities. Because of the nature of psychiatric impairments and disabilities, effective CSPs must offer comprehensive care and support to enable the chronically mentally ill to thrive in their communities. Programs must provide services that enable the patient and his or her family to compensate for a wide array of deficits in social, vocational, financial, medical, self-care, and psychiatric domains.

Effective CSPs have been shown to be successful alternatives to mental hospitals; however, they must be comprehensive in the range of services they provide (Bachrach 1982; 1980). Some of the attributes of successful community support programs include

1. Assertive outreach—This includes working with social and financial support systems and significant others for patients' needs. Because chronic mental patients have low motivation and difficulty in negotiating the system, they need flexible levels of support up to and including home treatment.
2. Individually tailored programs—Staff must set realistic goals to remediate skills deficits, social and financial needs, and family burden. Training in community living skills, opportunities to improve employability, appropriate living arrangements, and opportunities to develop social skills must be provided.

3. In vivo services—Staff must be available to work with patients in real-life community settings, such as jobs, stores, and homes. This promotes transfer of learning through prompting, modeling, and reinforcement.
4. Services that build on the strengths and assets of patients.
5. Attitudes that treat patients as responsible citizens who can advocate for their needs within our political system.
6. Crisis intervention that is available around the clock.
7. Coordination and advocacy with other community agencies and resources, including the patient's family. This includes assistance in applying for entitlement programs and protection of patients' rights.
8. Medical and mental health care.
9. Back-up support to families, friends, and community members.
10. Case management to ensure continuous availability of appropriate forms of assistance.

One of the most successful and emulated models of an effective community support program is the Program of Assertive Community Treatment (PACT) which was developed in Madison, Wisconsin as a partnership among the Mendota State Hospital, the Dane County Community Mental Health Department, and the University of Wisconsin Department of Psychiatry. PACT aims to maintain severely psychiatrically disabled persons in the community at a good quality of life by assertive outreach and training in community living.

PROGRAM OF ASSERTIVE COMMUNITY TREATMENT (PACT)

PACT is a community-based, comprehensive treatment service for chronically mentally ill persons that has had demonstrable success in reducing rehospitalization and improving the quality of life of participating patients (Stein and Test 1978). The PACT model provides in-vivo social support and training in community living to all severely psychiatrically ill patients in its county catchment area. Assertive provision of services; comprehensive, coordinated longitudinal provision of treatment; and individualized services are key attributes in its program philosophy.

PACT uses an assertive approach by taking the treatment to the patient rather than waiting for the patient to be motivated to participate. Patients are actively sought out and involved in treatment by mobile teams of professionals who work with patients primarily in community settings rather than in a clinic, office, or mental health center. Strong encouragement and support are provided for patients to participate in a range of therapeutic activities.

The in-vivo teaching of coping skills includes a) daily living skills, b) vocational skills, and c) social and recreational skills. The activities of daily living are taught in the environment specifically relevant to the patient; for example, staff will train and assist patients to do laundry in the laundromat closest to their living situation. Vocational rehabilitation involves assisting the patient with job seeking and developing good work and personal habits to maintain a job. Jobs can be competitive, sheltered, or volunteer experiences. Social and recreational needs of patients are met through activities that enhance social interaction and take advantage of community resources to fill free time in a satisfying manner.

PACT services are provided primarily by nurses, paraprofessionals, vocational rehabilitation counselors, occupational therapists, and social workers.

In addition to the work provided by the PACT staff, a strong emphasis is placed on involving other agencies in the process of providing for the needs of patients. PACT also has many volunteers who participate with patients socially and recreationally.

Patients are held responsible for their behaviors, as much as is realistic for them. This involves exposing patients to the same consequences for inappropriate behavior that are given to all citizens in the community. This approach has necessitated a close working relationship with legal and judicial agencies.

Each patient at PACT is involved in a practical and educational brand of individual psychotherapy. The goal of therapy is to help the patient come to terms with the fact that he or she has a significant illness and then focus on those specific areas of his or her life that can be changed for the better. Specific techniques are used to help patients manage symptoms as well as to develop ways of working toward specific behavioral goals. Patients are also treated with antipsychotic and antidepressant medications when indicated. The majority of the PACT patients are on antipsychotic medications for both treatment of acute psychotic states and prophylaxis of the occurrence of such states. PACT also provides minimal general medical care and evaluations for its patients and actively helps them obtain other more elaborate and specialized kinds of medical care that they need.

There is great variability in the frequency of contacts between PACT staff and patients, but daily contact is typical during the first two to four weeks the patient is in the program. For the next three to six months, contact is made every other day. Thereafter, treatment contacts are made according to the patient's needs, with many patients being seen daily indefinitely. Length of treatment is also according to the patient's needs, with most requiring involvement for many years.

A written individualized patient treatment plan is developed for each patient following assessment. The treatment plan covers 1) initial diagnosis and functional assessment of patient's problems, 2) clinical services needed by the patient, 3) treatment modalities to be used,

4) medications, 5) short-term goals, 6) long-term goals, 7) nutritional needs, 8) medical-surgical services, 9) educational needs, and 10) date of next review of treatment plan. Treatment implementation is documented in each patient's chart and covers response to treatment, problems encountered, and revisions.

Patient treatment at PACT is monitored and reviewed in the following ways:

1. Every six months each patient's treatment plan is comprehensively reviewed by his or her treatment team under the leadership of his or her case manager with changes in the plan made as they are appropriate. Treatment plans are also reviewed more often if a patient's status warrants it.
2. Staff meetings are held twice a day at PACT. The purpose of these meetings is to exchange clinical information, to review and adjust treatment plans, and to provide in-service training of an ongoing nature.

Each patient has a case management team consisting of either the PACT psychiatrist or social worker; one of the nurses, vocational rehabilitation counselors, or occupational therapists; and a psychiatric paraprofessional. The team is responsible for coordinating and supervising each patient's ongoing evaluation, treatment planning, and treatment implementation. Although this team carries out primary responsibility for the patient, other members of the PACT unit are usually involved in planning and carrying out treatment.

Treatment is provided by a multidisciplinary staff of 15 persons. Staff members have a background in basic clinical skills of assessment and treatment of mental illness, as well as experience in community treatment of chronically mentally ill persons. Ongoing education and training is provided to improve treatment knowledge and skills. The methods used include

1. Feedback, explanations and conceptualizations, and information presented regularly in the twice-a-day staff meetings in discussions of individual patients.
2. Once-a-month in-service programs done by either the PACT professional staff or by outside experts.
3. The offering to all PACT staff of attendance at outside conferences/ seminars/classes in topic areas related to PACT treatment.

The PACT program is very comprehensive. It provides nearly all of the services needed in a CSP. The program identifies the population requiring services; provides assistance in applying for entitlements; provides crisis services, psychosocial rehabilitation services, supportive services, and medical and mental health care; involves community members; protects patient rights; and provides case-management services.

Evaluation and Research of PACT

The clinically impressive program mounted by PACT has been substantiated in terms of its impact on patients and cost-benefit results through several rigorous research evaluations, both at PACT and at other sites replicating the procedures used by PACT. PACT maintains an active case load of 115 patients, with less than a five percent drop-out rate per year. Approximately 65 percent live independently, 25 percent live with parents, and 10 percent live in structured or semi-independent situations. In a carefully controlled study carried out in Madison, Wisconsin, Stein and Test (1980) randomly assigned acutely ill patients who were referred for inpatient care to either traditional hospitalization and aftercare or to PACT. Those patients assigned to PACT did not enter the hospital, despite their acute symptoms. Over a one-year period, patients in PACT had better vocational and social outcomes without a cost of greater psychopathology. The PACT patients were not an increased burden on their families or to the general community. Most revealing was the reduction in rehospitalization: As shown in Figure 23, only 18 percent were rehospitalized from PACT, compared with 89 percent from the traditional program.

PACT was replicated in Sydney, Australia by Hoult and his colleagues, who found similar benefits in a controlled study with one-year follow-up. One hundred and twenty patients presenting for admission to a state psychiatric hospital were randomly allocated to standard hospital and after-care or to comprehensive community treatment with a 24-hour crisis service. While 96 percent of the patients receiving standard treatment were admitted—51 percent more than once—only 40 percent of the community-treated patients were admitted, with only 8 percent more than once. Patients from the PACT-type program spent an average of 8.4 days in the hospital, compared with the 53.5 days for patients from the standard program. The community-based treatment did not increase the burden upon the community or relatives, was considered to be significantly more satisfactory and helpful by patients and their relatives, achieved a clinically superior outcome, and cost less than standard care (Hoult et al. 1984: Hoult and Reynolds 1984).

Another replication of the PACT services has also been shown to be effective, this one adapted to the urban setting of Chicago in the context of an existing psychosocial rehabilitation program based on the Fountain House model. In this setting, where less control over patients' movements and treatments is possible, rehospitalization among patients participating in the assertive outreach program dropped from 3.3 in the year before intake to 2.0 during the year of participation, with the av-

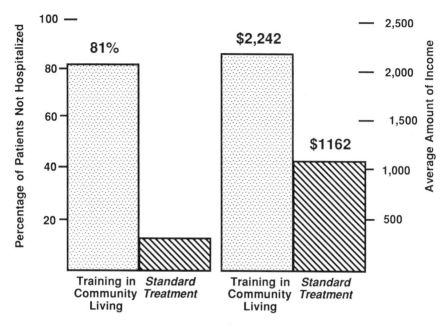

FIGURE 23: Comparison of community tenure and employment income during the first year after entry into either a standard program of mental hospital and aftercare services or a program of Training in Community Living. Patients had chronic mental disorders and all were considered suitable for hospital treatment at the time of random assignment to the two programs. The differences between the two programs was highly statistically significant. Adapted, with permission, from Stein LI, Test MA (Editors): Alternatives to Mental Hospital Treatment. New York, Plenum Press, 1978.

erage number of days hospitalized reduced from 134 to 52 (Bond 1984). The reduced hospital use by patients who received the assertive outreach services in the community is translated into an estimated savings in total treatment costs of $5,700 per patient per year. The adaptation of PACT to the more complex service delivery requirements of an urban area has led to some modifications of program design; however, the methods have been documented to be effective with a wide range of severely disabled and recidivistic patients (Witheridge and Dincin 1985).

SUMMARY

Responsibility for the continuing, long-term care of the chronically mentally ill has shifted from state hospitals to the communities into which they have been released. The National Institute of Mental Health began the Community Support Program to assist states and localities in developing a spectrum of community-based services. Key services include case management, residential alternatives, and crisis intervention.

Case management assists chronic mental patients in maximizing their use of existing resources. The residential continuum includes all of the following alternatives—hospital, group home, halfway house, board and care homes, supervised apartment, and satellite apartment. Crisis services are short-term, and are frequently medically oriented and utilize a multifaceted intervention.

The Program of Assertive Community Treatment (PACT) is a community-based, comprehensive treatment service for the chronically mentally ill. The model provides in-vivo social support; training in community living; assertive provision of services; comprehensive, coordinated, longitudinal provision of treatment; and individualized services. Studies conducted on the PACT program have demonstrated that it is cost effective and reduces rehospitalization rates.

REFERENCES

Bachrach LL: The homeless mentally ill and mental health services, in The Homeless Mentally Ill. Edited by Lamb HR. Washington, DC, American Psychiatric Press, 1984a

Bachrach LL: Research on services for the homeless mentally ill. Hosp Community Psychiatry 35:910–913, 1984b

Bachrach LL: Assessment of outcomes in community support systems: results, problems, limitations. Schizophr Bull 8:39–61, 1982

Bachrach LL: Overview of model program for chronic mental patients. Am J Psychiatry 137:1023–1031, 1980

Beard JH, Malmud TJ, Rossman E: Psychiatric rehabilitation and long-term rehospitalization rates: the findings of two research studies. Schizophr Bull 4:622–635, 1978

Bond ER: An economic analysis of psychological rehabilitation. Hosp Community Psychiatry 35:356–362, 1984

Goldman HH, Gatozzi J, Taube R: The national plan for the chronically mentally ill. Hosp Community Psychiatry 32:16–28, 1981

Grusky O: Report on the Clackamas County Community Support Site. Department of Sociology, University of California at Los Angeles, August 1983

Hammer M: Influence of small social networks as factors on mental hospital admission. Human Organizations 22:243–251, 1963–64

Heller K, Swindle RW: Social networks, perceived social support, and coping with stress, in Preventive Psychology: Theory, Research and Practice. Edited by Felner RD, Jason LA, Moritsugu JN, et al. New York, Pergamon Press, 1983

Hoult J, Reynolds I: Schizophrenia: a comparative trial of community oriented and hospital oriented psychiatric care. Acta Psychiatr Scand 69:359–372, 1984

Hoult J, Rosen A, Reynolds I: Community oriented treatment compared to psychiatric hospital oriented treatment. Soc Sci Med 18:1005–1010, 1984

Intagliata J, Willer B, Egri G: The role of the family in case management of the mentally ill. Schizophr Bull 12:699–708, 1986

Kemp B: The case management model in human service delivery, in Annual Review of Rehabilitation (Volume 2). Edited by Pan E, Backer TE, Vash CL. New York, Springer, 1981

Kuehnel TG, DeRisi WJ, Liberman RP, et al: Treatment strategies that promote deinstitutionalization of chronic mental patients, in Programming Effective Human Services: Strategies for Institutional Change and Client Transition. Edited by Christian WP, Hannah GT, Glahn TJ. New York, Plenum Press, 1984

Lamb HR: Guiding principles for community survival, in Community Survival for Long-Term Patients. Edited by Lamb HR. San Francisco: Jossey-Bass, 1976

Lamb HR: The new asylums in the community. Arch Gen Psychiatry 36:129–134, 1979

Liberman RP, Falloon IRH, Wallace CJ: Drug-psychosocial interventions in the treatment of schizophrenia, in The Chronically Mentally Ill: Research and Services. Edited by Mirabi M. New York, SP Medical and Scientific Books, 1984

Liberman RP, Wallace CJ, Vaughn CE, et al: Social and family factors in the course of schizophrenia, in The Psychotherapy of Schizophrenia. Edited by Strauss J, Bowers M, Downey TW, et al. New York, Plenum Press, 1980

National Institute of Mental Health, Division of Biometry and Epidemiology: Data Sheet on State and County Mental Hospitals. Rockville, MD, NIMH, 1977

National Institute of Mental Health: Comprehensive Community Support System for Severely Mentally Disabled Adults: Definition, Components and Guiding Principles. Rockville, MD, NIMH, 1977

Peterson R: What are the needs of chronic mental patients? in The Chronic Mental Patient. Edited by Talbott J. Washington, DC, American Psychiatric Association, 1978

Sokolovsky J, Cohen C, Berger D, et al: Personal networks of ex-mental patients in a Manhattan SRO hotel. Human Organization 37:5–15, 1978

Stein LI, Test MA: Alternatives to Mental Hospital Treatment. New York, Plenum Press, 1978

Stein LI, Test MA: Alternatives to mental hospital treatment. Arch General Psychiatry 37:392–397, 1980

Wallace CJ, Boone SE, Donahoe CP, et al: Psychosocial rehabilitation for the chronic mentally disabled: social and independent living skills training, in Behavioral Treatment of Adult Disorders. Edited by Barlow D. New York, Guilford Press, 1985

Witheridge TF, Dincin J: The Bridge: an assertive outreach program in an urban setting, in The Training in Community Living Model. Edited by Stein MI, Test MA. New Directions for Mental Health Services, No. 26. San Francisco, Jossey-Bass, 1985

INDEX